DISCLAIMER

This book is not intended to replace the fetal monitor manual. You are encouraged to read the manual before using the fetal monitor.

This book does not include directions on setting the monitor clock or specific features that are unique to only one or two monitors. Therefore, you are encouraged to work with a skilled clinician who will assist you in setting the clock and using the unique features of your monitor. Since clocks are battery-backed, you should only have to set the clock when there is a change in daylight savings time. If you plug in the monitor and there is a message, e.g., "set time/date," the battery must be replaced. Tag the fetal monitor with a note to replace the clock battery and send it to the Biomedical Department.

Lastly, content of the book is based on references from Antepartal and Intrapartal Fetal Monitoring, Second Edition ©1997 and common knowledge in the field of obstetrics and fetal monitoring. Any questions or concerns you have about content should be sent to Learning Resources International, Inc.

INTRODUCTION

The fetal heart rate (FHR) may be evaluated to predict fetal status. Choosing auscultation or the electronic fetal monitor to evaluate the FHR depends on maternal and fetal risk factors, the number of nurses available to monitor, and protocol. If you use the fetal monitor, you will be expected to identify FHR pattern components and determine the significance of the FHR and uterine activity patterns. Although interpretation is subjective, no one can argue with the *absence of any sign of fetal well-being*. Therefore, this book will prepare you to identify the signs of fetal well-being and the more common signs of fetal compromise.

The goals of this workbook are to:

- help you identify maternal and fetal assessment techniques
- prepare you to recognize the most common FHR patterns
- teach you the names of each part of the FHR pattern
- help you select actions to improve fetal oxygenation
- help you evaluate changes in maternal and/or fetal status as a result of your actions
- provide you with information to identify ineffective actions that delay timely intervention when there is a nonreassuring FHR pattern, and
- suggest how to document your assessments, actions, evaluations, and communications that reflect the standard of practice.

Learning is a journey. This is just the beginning. Knowledge of concepts in fetal monitoring is cumulative. We strongly recommend you plan to attend at least one advanced fetal monitoring course every two years and as many inservice programs as you can to give you more exposure and insight into the fetal condition. Fetal monitors cannot replace hands-on care. They are an adjunct to your care. Therefore, it is important that you touch your patients to palpate contractions and fetal movement.

Michelle L. Murray, PhD, RNC

Trish Urbanski, MSN, CNM, RNC

ESSENTIALS OF FETAL MONITORING

By MICHELLE L. MURRAY, PhD, RNC
Perinatal Clinical Nurse Specialist
Clinical Associate
University of New Mexico
Health Sciences Center
College of Nursing
Albuquerque, New Mexico

PATRICIA URBANSKI, MSN, CNM, RNC, CCE
Perinatal Clinical Nurse Specialist
Clinical Educator
Education and Consulting Services
University Hospital
Albuquerque, New Mexico

PUBLISHED BY LEARNING RESOURCES INTERNATIONAL, INC.

"I have found it helpful to recover a sense of my work not as a career but as a calling."

Smith, D.H. (June 1994). How to be a good doctor in the 1990s: Stand and deliver, American Journal of Obstetrics and Gynecology, 170 (6), 1724-1728, p. 1725.

ISBN: 0-942835-02-6 Second Printing November 1999

The information, guidelines, and techniques of practice included in this book are not intended to dictate a plan of care. Publication should not be construed as excluding other acceptable approaches to clinical management. Medication dosages are provided in this book, but it is possible they may change. The reader is urged to review the formulary or manufacturer's package information prior to drug administration.

Production Supervisor: Michelle L. Murray, PhD, RNC
Production Assistant: Patricia Garibay
Production Designer: Nancy Denker, MS, Focus Ink, Incorporated, Albuquerque, NM
Cover Design: Gaye Roth, Paper Graphiti, Albuquerque, NM

Printed in the United States of America

Learning Resources International, Inc.
PO Box 92050
Albuquerque, NM 87199-2050
1-505-822-8951 Fax 505-822-0326

TABLE OF CONTENTS

SECTION 1
Systematic Assessment of the Pregnant Woman

SYSTEMATIC ASSESSMENT

The maternal condition can affect fetal status. Therefore, it is critical to systematically gather important maternal information prior to interpretation of the fetal heart rate (FHR) pattern. If it is available, review prenatal and historical information prior to approaching the pregnant woman. If the prenatal record is not complete, obtain additional information by interviewing the patient. If possible, obtain a complete prenatal record from the clinic or physician's office. The choice of monitoring methods depends on the practitioner's orders, the institution's policies and procedures, and patient requests or needs. Before approaching the patient, you must know if auscultation and palpation are going to be the only monitoring methods or if fetal monitoring will be intermittent, continuous, or a combination of both auscultation and electronic fetal monitoring.

Utilize the fetal monitor to complete your assessment of the maternal/fetal dyad. Use a systematic approach to evaluate the pregnant woman and fetus. You may choose to do all or part of this assessment prior to monitor use.

Maternal/Fetal Assessment

- Perform Leopold's Maneuvers
- Estimate fetal weight
- Palpate fetal movement
- Evaluate fetal heart tones by fetoscope
- Assess maternal vital signs and risk factors
- Perform a maternal head to toe assessment
- Determine fundal height – is it appropriate for gestational age?
- Determine uterine activity
- Assess the cervix if there are no contraindications
- Determine the presence of labor

Leopold's Maneuvers

Preparation

Place the woman on her back in a semi-Fowler's position. You may wish to place a pillow under her right hip to displace the uterus off the inferior vena cava and aorta.

You will be inspecting and palpating the maternal abdomen to determine fetal lie and presentation. This will also help you locate the fetal back for external ultrasound transducer placement.

First Maneuver: What is in the Fundus?

Stand at the woman's side and palpate the content of the fundus using both hands.

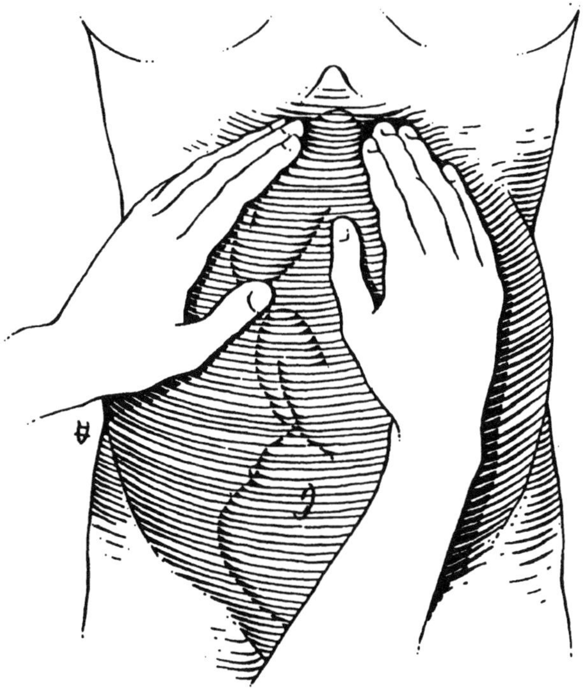

1.1 ***First Maneuver - Identify what is in the fundus.*** (Reproduced with permission of Appleton & Lange from Oxorn, H. (1986). Human labor and birth, 5th ed. Stanford, CT.)

- *the head feels hard and moves when you push against it*
- *the buttocks feels soft and round*

Second Maneuver: Where is the Fetal Back?

Face the woman and place both hands on either side of her abdomen. While holding one hand still, push on the fetus and feel for the arms and legs and the curve of the fetal back. Now hold the opposite hand still while pushing with the other hand. Can you feel the fetal back? Did the fetus move? You can document fetal movement as "FM palpated" or "FM +." It is especially important to keep one hand still so that if the fetus has died you do not mistake pushing the fetus towards the other hand as fetal movement.

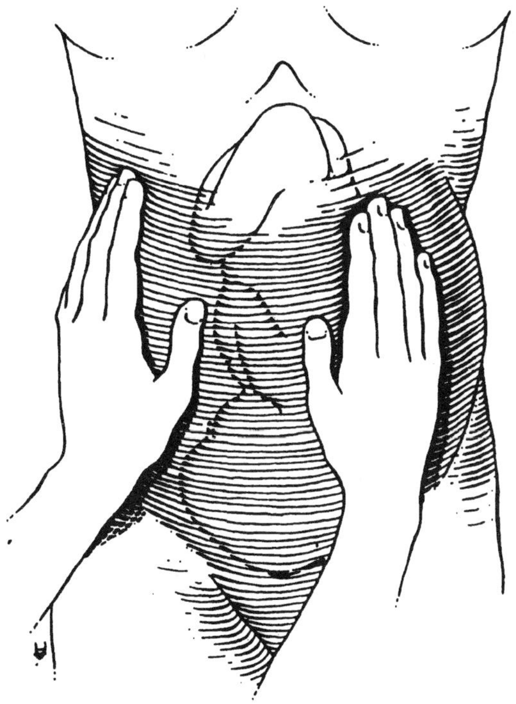

1.2 ***Second Maneuver - Find the fetal back.***
(Reproduced with permission of Appleton & Lange from Oxorn, H. (1986). Human labor and birth, 5th ed. Stanford, CT.)

- *the back feels firm, curved, and smooth*
- *the legs, feet, arms, and hands feel irregular*

Third Maneuver: What is the Presenting Part?

Grasp the lower uterine segment by pushing in above the pubic bone. Palpate for a hard or soft mass. If in doubt, the vaginal examination may be used to help you confirm the fetal presenting part.

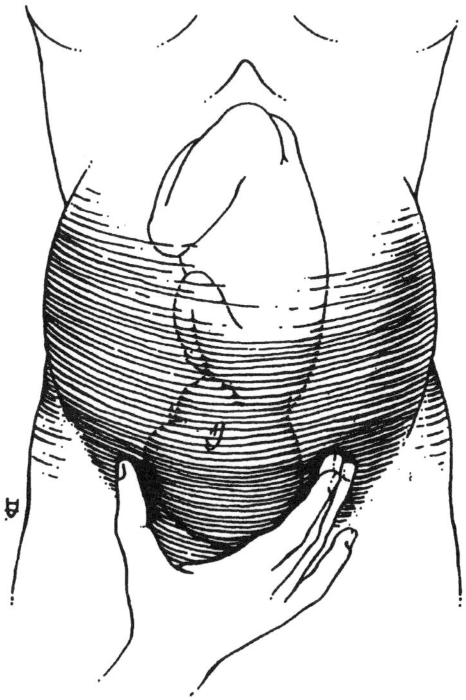

1.3 ***Third maneuver - Identify the presenting part.***
(Reproduced with permission of Appleton & Lange from Oxorn, H. (1986). Human labor and birth, 5th ed. Stanford, CT.)

- *the fetal buttocks feels soft and round*
- *the head feels hard and round*

Once you have located the fetal back, what's in the fundus, and the presenting part, you should be able to determine the fetal position. If the back of the baby is on the maternal left (L) side, the occiput (O) is also on the left. The baby will be LOA, LOP, or LOT were A means anterior, P means posterior, and T means transverse.

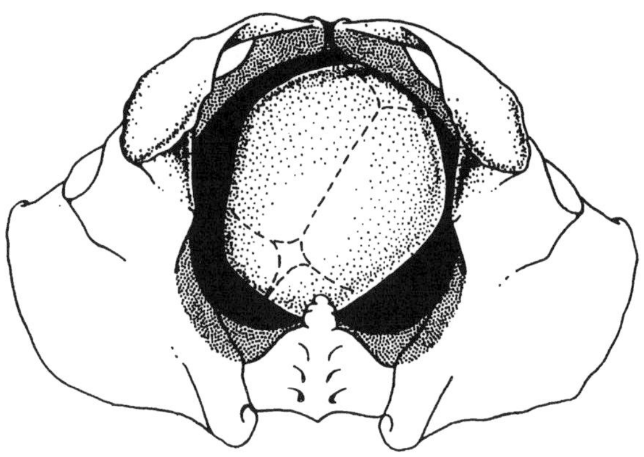

1.4 ***This baby is in a left occiput anterior position.*** (Reproduced with permission of Appleton & Lange from Oxorn, H. (1986). Human labor and birth, 5th ed. Stanford, CT.)

Fourth Maneuver: Where is the Cephalic Prominence?

When the fetal head is the presenting part, the fourth maneuver will identify the cephalic prominence, which is the back of the baby's head.

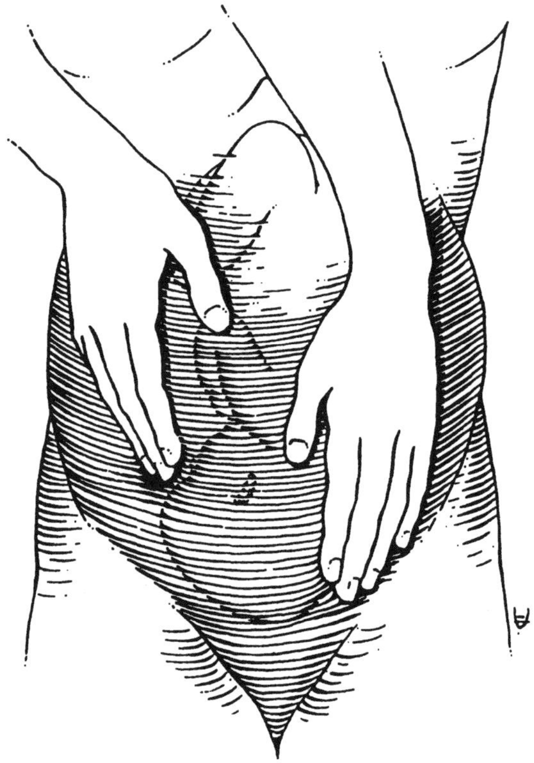

1.5 ***Fourth maneuver - Identify the cephalic prominence.*** (Reproduced with permission of Appleton & Lange from Oxorn, H. (1986). Human labor and birth, 5th ed. Stanford, CT.)

Face the woman's feet and slide your hands down the sides of her uterus until your fingers on one hand meet resistance. This is the cephalic prominence. It may be the baby's forehead or back of the head. If the cephalic prominence is opposite the baby's back, the head is flexed. This is what you want to find. If the occiput is the cephalic prominence, the baby's head is in extension which can impede fetal descent.

ESTIMATE THE FETAL WEIGHT AND PALPATE FETAL MOVEMENT

Estimate the Fetal Weight and Palpate Fetal Movement

When doing Leopold's Maneuvers, you can also estimate the fetal weight. A way to practice is to close your eyes while palpating a 4 pound sack of sugar, a 5 pound sack of sugar, and a 10 pound sack of sugar which are flat on a table. Feel the difference in the density of the bags. Note the difference between the 4 pound and 5 pound bag. Is the fetus more like the 5 pound sack of sugar or the 10 pound sack of sugar? As you become more comfortable in estimating fetal weight, it may become easier to predict how well the fetus will fit through the pelvis. Review the maternal obstetric history. Look at the clinical pelvimetry findings in the prenatal record. Does the fundal height suggest a large or small baby? Estimation of fetal weight is important if a 40 or more pound weight gain has occurred, as the risks of macrosomia and fetopelvic disproportion increase especially when your patient also has gestational diabetes. Gently place your hand on the maternal abdomen to feel for spontaneous fetal movement.

AUSCULTATION

Evaluate Fetal Heart Rate by Auscultation

Before you assess the FHR, confirm the rate from previous monitoring strips or documentation in the prenatal record. For example, a nonstress test result may be written in the prenatal record or the actual FHR may be recorded by the practitioner during prenatal visits. The FHR drops 1 beat per minute (bpm) per week for every week of gestation beginning at 16 weeks. The FHR stabilizes at 35 weeks of gestation. Auscultation is ideally used to confirm fetal life and the FHR prior to placement of the external ultrasound transducer. It is also used to intermittently monitor the fetal condition in the low-risk woman during labor.

You can confirm fetal life by auscultating the fetal heart tones with a fetoscope prior to ultrasound transducer application. The FHR can also be determined by a hand-held Doppler device. A fetoscope or stethoscope allows you to hear *tones* or the actual sound of the ventricles. The Doppler is a motion detector which determines a *rate*. If a hand-held Doppler is used, it is best to simultaneously assess the maternal pulse to differentiate it from the FHR. Record both the maternal pulse and the FHR. The fetoscope, stethoscope, or Doppler are placed over the fetal back near the baby's head. Listen for at least 30 seconds following a contraction to detect any decelerations. You may want to listen and record a rate every 6 seconds for 30 seconds to a full minute. Then add a zero to see the beats per minute rates. Accelerations and decelerations are easier to detect. For example, if you count 5 rates for 6 seconds each over 30 seconds and record 10, 11, 12, 11, 10, the FHR was 100, 110, 120, 110, 100. In a term or postterm fetus, 100 to 110 bpm would be in the normal baseline range.

CONFIRM FETAL LIFE

Confirm Fetal Life

Do **NOT** apply the fetal monitor ultrasound transducer until you are sure the fetus is alive. The printout can be 100% maternal. The woman's heart rate or doubling of her heart rate can appear on the fetal monitor paper (see 1.6). The maternal heart rate (MHR) doubles at times due to the monitor's software analysis that counts systole and diastole as two separate beats.

By listening to actual fetal heart sounds with a fetoscope or stethoscope **before** applying the fetal monitor, you can avoid mistaking the MHR for the fetal heart rate. The hand-held Doppler device is a motion, not a sound detector. If you use a hand-held Doppler device to assess the fetal heart rate, you **must** take the MHR **simultaneously** to identify and differentiate the fetal rate from the maternal rate.

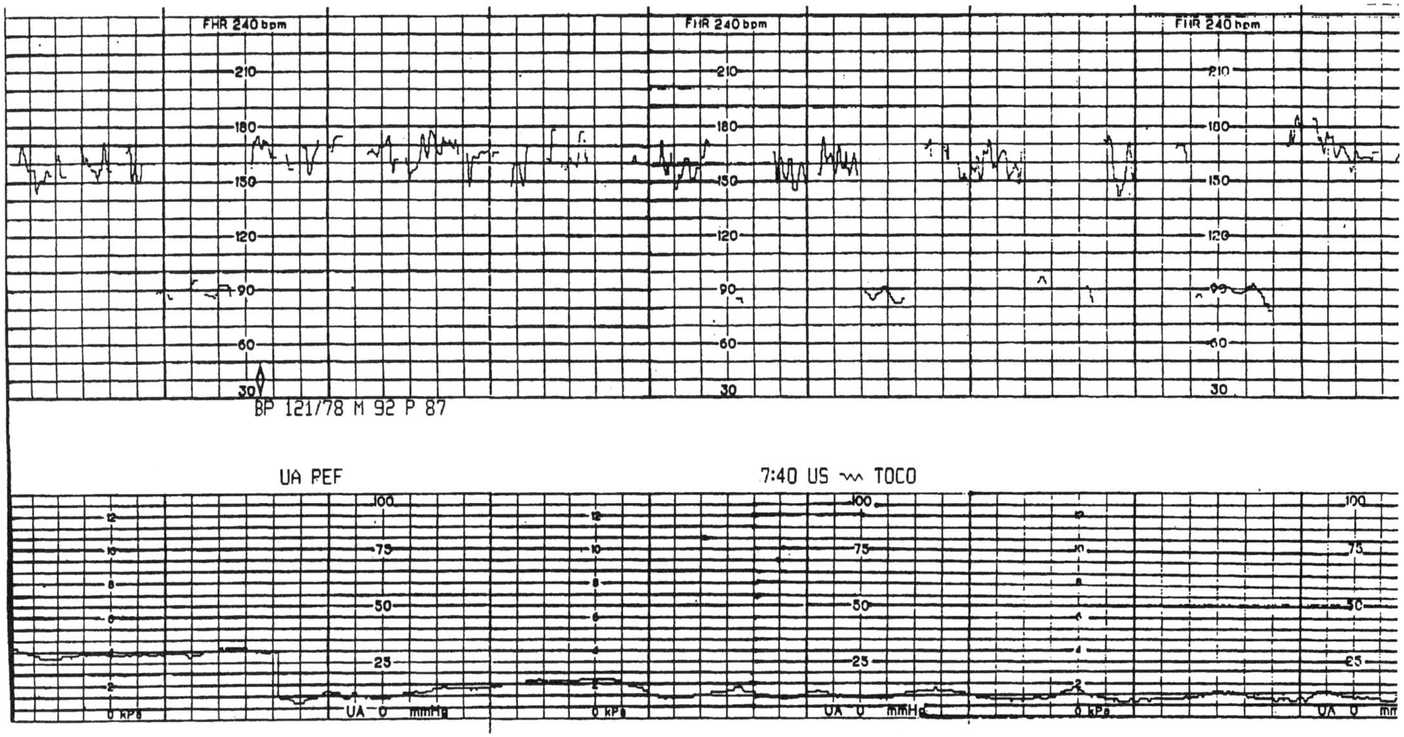

1.6 Maternal heart rate near 87 beats per minute and doubling near 174 beats per minute. The fetus was dead yet the nurse never confirmed fetal life prior to application of the fetal monitor.

APPLY THE MONITOR

Apply the Monitor

To apply the external ultrasound transducer, place the belt under the woman. Locate the fetal back. Apply ultrasound transmission gel to the transducer. Place the transducer over the fetal back. If you have difficulty finding the FHR, move the ultrasound device slightly to the left or right or use the second maneuver to again locate the fetal back.

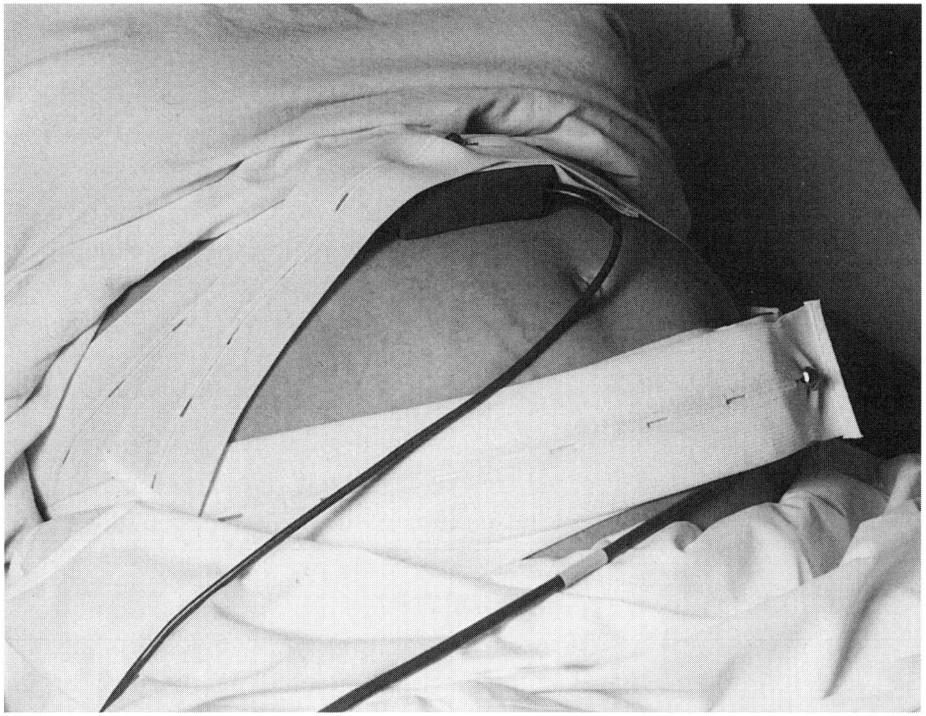

1.7 The ultrasound transducer is placed on the maternal left, over the baby's back and below the umbilicus. The tocotransducer is at the top of the uterus.

FETAL WELL-BEING

The presence of a stable FHR, an acceleration, and the absence of a deceleration, during the period of time the patient is auscultated indicates fetal well-being. The lack of fetal well-being requires prompt communication. *Prompt communication to the midwife or physician of changes in the maternal or fetal status is the nurse's role.*

Auscultation can be used during labor when a one to one nurse to patient ratio is available. Documentation should include the FHR, the presence of accelerations, the absence or presence of decelerations, and if possible, how high the FHR rose or how low it fell in bpm. For example, you might mention "no decelerations heard." Also, document any fetal movement palpated.

AUSCULTATION: ABNORMAL FINDINGS

Auscultation: Abnormal Findings

A FHR greater than 160 bpm, less than 120 bpm if the fetus is preterm, and less than 100 bpm if the fetus is term or post term, or an irregular rhythm should be reported to the midwife or physician as soon as possible. Also, report any FHR which is greater than 20 bpm above or below the baby's expected rate based on previous monitoring during the pregnancy. Apply the electronic fetal monitor if you hear a rate greater than 160, less than 100, or an irregular rhythm.

MATERNAL VITAL SIGNS AND RISK FACTORS

Assess Maternal Vital Signs and Risk Factors

BLOOD PRESSURE

Take the woman's blood pressure (BP) and pulse. The cuff must be an appropriate size and should be approximately 20% wider than the width of her arm. The woman should have her BP taken in a semi-Fowler's or side-lying position versus supine. It is best to take BP between contractions as BP rises during contractions. Compare the readings with her baseline BP from her prenatal record. If it is elevated, pay special attention to her urine protein, edema, and reflexes. Also assess visual disturbances, headache, and epigastric pain. Could she have preeclampsia?

RESPIRATORY RATE

Respiratory Rate

Assess maternal respirations. Are they rapid and labored? Quiet and slow? An unusually fast rate (> 24/minute) may suggest anxiety with hyperventilation or a compromised respiratory system requiring further assessment of her pulmonary or hemodynamic status and her temperature.

TEMPERATURE

Temperature

If her temperature is elevated, look for signs of infection such as skin that is warm to the touch, foul smelling vaginal discharge, a tender uterus, fetal tachycardia (>160 bpm), and/or maternal tachycardia (>100 bpm). Assess skin turgor, mucous membranes, and her lips for dryness. If she is febrile, she may also be dehydrated. Assess her urine for ketones.

HEAD TO TOE ASSESSMENT

Perform a Maternal Head to Toe Assessment

	FINDINGS
HEENT (head, eyes, ears, nose, and throat)	headache, blurred vision, tinnitus, nasal congestion, airway, dizziness?
Heart	regular rate and rhythm, murmur, chest pain, palpitations?
Lungs	clear breath sounds bilaterally, unlabored respirations? absence of wheezing, grunting, adventitious sounds?
Abdomen	tenderness, pain, rigidity, distention, heartburn? quality and quantity of contractions? fetal movement?
Extremities	edema, reflexes, clonus? negative Homan's sign?
Genitourinary	urine protein, ketones, glucose, blood? genital vesicles or warts?

COMPLETING YOUR ASSESSMENT

Inspection, palpation, and auscultation are used to complete your initial maternal assessment. Observe her general appearance and body language which provide clues of any underlying physical or psychological problems. Ask when she last ate and what she ate. When she is alone, ask if she has been hit, slapped, kicked, or punched any time during this pregnancy. Ascertain if she has had any bleeding problems, a history of previous hemorrhage with birth, or transfusions. This may prepare you for the possibility of a postpartum hemorrhage or a newborn with hemolysis as a result of an antibody-antigen reaction. Record your findings. Ask her to urinate prior to her cervical examination. If membranes are ruptured, record the color, estimated amount, and odor of the fluid (**1 milliliter (ml) of fluid weighs 1 gram (gm)**). Determine if there is a vaginal discharge or foul odor. The odor may be recorded as foul or not foul. To prevent infection, a sterile speculum examination should be done if membranes are ruptured but she is not in labor.

FUNDAL HEIGHT AND FETAL GROWTH

Determine Fundal Height — Is it Appropriate for Gestational Age?

What is the estimated date of delivery (EDD)? If fundal height has not been measured in the last week, or you are concerned her placenta may be abrupting, measure the fundal height by placing a tape measure at the top of the symphysis pubis stretching it to the top of the fundus. Mark the top of the fundus using a ballpoint pen if you plan to measure and compare findings at a later time.

After the 20th week of pregnancy, the fundal height is similar to the weeks of gestation. If there is a 3 or more centimeter difference, e.g., she is 26 weeks of gestation, but the fundal height is 23 centimeters (cm) or 29 cm, further tests are needed.

When the fundal height is smaller than expected and not within three cm of the gestational age, review the medical and prenatal history for persistent vomiting, poor weight gain, hypertension, the use of street drugs, and smoking. All of these could diminish oxygen and nutrient delivery to the uterus, placenta, and fetus.

Polyhydramnios, macrosomia, fibroids, and diabetes, may be associated with a larger than expected fundal height.

UTERINE ACTIVITY

Determine Uterine Activity

Palpate the woman's uterus. Assess the symmetry of the abdomen during contractions. During normal labor, the uterus begins to contract at the fundus and the fundus moves forward. Record "mild," "moderate," or "strong" uterine contractions. If some are mild and others are moderate, record "UCs mild–mod" or "ctx mild to mod." Feel your cheek. It's indentable. That's how a mild contraction feels. Feel your nose. A little harder, but slightly indentable is how a moderate contraction feels. Feel your forehead. This is how a strong contraction feels to palpation.

LABOR

Determine the Presence of Labor

Labor is defined as regular uterine contractions accompanied by a change in dilatation. Determine the presence of contractions. Evaluate maternal pain by observing the woman's face, hands, and toes. Is she curling her toes or tightening her grasp? Perhaps she is focused inwardly, suggesting advanced labor progress. Is her pain response what you would anticipate with the contractions you are feeling? What impact does her culture have on her display of pain?

Prior to applying the fetal monitor

- assess comfort or pain
- identify and address concerns about the electronic fetal monitor (EFM)
- adapt the monitoring belts as needed for the obese patient, e.g., attach one belt to another one or hand-hold the ultrasound transducer
- do not use the ultrasound transducer or spiral electrode if the fetus is not viable (≤23 weeks) or has died
- do not apply the monitor if the woman refuses it

If a women refuses EFM for an admission test, the physician or midwife should be informed immediately and the nurse must document the patient's refusal for the use of EFM. Record her words in quotation marks.

PLACEMENT OF THE TOCO-TRANSDUCER

Secure the tocotransducer (toco). Correct placement of the toco should detect uterine contractions not maternal breathing movements. Placement of the toco depends on gestational age. If the fetus is less than 30 weeks of gestation, place the toco under the umbilicus. Place it above the umbilicus if the fetus is greater than 30 weeks of gestation.

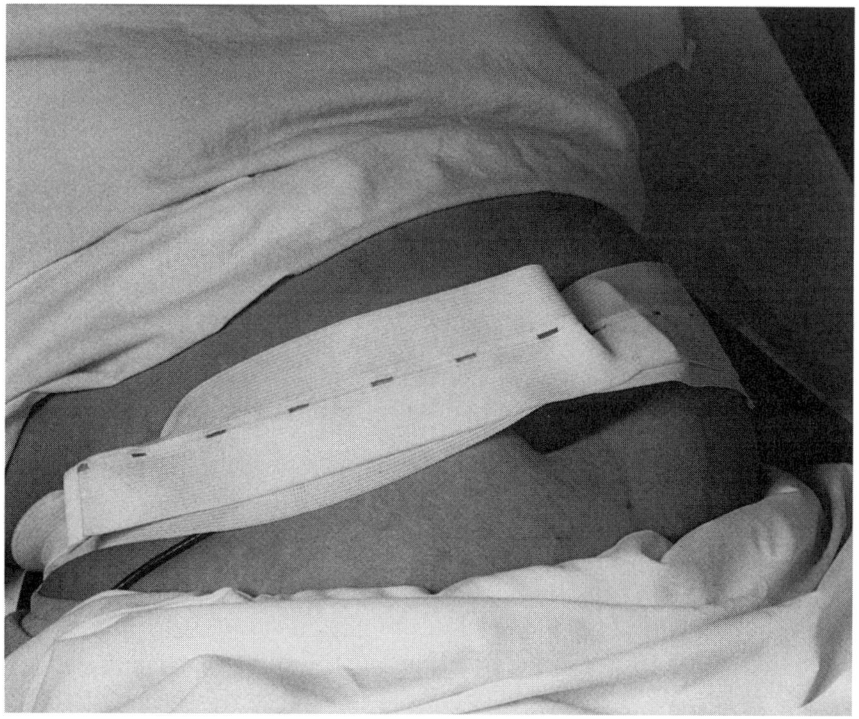

1.8 Preterm pregnancy tocotransducer placement.

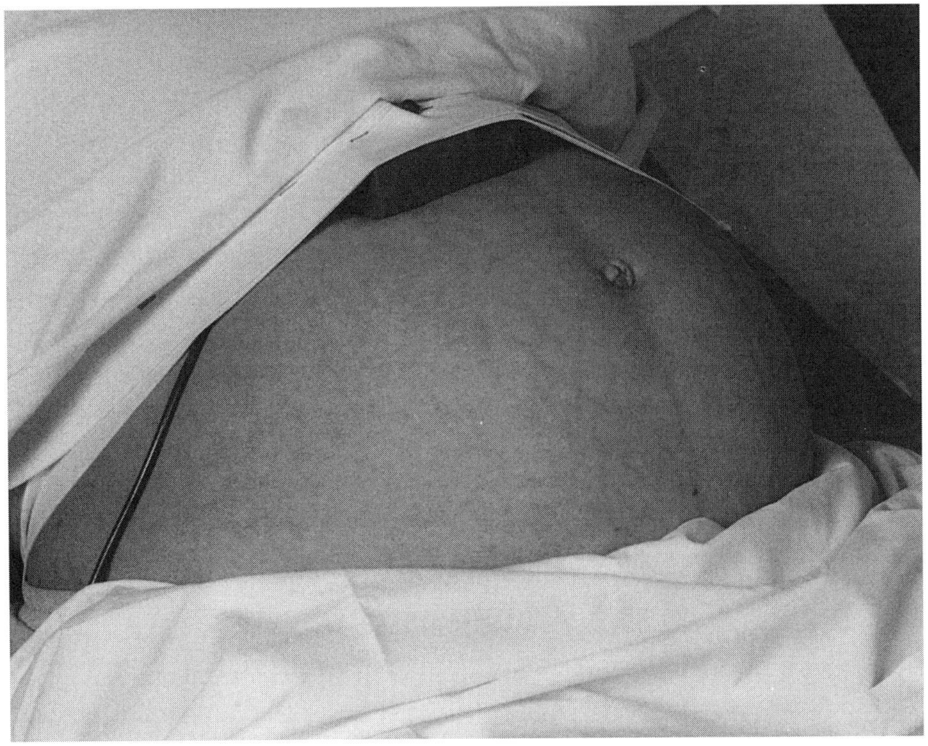

1.9 Term pregnancy tocotransducer placement.

THE CERVIX

Assess the Cervix

Defer cervical examinations when bleeding is present until you know the location of the placenta. Follow protocols that state who should examine the woman. If membranes are ruptured preterm, the cervix may be examined visually using a sterile speculum.

During cervical examination, assess

- presentation — vertex, breech, or other, e.g., face, brow, shoulder. Is there caput or molding? cord or compound presentation, e.g., head and hand?
- station — determine presenting part in relation to the level of the ischial spines. When the tip of the baby's skull is at the level of the ischial spines, that is zero (0) station. Use centimeters: -1, -2, -3, ballottable (all are above the spines), +1, +2, +3, +4, +5 (below the spines)

- effacement — at term the cervix is approximately 2.5 to 3 cm long. It may be firm or soft. Measured in percent e.g., 70%, how thin is the cervix?

- location — locate the cervical os, is it posterior, in a midposition, or anterior.

SUMMARY

Summary

Establish a data base that includes maternal, FHR, and fetal movement information. Continue to evaluate the woman and fetus. The nurse, midwife, and/or physician should discuss the plan of care. Once the plan of care is determined, the midwife or physician usually shares this with the woman and her family. Assessment of her initial and ongoing status and behavior helps you recognize normal or abnormal progress which may influence the FHR. *Always try to respond to the maternal and fetal physiology.* Think beyond the paper printout.

SECTION 1: SYSTEMATIC ASSESSMENT OF THE PREGNANT WOMAN

QUESTIONS

QUESTIONS

Directions: Circle T if the statement is true, F if it is false.

T F 1. A systematic approach for patient assessment includes Leopold's Maneuvers.

T F 2. The choice of monitoring methods depends on the number of registered nurses.

T F 3. Auscultation of the fetal heart rate is necessary prior to fetal monitor application.

T F 4. When a fetoscope is used, document the fetal heart rate, accelerations, and decelerations.

T F 5. The initial assessment may include fundal height to rule out intrauterine growth restriction or macrosomia.

T F 6. A cervical examination can be used to confirm the fetal presenting part.

T F 7. At 26 weeks of gestation, the tocotransducer should be placed above the umbilicus.

T F 8. It is important to consider the impact of maternal and fetal physiology on the FHR.

SECTION 2
The Paper

STRIP OR TRACING

You may recall from Section 1 that it is best to observe and respond to the fetal and maternal physiology that produces the FHR printout. The printout is also called a *strip or tracing.*

PAPER SPEED

The tracing flows out of the fetal monitor at 3 centimeters (cm) per minute. In some countries this speed is reduced to 1 or 2 cm/minute. In the United States the standard is 3 cm/minute. **Find the paper speed switch on your fetal monitor.** If it is set at 1 or 2 cm/minute, the image will be compressed and may be misinterpreted. Change it to 3 cm/minute.

HEAT-SENSITIVE PAPER

The tracing is printed on *heat-sensitive* paper. It turns black when a hot printer touches it. The paper is printed with two channels. The upper portion or fetal heart rate channel is 30 to 240 beats per minute (bpm) or 50 to 210 bpm. The lower portion or uterine activity channel is usually 0 to 100 mm Hg or 0 to 90 mm Hg.

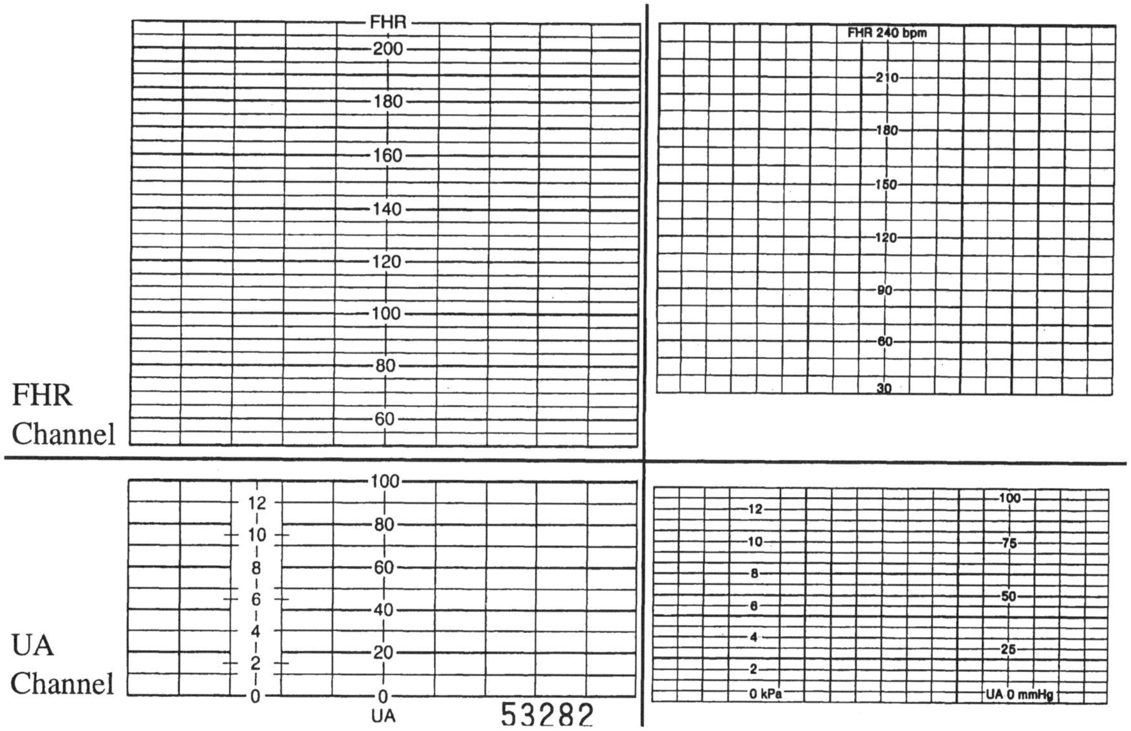

2.1 The fetal heart rate channel is always at the top of fetal monitoring paper and the uterine activity channel is at the bottom.

INK

The color of the grid on the paper is *not* significant. What is important is the numeric scale on the FHR channel.

USA-SCALED PAPER

Look again at the paper on the left. It is 30 to 240 bpm. Each ascending line is 10 bpm above the line below it. This is called USA-scaled paper.

EUROPEAN-SCALED PAPER

The paper on the right is 50 to 210 bpm and each ascending line is 5 bpm above the line below it. This is called European-scaled paper, to differentiate it from USA-scaled paper. Some European-scaled paper has a range of 60 to 200 bpm. Both types of paper may be used in any fetal monitor *provided the machine is adjusted to print to that scale.*

REVIEW QUESTION

All fetal monitor paper, whether USA-scaled or European-scaled, should roll out of the electronic fetal monitor at the same speed. What is that speed?

If you said 3 cm/minute you're right! Now look again at the fetal monitor paper. Notice the vertical lines on the FHR channel. As your eye moves from left to right, count 6 small squares on the paper on the left. Each square is 10 seconds in duration. Six squares are equal to one minute of time. Each minute is 3 cm in length. The paper on the right has 20 seconds between each vertical line. On both types of paper, 1 cm equals 20 seconds and 3 cm equals 1 minute.

So, whether or not you have European-scaled or USA-scaled paper in the machine, they both should be moving out of the fetal monitor at 3 cm/minute. If your hospital changes from USA to European-scaled paper or vice versa, a biomedical technician must adjust the fetal monitor printer or the printed image of the FHR will be erroneous.

LOADING THE PAPER

Loading the Paper

When you load the fetal monitor paper, the *FHR* channel should appear on the *left* and the UA channel will be on the *right*. **Practice loading and removing the paper**. Read any directions on the paper package so that you follow any guidelines. Some paper loads with the first sheet on the bottom of the paper pack. Each paper pack lasts at least 8 hours when the paper speed is 3 cm/minute.

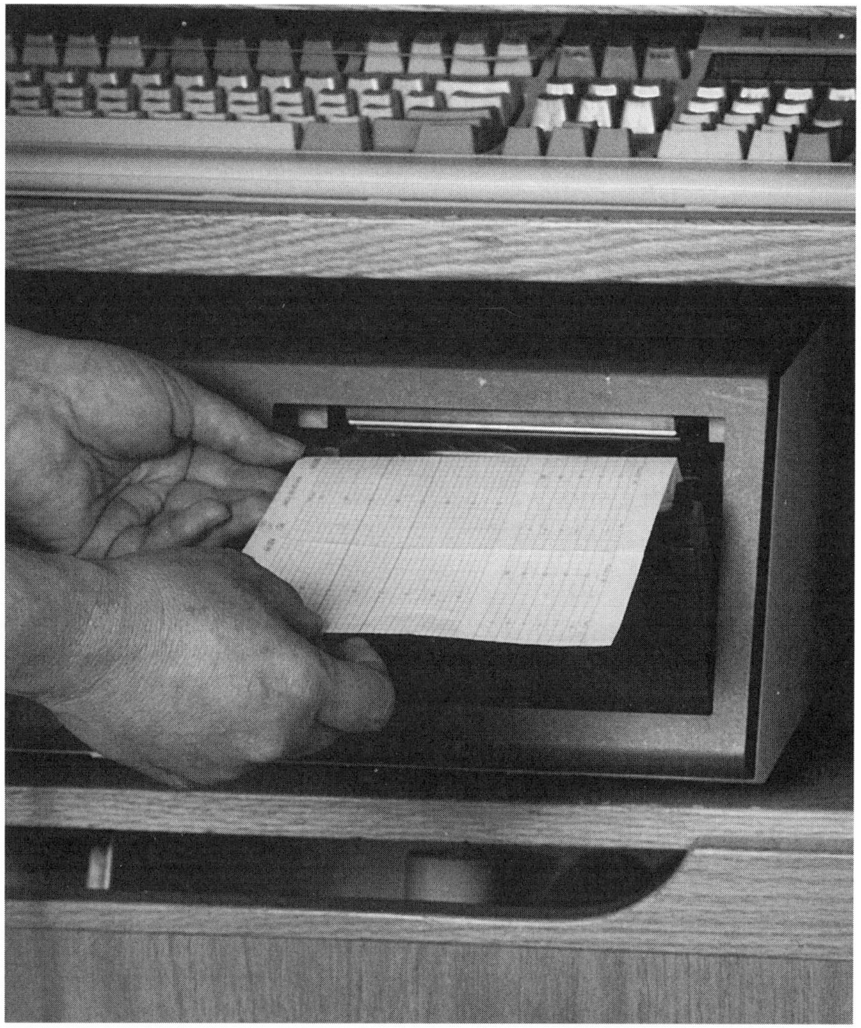

2.2 ***When the fetal monitor paper is loaded properly, the FHR will print on the channel on the left and uterine activity will print on the channel on the right.*** (Photograph by Pam Barncastle, Castle Studio, Albuquerque, New Mexico).

DOCUMENTATION

Documentation When You Begin Monitoring

Your facility may have a specific policy on what should be written on the first square of the fetal monitor paper. If not, it is best to write patient identifying information. If the fetal monitor does not print the date on the tracing and the monitoring start time, it should be written. Any additional information, e.g., the admitting practitioner, may be added to help identify this legal document.

Strip with Initial Documentation

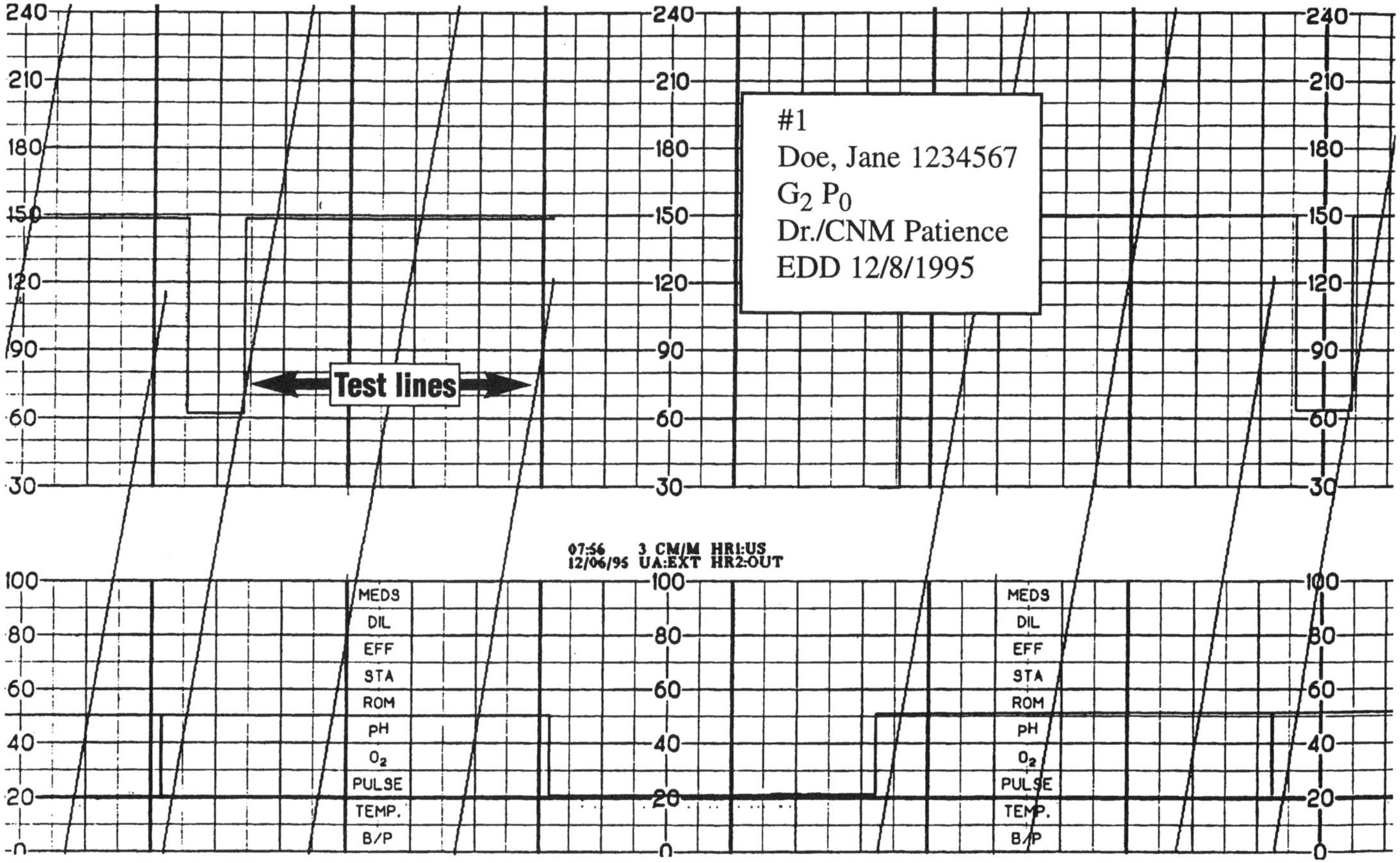

2.3 Label the tracing with patient identifying information and the number of the strip. Also note diagonal lines are printed as a monitor/printer test when the monitoring begins. See test lines.

NUMBER THE TRACING

Number 1 signifies this is the first tracing generated in Jane Doe's visit. If for any reason the tracing should be torn off (pages are perforated), or the paper is changed, each consecutive tracing should be numbered, e.g., #2, #3. This will help you put the tracings in order before they are submitted to the Medical Records Department.

Also included in this initial labeling of the strip are Jane's name and medical record number, the number of this pregnancy (gravida), parity (para) or the number of babies delivered who weighed at least 500 grams or who had a gestational age of 20 weeks, her physician or midwife's name, and her estimated date of delivery at 40 weeks of gestation. Record patient identifying information on consecutive strips.

Testing the Fetal Monitor

AUTO TEST

Now that the paper is in the machine and it is properly labeled, turn the fetal monitor on. Be sure the paper is moving. Is the record button on? The **auto test** feature should be automatically activated. The printer will print and the digital display will be illuminated. Look at the lines printed on the paper as the paper advances. There should be no gaps. Look at the lighted display, are the numbers totally illuminated? If there are gaps on the test lines or if the printer is not printing on the paper lines, the printer needs to be repaired or perhaps the paper feed needs to be adjusted. Tag the fetal monitor "printer not properly printing," include a sample of the misprinted paper, and send the monitor to the Biomedical Department.

MANUAL TEST

If you wish to see the test strip again, or if the monitor does not perform an auto test, push the **test** button for a **manual test**. If the fetal monitor does not record an auto test strip after it is turned on, perform a manual test to document the monitor printer was functioning normally prior to use.

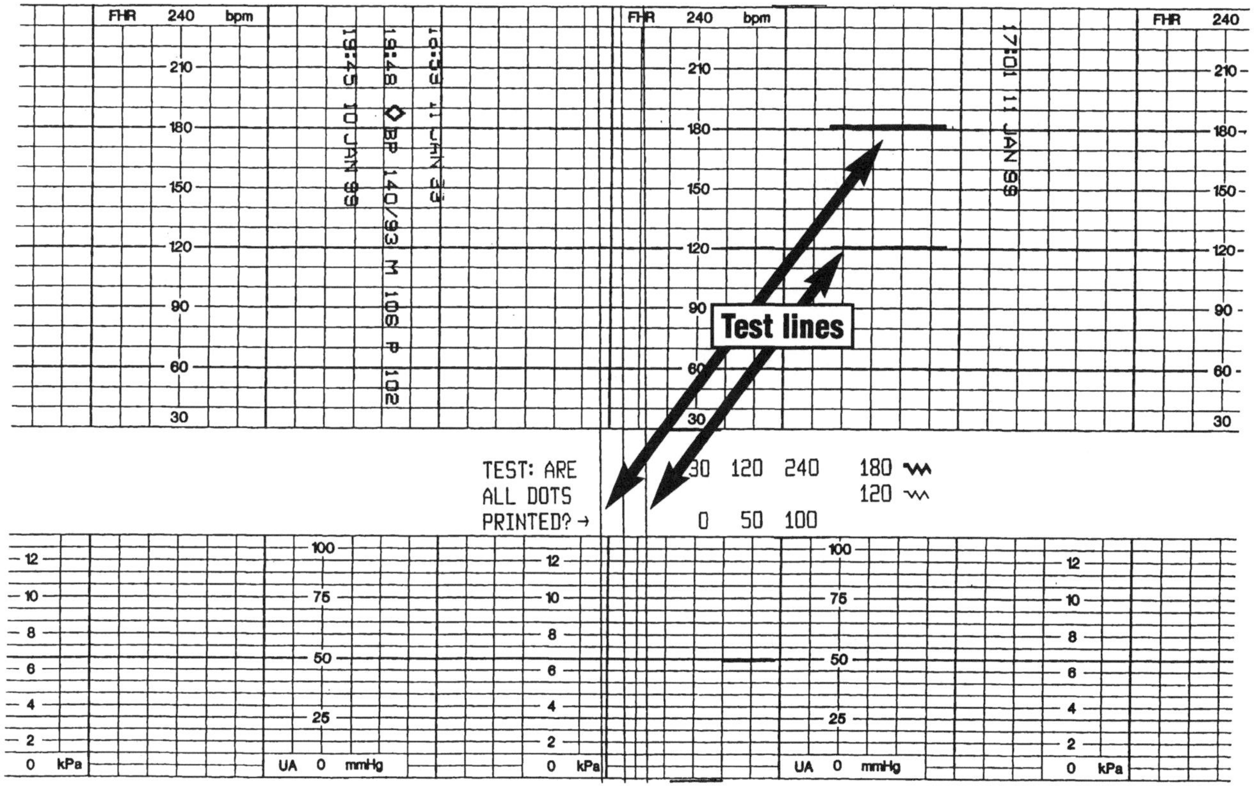

2.4 All the printed lines should be continuous and on the paper lines. If the test lines are not on the paper lines, the printer or paper feed needs to be adjusted by biomedical personnel.

You can also test each internal and external FHR and uterine activity component that plugs into the fetal monitor. These specific tests will be discussed in Section 3: External and Internal Fetal Monitoring.

THE CLOCK

A battery backs up the monitor clock so that even when it is unplugged the date and time will remain set. If you plug in and turn on the fetal monitor and a message is printed on the paper such as "set time/date," the battery is dead. Label the fetal monitor with a note, "replace clock battery" and send the monitor to the Biomedical Department.

Alternatively, your Biomedical Department may be able to send a technician who can replace the battery without removing the monitor from service. **Learn how to set the time and date**. All monitors should be set to identical times. One watch should be set to the main operating room clock. Each monitor clock is then set using that watch. Set your watch to the monitor time. When you care for more than one woman, documented events will then reflect the time on the fetal monitor in every room.

EXERCISES

EXERCISES

1. What is the FHR range of USA-scaled paper?
   a. 50 to 210 bpm
   b. 30 to 240 bpm
   c. 30 to 200 bpm

2. What is the FHR range of most European-scaled paper?
   a. 50 to 210 bpm
   b. 30 to 240 bpm
   c. 30 to 200 bpm

3. What is the paper speed in the United States?
   a. 1 cm/minute
   b. 2 cm/minute
   c. 3 cm/minute

4. What does it mean when the print-out on the paper is "set time/date?"
   a. the time is wrong and needs to be reset
   b. The clock back-up battery needs to be replaced
   c. This message always appears when the monitor is turned on

5. Which of the following is not needed when the fetal monitor is initiated?
   a. woman's name
   b. identification number
   c. maternal diagnosis

See page 29 for the correct responses.

MATERNAL HEART RATE

Maternal Heart Rate (MHR)

Since women have variability or fluctuations of their heart rate it is possible that the MHR will print when the fetus has died or the external ultrasound transducer is over the maternal aorta. By comparing maternal pulse **simultaneously** with the printed rate, you should be able to confirm you are not recording the MHR. If you are concerned, confirm the fetal heart rate by listening to fetal ventricular heart sounds with a fetoscope or apply the **maternal 3-lead ECG cable** (see figure 2.5). This device is sold by all fetal monitor companies. You can also apply a maternal pulse oximeter and compare the pulsation sound with sound generated by the fetal monitor. They should differ. Some fetal monitors have a maternal pulse oximeter finger probe that plugs into the fetal monitor. The MHR will be continuously printed (see figure 2.6). If the MHR and printout coincide, the FHR is not being recorded. Use a fetoscope or real-time ultrasound to confirm fetal cardiac motion and the FHR.

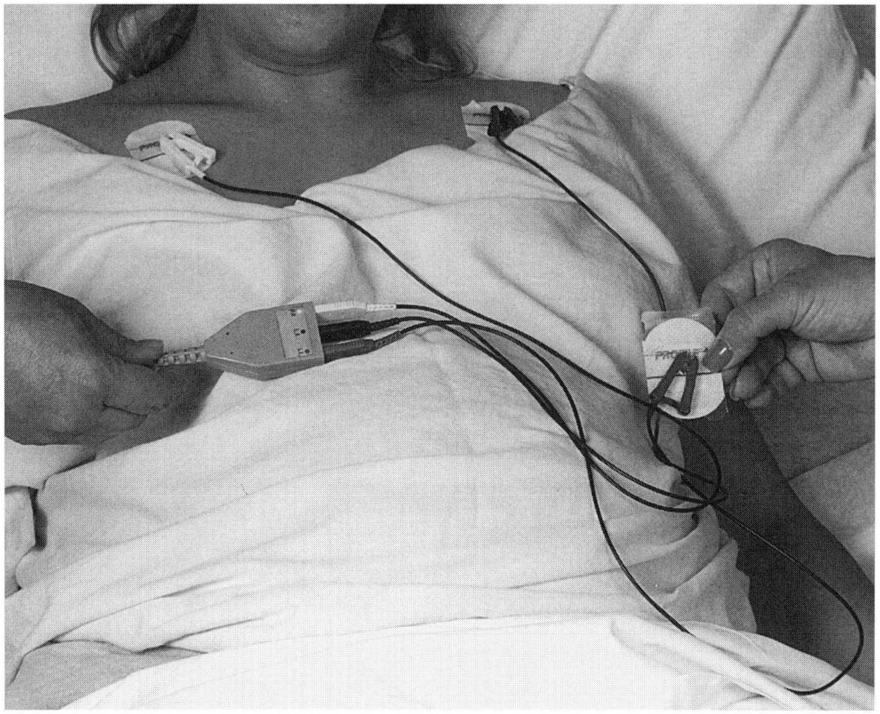

2.5 Maternal 3 lead ECG cable for the fetal monitor. (Photograph by Pam Barncastle, Castle Studio, Albuquerque, New Mexico).

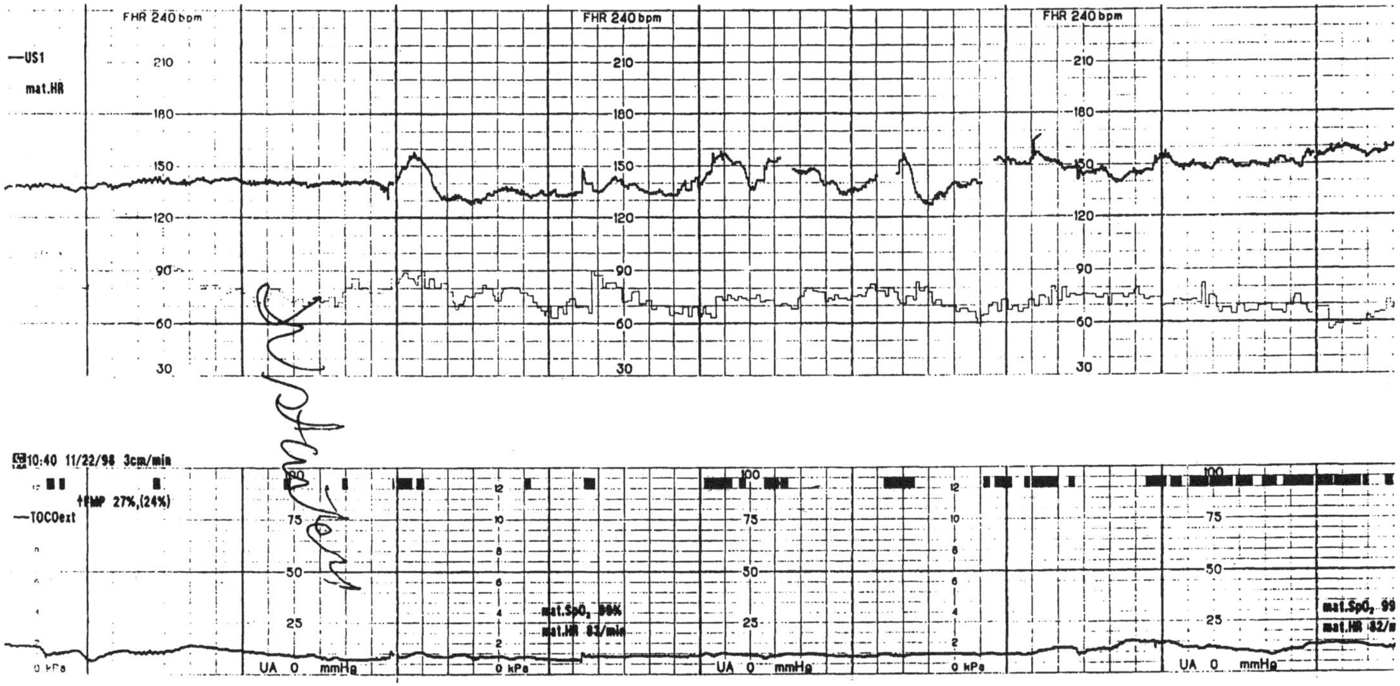

2.6 Fetal heart rate demonstrating fetal well-being. The baseline is initially near 140 bpm with spontaneous accelerations. Maternal heart rate is 65-85 bpm. Note there is variability. Fetal movement is indicated by black marks on the top of the uterine activity channel and maternal SpO_2 is 99%.

TWIN MONITORING

Twin Monitoring

Fetal monitors may record the same fetus twice when both external ultrasound transducers are directed towards the same fetus or the spiral electrode (internal monitor) and ultrasound (external monitor) are on the same fetus. Depending on the manufacturer, there may be an indication this is happening, e.g., Hewlett Packard series 50 monitors will print a ? on the top of the FHR channel. This is called **cross-channel verification.** If this occurs, locate the other fetus by palpation and reposition the ultrasound. A fetoscope or real-time ultrasound may be needed to confirm fetal life.

CROSS-CHANNEL VERIFICATION

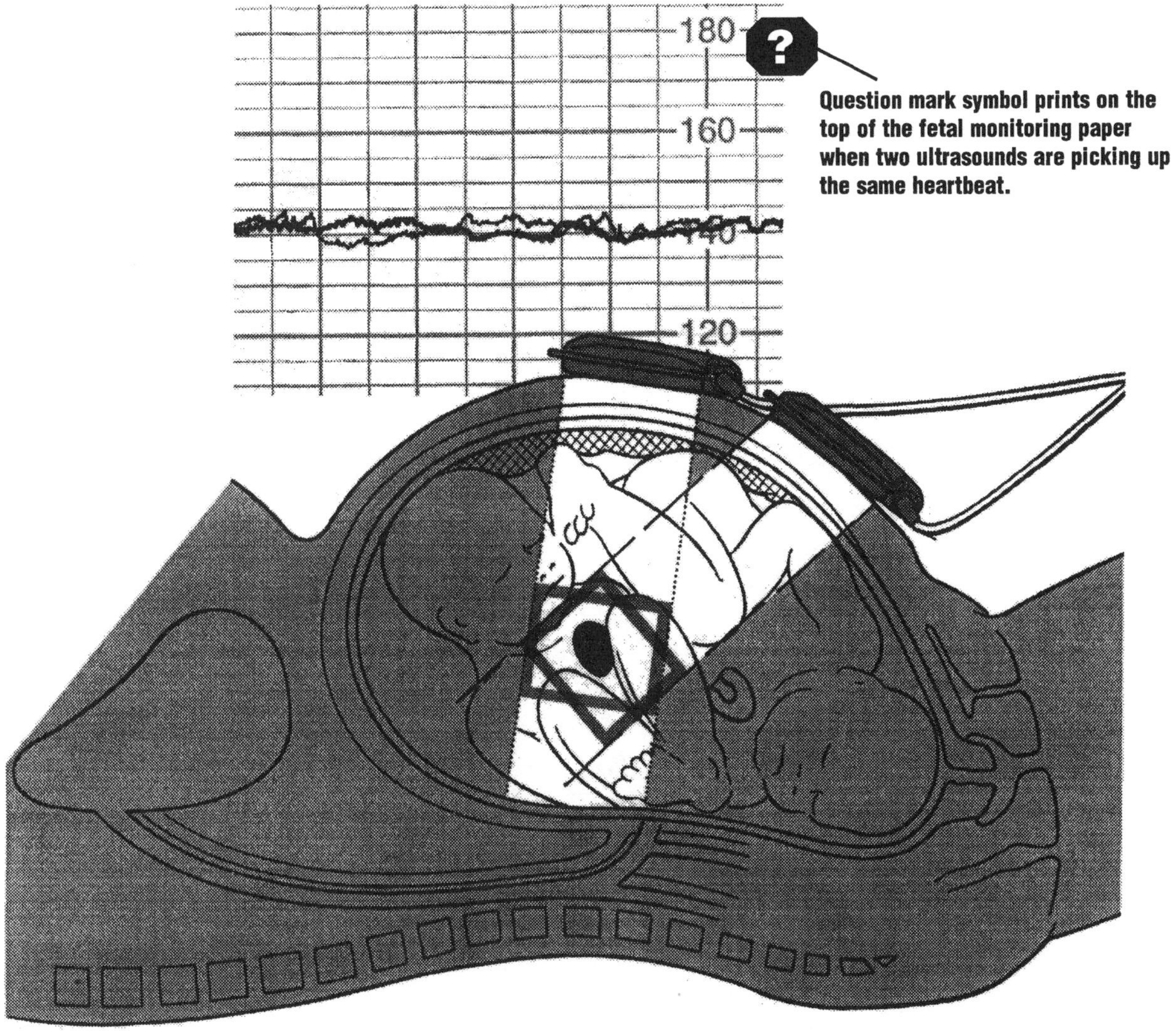

2.7 ***Series 50 fetal monitor with cross-channel verification*** (provided with permission of Hewlett-Packard® Company).

BASELINE OFFSET

Sometimes the fetuses are clearly recorded but the FHR patterns are in the same range, making it difficult to see each FHR. By pushing a button, e.g., the *mark* button on the *Corometrics*® 116, 118, or 120 series monitors, the twins will be separated by 20 bpm. This is called a **baseline offset** (see figure 2.8). The baseline offset of the Spacelabs fetal monitor is 30 bpm. *Toitu*® monitors label each fetus and each fetus' activity (see book cover).

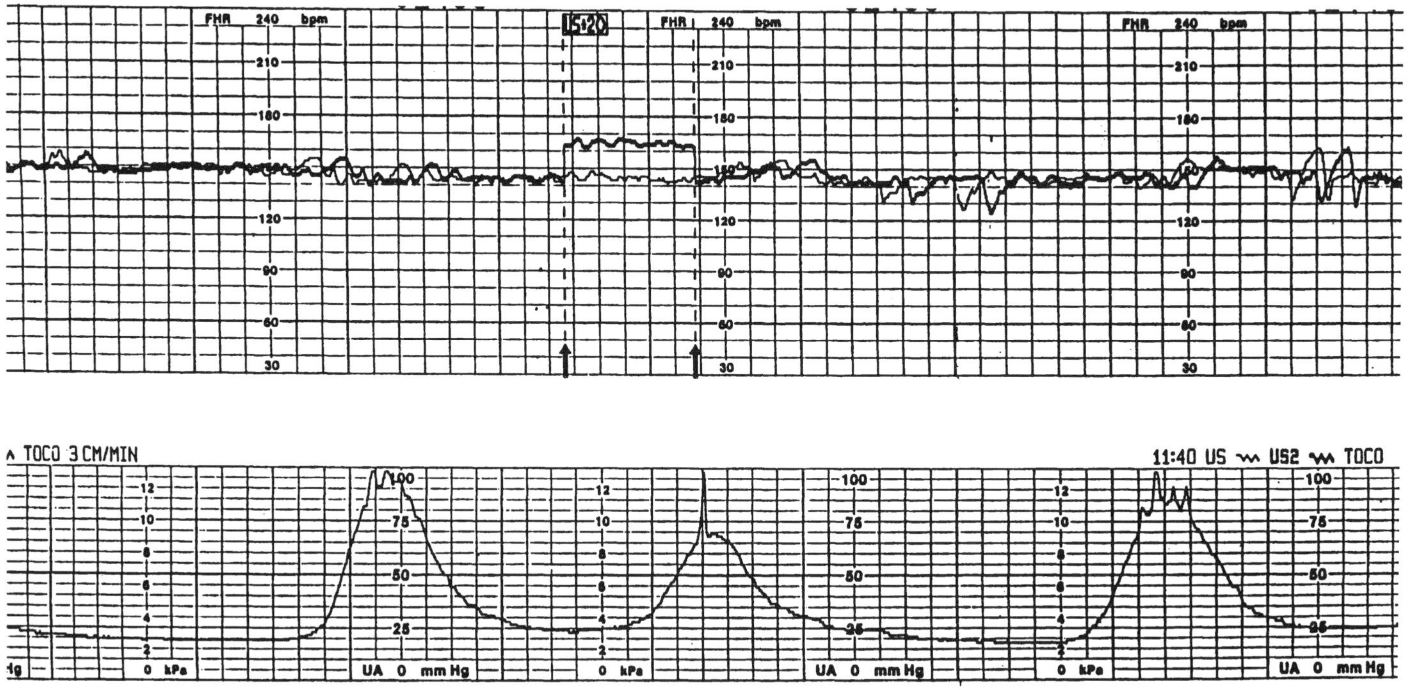

2.8 Baseline offset of Corometrics® fetal monitor. Pushing the mark button for 3 seconds elevates one twin's rate. Pushing the mark button again returns it to its normal level.

DOCUMENTATION OF TWINS

Documentation of Twins

If you are not sure that both twins are alive, listen for two different heart rates using a fetoscope or ask the appropriately skilled clinician to assess fetal cardiac motion using a real-time ultrasound machine.

When you begin monitoring, label each respective tracing "Twin A" and "Twin B" (see figure 2.9). This can be repeated from time to time, e.g., every half hour to hour. If twin B should deliver first, the note on the delivery summary should read "First twin (B), second twin (A)." If you are performing an antepartal test, such as a nonstress test, note twin A's and Twin B's average heart rate in the prenatal record. Try to keep A as A and B as B in subsequent monitoring. The FHR drops 1 bpm per week of gestation beginning at 16 weeks of gestation. The FHR stabilizes at 35 weeks. If each twin has a different average FHR, e.g., 130 bpm and 150 bpm, it should be easy to keep them as A and B throughout the pregnancy.

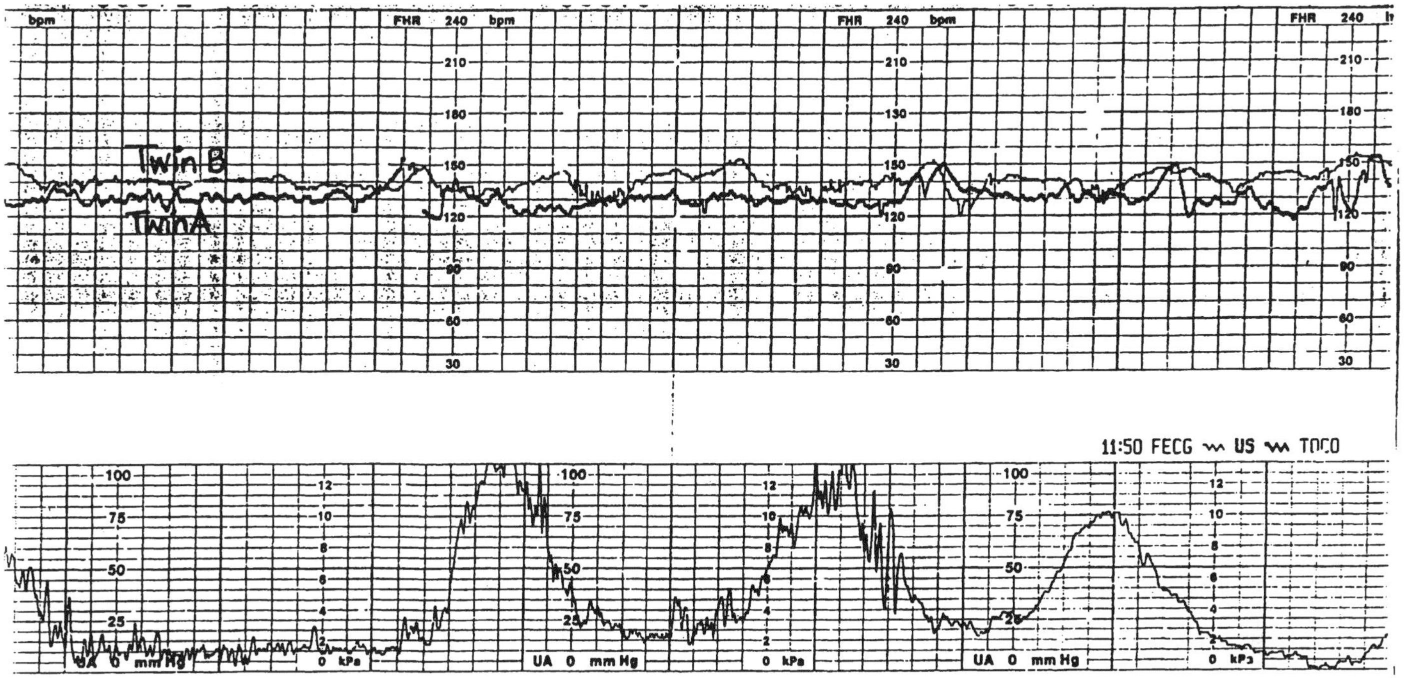

2.9 Label the FHR of each twin every ½ to 1 hour. This helps anyone who reviews the strip to easily verify fetal status.

MATERNAL HEART RATE DOUBLING

Maternal Heart Rate Doubling

The maternal heart rate can be recorded when the fetus is dead or the ultrasound transducer is over the maternal aorta. The maternal heart rate may double for short periods of time (see figure 2.10). The fetal heart rate **never** doubles with second-generation monitors. However, if the fetal heart rate exceeds the paper scale, it will halve, e.g., a rate of 300 bpm will print at 150 bpm. This occurs when the fetus has supraventricular tachycardia.

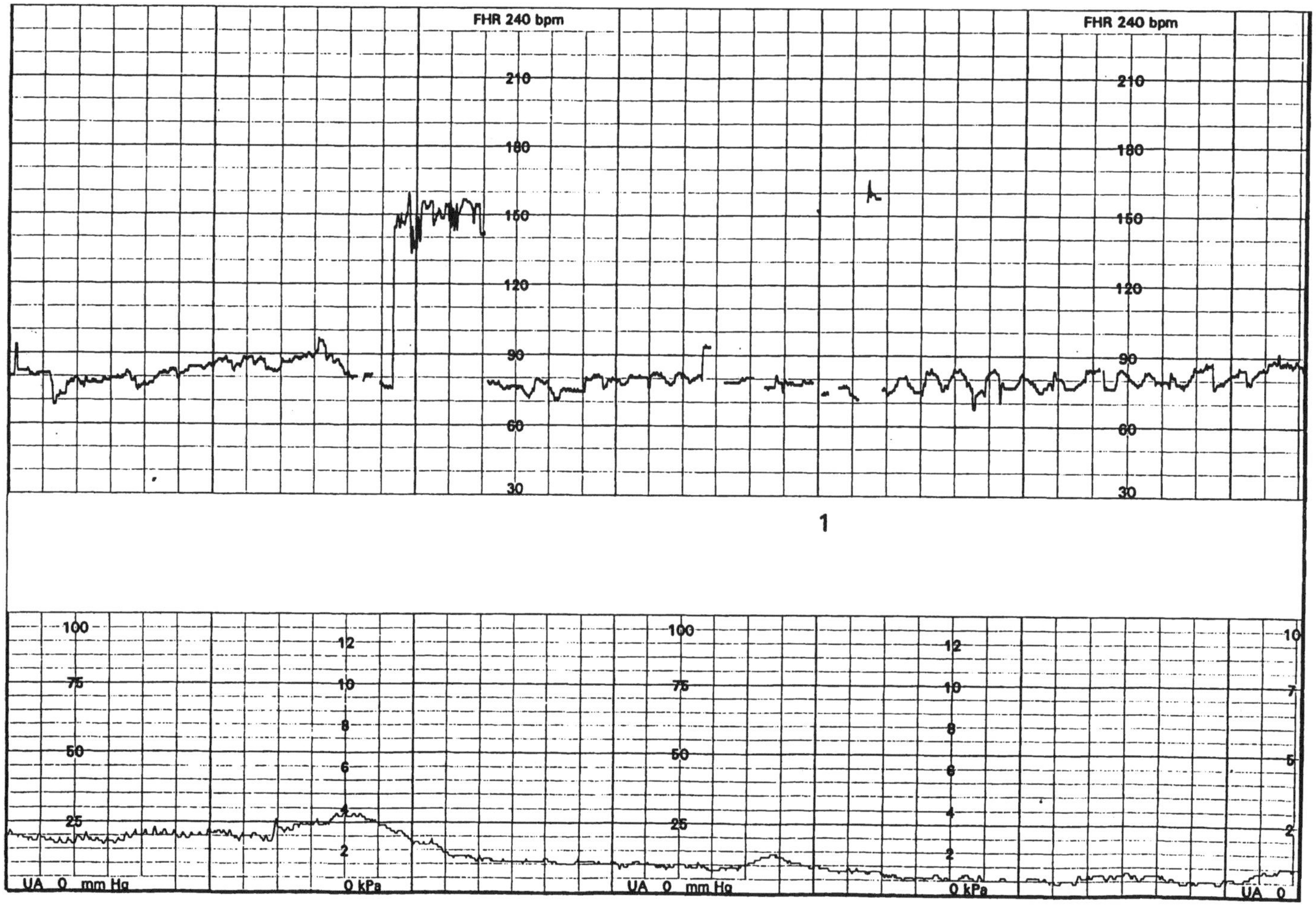

2.10 Doubling of the maternal heart rate can occur. However, second-generation fetal monitors **never** *double the fetal heart rate. Most monitors created in the1980s and beyond are second-generation monitors.*

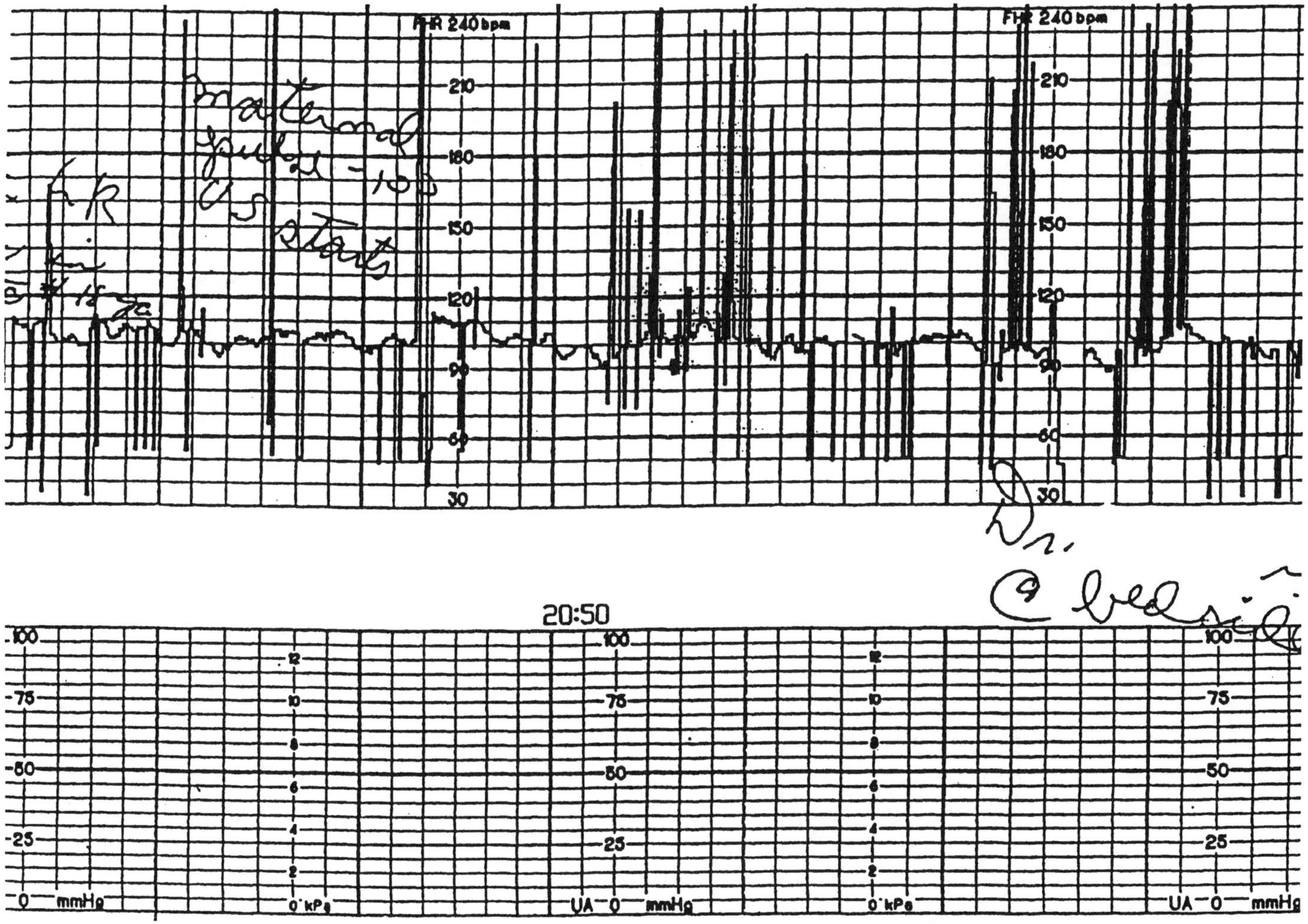

2.11 The maternal heart rate averages 100 bpm in this tracing. A spiral electrode was on the fetus and it transmitted the maternal ECG signal. Note lines called artifact. Artifact is due to signal interruption.

Healthy women have short-term and long-term variability. Artifact appears as lines of various lengths due to signal transmission interruption through the spiral electrode.

MATERNAL ACCELERATIONS

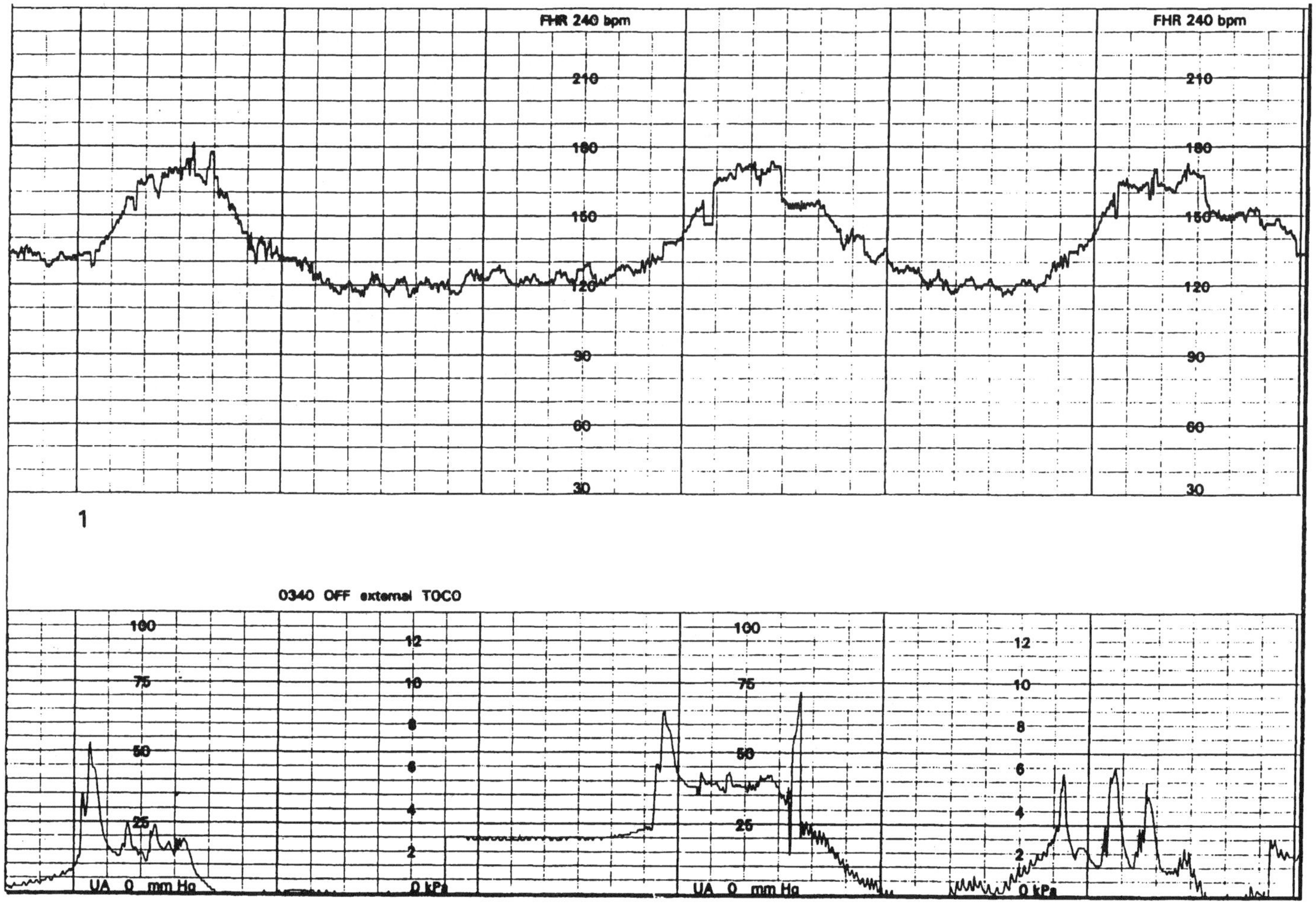

2.12 Maternal heart rate accelerations with pushing.

The maternal heart rate will accelerate in response to pain, especially during pushing (see figure 2.12). Sometimes the maternal heart rate decelerates during contractions, but this is rare.

ANSWERS TO EXERCISES

1. b
2. a
3. c
4. b
5. c

SUMMARY

Summary

USA-scaled paper has a range of 30 to 240 bpm. Each ascending line is 10 bpm higher than the line below it. Each square moving from left to right represents 10 seconds of time. Six boxes represent a minute of time. The paper speed is 3 cm/minute. When utilizing a fetal heart monitor start by testing the equipment. Label the fetal heart rate tracing with identifying information. Determine if the tracing represents a maternal or fetal heart rate by comparing the print-out simultaneously with the maternal rate. Label twins on the monitor tracing as Twin A and Twin B every 1/2 to 1 hour.

SECTION 2: THE PAPER

QUESTIONS

QUESTIONS

Directions: Circle T if the statement is true, F if it is false.

T	F	1.	European-scaled paper speed is 1 cm/minute.
T	F	2.	Each 20 seconds equals 1 cm in length on the fetal monitor paper.
T	F	3.	If the paper is loaded correctly, the fetal heart rate channel is on the right.
T	F	4.	Parity is the number of live babies delivered after 20 weeks of gestation.
T	F	5.	It is acceptable to use a fetal monitor even if the printer test strip lines are misaligned with the paper grid.
T	F	6.	The maternal heart rate can print on the fetal monitor paper.
T	F	7.	If twin B delivers first, the baby becomes twin A.
T	F	8.	Fetal heart rates can double with second-generation monitors.
T	F	9.	Maternal pain may be related to accelerations of the maternal heart rate.
T	F	10.	The maternal heart rate may decelerate.

SECTION 3
External and Internal Fetal Monitoring

ULTRASOUND TECHNOLOGY: EXTERNAL FHR MONITORING

PEAK DETECTION

Peak Detection

Fetal monitors have changed over the last thirty years. You are probably not using fetal monitors made in the 1970s and early 1980s. The first generation machines determined the fetal heart rate (FHR) by detection of the ultrasound waveform peaks, thought to represent systole of the heartbeat. The beat-to-beat interval was estimated. A beats per minute (bpm) rate was determined and was printed. Some of the old sayings when these monitors were used were:

FIRST GENERATION MONITOR SAYINGS

- *"If it looks bad on external, its worse on internal."* (meaning the ultrasound tracing that looked nearly smooth, would be even smoother when a spiral electrode was used)
- *"Don't document beat-to-beat variability when an external is used."*(meaning if the printout generated by the external ultrasound is bumpy, when a spiral electrode is used, it might be smooth)

AUTO-CORRELATION

Autocorrelation

A change and improvement in ultrasound hardware and software in the 1980s improved analysis of the ultrasound signal. The new software uses a process called autocorrelation to analyze the ultrasound waveform created by the movement of the fetal heart valves. Monitors that use autocorrelation are called second-generation monitors. With autocorrelation, the printed rate is within 2.5 bpm of the true rate. A high-speed data processor analyzes each incoming nonrandom ultrasound signal generated by fetal mitral and tricuspid valve movement. After 0.5 to 1.2 seconds are evaluated, the FHR is calculated and printed. The printed rates, when connected, create a FHR baseline, accelerations, and decelerations.

Ultrasound (US) Principles

- The US detects movement, not electrical energy or sound.
- Movement of the heart valves creates US waveforms for counting.
- Analysis of the US signal depends on the software capabilities of the fetal monitor.
- Very little additional clinical information will be gained by the application of a spiral electrode when compared with a consistent ultrasound-derived FHR pattern.

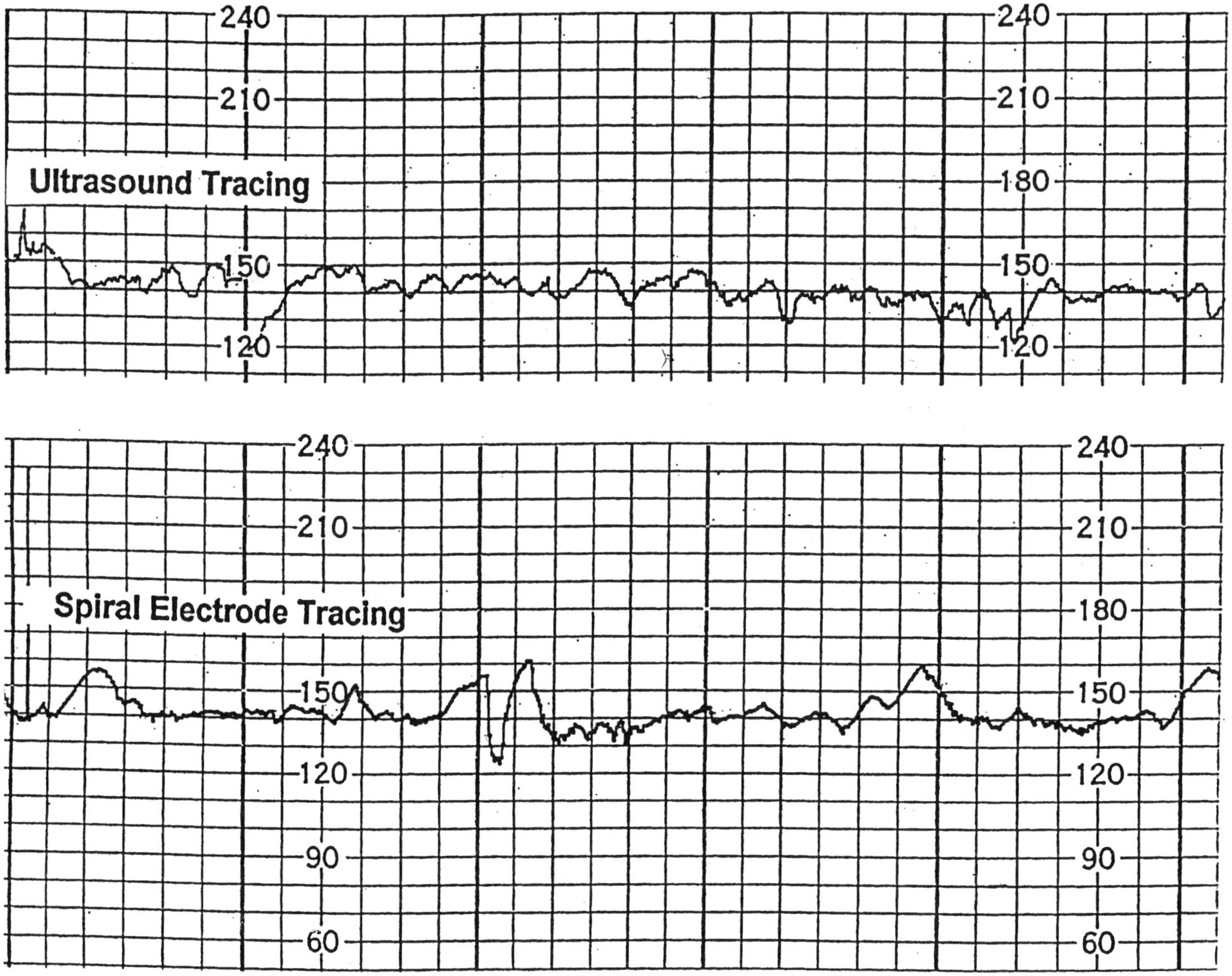

3.1 ***With second-generation monitors, the ultrasound tracing is nearly identical in appearance to the spiral electrode tracing. These examples of the fetal heart rate pattern of the same fetus illustrate the similarity before and after spiral electrode use.***

SECOND GENERATION MONITOR SAYINGS

Current sayings about second-generation monitors are:

- *"If it looks GOOD on external, it's probably GOOD on internal."*
- *"If it looks BAD on external, it may be better on internal." "Bad on external" means a smooth tracing which suggests the absence of short-term variability.*
- *"If long-term variability (LTV) and a reactive acceleration are present on external, metabolic acidosis is ruled out and short-term variability (STV) is (conceptually) present."*

ULTRASOUND TRANSDUCER

Ultrasound Transducer (US)

Ultrasound transducers emit high frequency sound waves. These sound waves cannot be heard by the clinician but are interpreted by the computer periodically within the FHR monitor. What you hear is an artificial sound generated by the monitor and you see a digital rate that is printed on moving graph paper. The pattern in then visually interpreted by the clinician to determine the baseline, accelerations, decelerations, shot-term and long-term variability.

COUPLING GEL

Coupling transmission gel (one example is Aquasonic® gel) is applied to the US transducer to promote transmission of the US waves. This gel will need to be replaced if the transducer face dries out. Inspect it periodically, especially if gaps occur in the printout.

AUTOMATIC GAIN CONTROL

Automatic gain control is an electronic feature of electronic fetal monitors that strengthens weak signals transmitted by the US transducer or spiral electrode. This feature can strengthen the maternal heart rate signal from aortic pulsations and bloodflow. In that case, the maternal heart rate (MHR), not the FHR will be printed.

ARTIFACT

Gaps in the FHR printout generated when a US is used occur when there is a weak or inadequately transmitted signal. The gaps and dots are called artifact (see 3.2).

TESTING THE ULTRASOUND TRANSDUCER

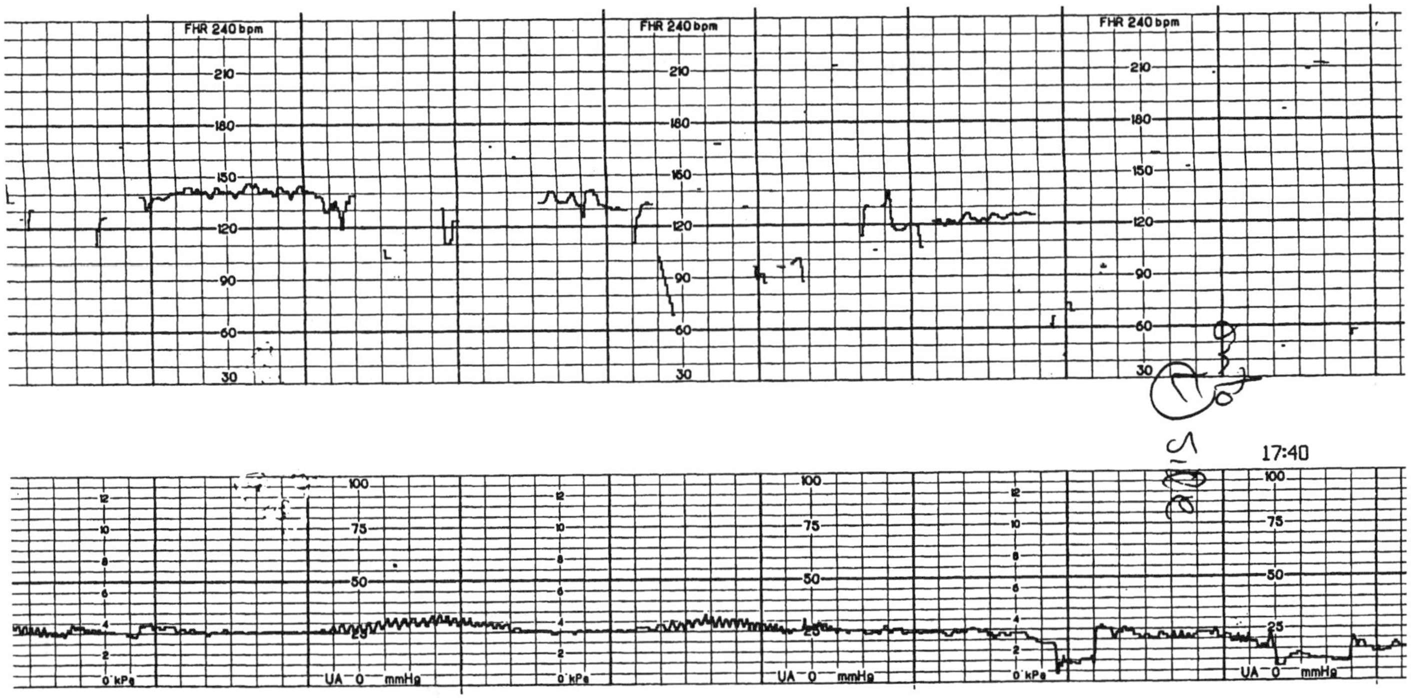

3.2 Ultrasound tracing with gaps and dots or artifact.

Testing the US Transducer

To test the US transducer, plug the cable into the monitor, turn the power on, and turn up the sound volume. Apply aquasonic gel to the transducer face then gently rub the transducer face in small circles, moving in a clockwise direction. Alternatively, you can hold the dry transducer against your left palm while tapping fingers of your right hand on the top of your left hand. Do you hear static on the fetal monitor? Static means the transducer is working.

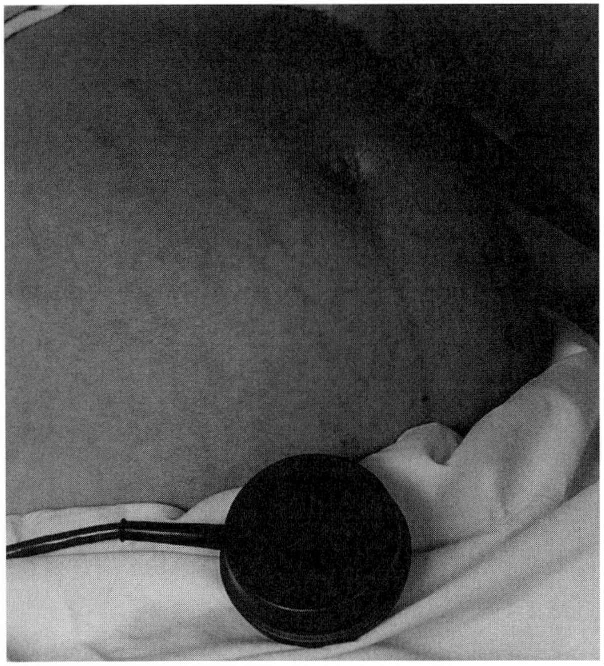

3.3 Ultrasound transducer without aquasonic gel. (Photograph by Pam Barncastle, Castle Studio, Albuquerque, New Mexico).

The lack of static suggests the sensitive crystals in the transducer do not work. If that is the case, that transducer should be sent to the Biomedical Department. It may be unrepairable and will be discarded. Since each fetal monitor component costs hundreds of dollars handle and store them carefully to prevent damage.

Tocotransducer (toco): External Uterine Activity Monitoring

External monitoring of uterine contractions with a tocotransducer reflects uterine activity when the toco is placed correctly on the abdomen. There are no known risks in the application of a toco, however, some women find the belts uncomfortable.

TOCOTRANSDUCER TEST

Testing the Tocotransducer

To test the tocotransducer, plug the cable into its port on the fetal monitor and turn the monitor on. Push the toco's pressure-sensitive surface and look at the digital readout on the monitor screen. It is usually +199 on Corometrics® monitors and +127 on Hewlett-Packard® monitors. Consult the manufacturer's manual for your monitor. Anything less suggests the toco is malfunctioning. When you begin recording, you may reset the toco baseline to the level of 10 mm Hg. This is done by pressing the UA ref button or uterine reference button. Review all the buttons on the face of the fetal monitors you will be using. When you use a tocotransducer, the numbers on the fetal monitor paper are insignificant. The exact duration and strength of the contraction cannot be determined. Instead, the uterine activity waveform is examined to determine contraction frequency. Duration is estimated. Palpation is required to determine contraction strength and uterine relaxation between contractions.

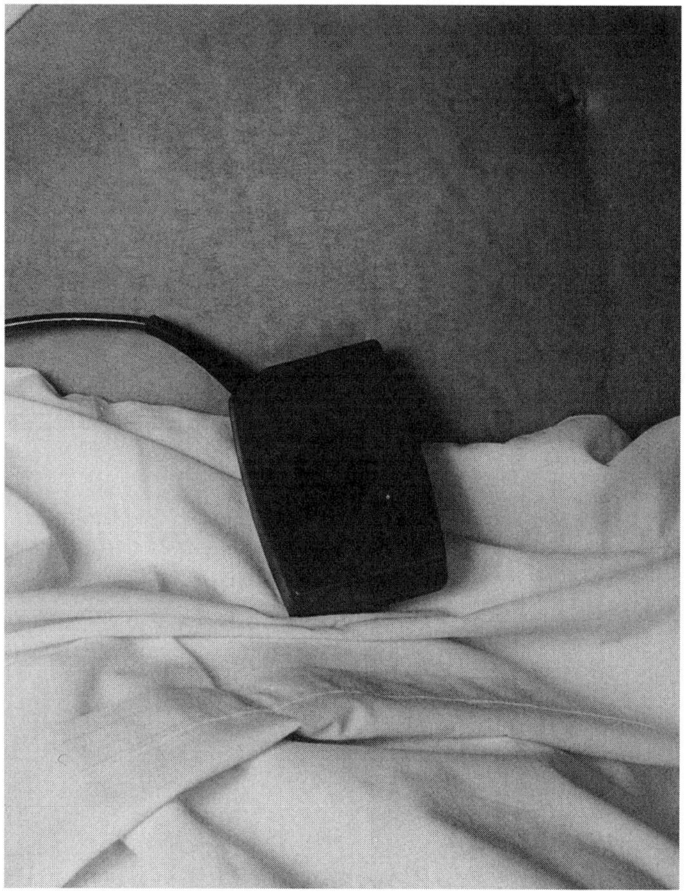

3.4 ***The tocotransducer is a pressure-sensitive device that does not require aquasonic gel. Pressure on the button creates a waveform in the uterine activity channel on the tracing.*** (Photograph by Pam Barncastle, Castle Studio, Albuquerque, New Mexico).

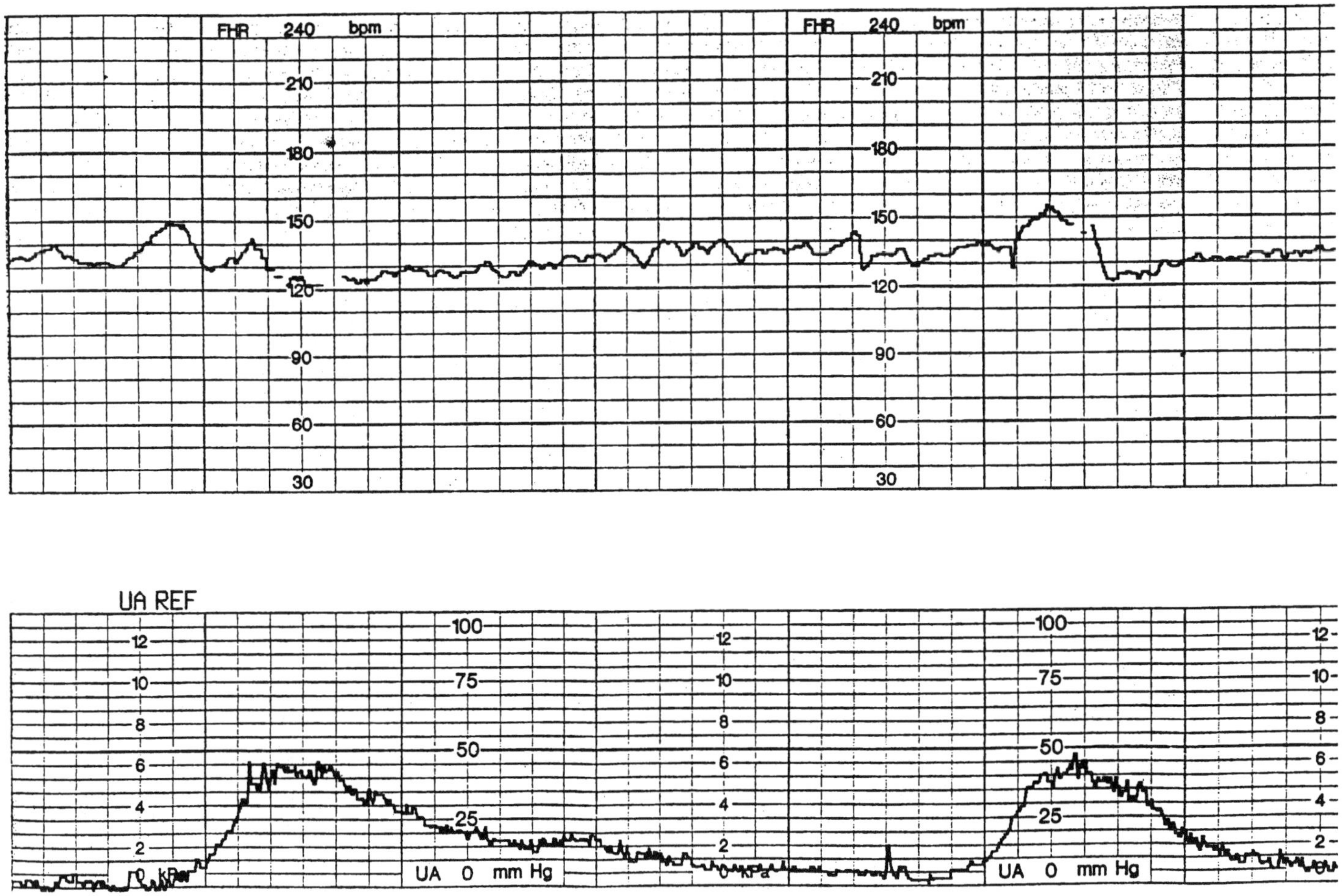

3.5 UA Ref indicates the fetal monitor automatically adjusted the uterine activity baseline. Frequency and duration are considered relatively accurate when a tocotransducer is used. Duration is 90 to 120 seconds. Palpation of contractions is needed to confirm contraction duration and strength plus resting tone between contractions.

SPIRAL ELECTRODE AND REFERENCE ELECTRODE

Internal Monitoring of the Fetal Heart Rate – The Spiral Electrode (SE)

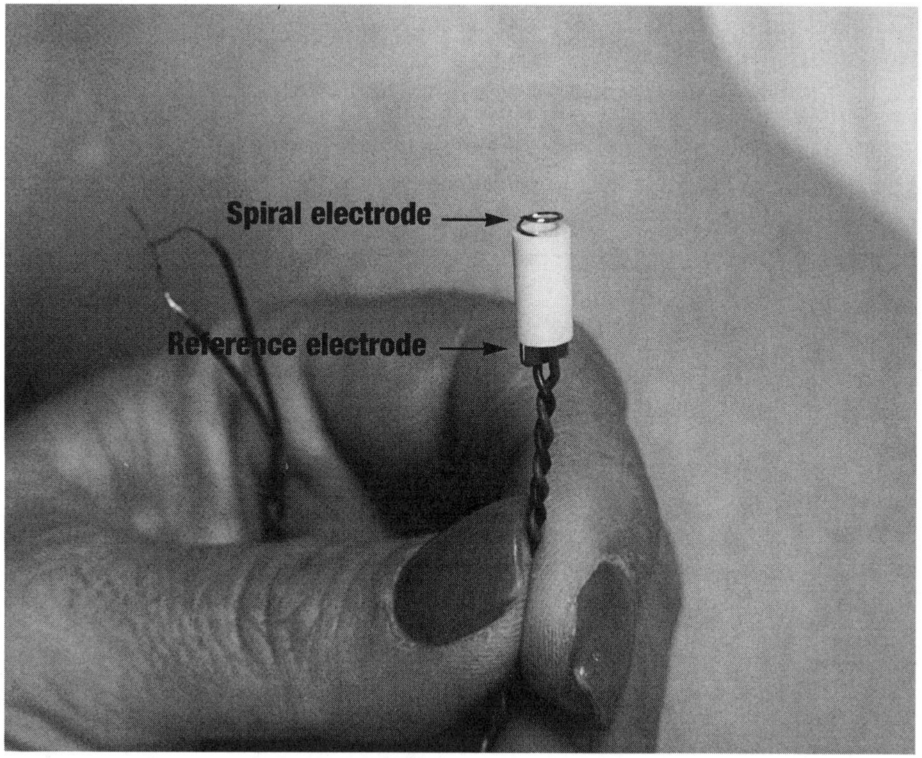

3.6 ***Spiral electrode. The helix is called a spiral electrode. The metal plate on the opposite side of the plastic is called the reference electrode.*** (Photograph by Pam Barncastle, Castle Studio, Albuquerque, New Mexico).

When ultrasound information is inadequate to make clinical decisions, the application of a spiral electrode to the fetal scalp or buttocks may be needed after weighing risks and benefits. Keep the US transducer on but unplug it. When the spiral electrode is in and working properly the US may be removed. The spiral electrode (SE) is used to acquire a direct fetal electrocardiogram signal (DECG) which is transmitted to the fetal monitor along the green wire. On the opposite side of the SE's white plastic tip is a square metal plate or wire. This is the reference electrode. When the reference electrode is in maternal secretions, the maternal electrocardiogram (ECG) is transmitted to the fetal monitor via the red wire. So, the green wire transmits the fetal ECG and the red wire transmits the maternal ECG. If the fetus is dead, the maternal ECG will be conducted through the fetus and the green wire, and the maternal heart rate will appear on the electronic fetal monitor's printout. That is why it is best to confirm fetal life and the maternal heart rate prior to placement of the spiral electrode or ultrasound transducer. Naturally, the recorded FHR should be different than the maternal pulse.

The benefit of SE application is the accurate measurement of the fetal heart rate and short-term variability.

BENEFIT AND RISK OF SPIRAL ELECTRODE USE

Therefore, a SE is needed when accelerations are not evident and fetal well-being is questioned. Risks of SE application are related to consequences of rupture of membranes such as cord prolapse, infection, and scalp abscess or transmission of maternal infection to the fetus, e.g., herpes or human immunodeficiency virus.

CONFIRM FETAL LIFE

Prior to spiral electrode application, confirm fetal life. Palpate fetal movement or auscultate fetal heart sounds *with a fetoscope*. A hand-held Doppler is no better than an external ultrasound transducer, as both detect motion. When heart sounds are heard, you are hearing the ventricular not atrial rate. Other devices, such as a Pinard, a stethoscope, and even an empty cardboard toilet paper roll, have been used to auscultate fetal heart sounds. Of course, a toilet paper roll is not recommended, unless you are in the field without equipment.

DYSRHYTHMIAS

If you auscultate an irregular rhythm, perhaps there is a dysrhythmia such as premature atrial contractions (PACs), premature ventricular contractions, or a second-degree heart block. Since there is a small (< 10%) chance of a fetal cardiac defect, the physician should be notified of an irregular rhythm. An ultrasound may be done to evaluate fetal cardiac anatomy. When an irregular rhythm was heard, the FHR pattern looked like this:

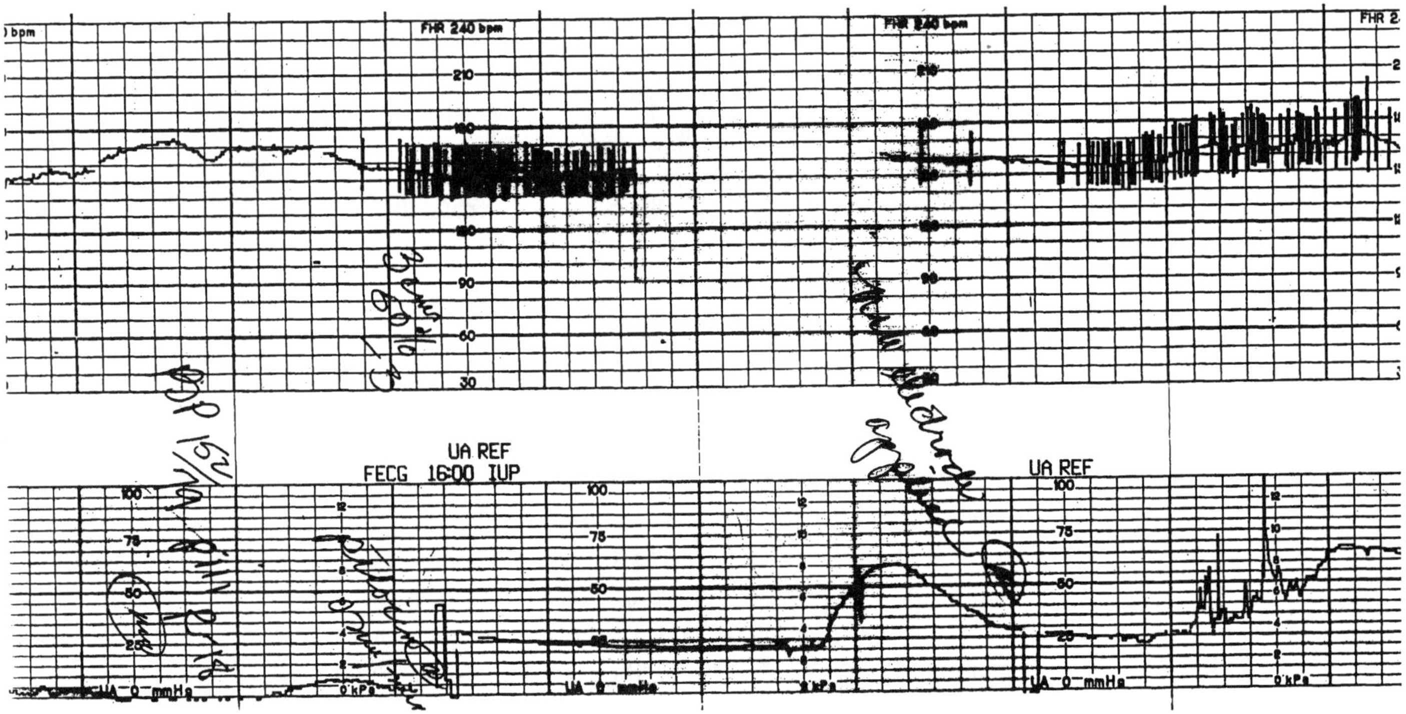

3.7 Fetal heart rate tracing indicative of premature atrial contractions (PACs) (lines up and down).

This was generated as a result of multiple fetal PACs. PACs are the most common fetal arrhythmia. No treatment or interventions are required. PACs usually resolve after delivery. However, a pediatrician should be informed of the suspected fetal arrhythmia.

ARTIFACT

Artifact appears when the maternal and fetal ECG signals are interrupted in their transmission. This is especially common with maternal pushing as the electrode wires bounce against the vaginal walls.

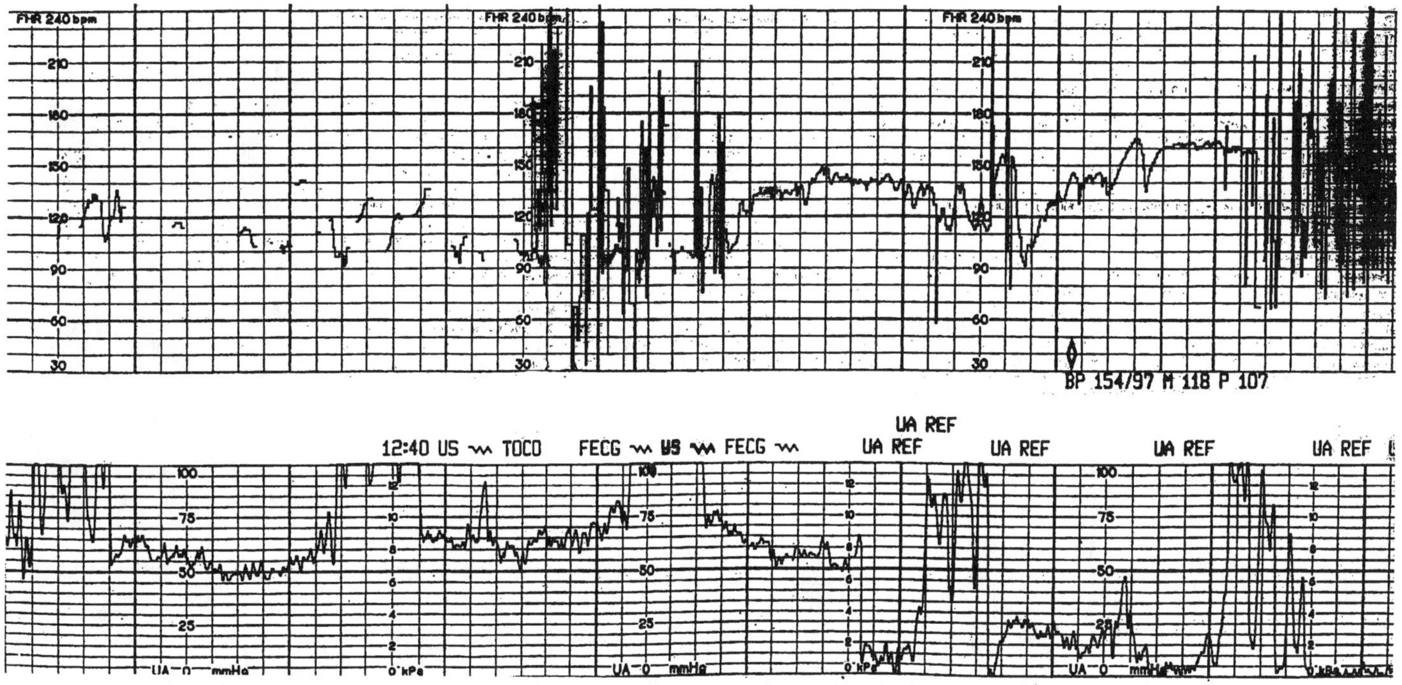

3.8 ***When a spiral electrode is applied, irregular lines or artifact indicate signal transmission is interrupted.***

If artifact persists, pull gently on the electrode wires to determine if the electrode fell off. You may need to reapply the ultrasound transducer while a new SE is being applied or auscultate the FHR to reconfirm fetal life. Also, look under the sheets. The fetus may now be a newborn!

LEG PLATE

Once the electrode is clearly attached to the fetal scalp, the red and green wires are inserted into a leg plate. Some leg plates have push pins into which each wire is inserted. Others have a hole into which the combined green and red wires are inserted.

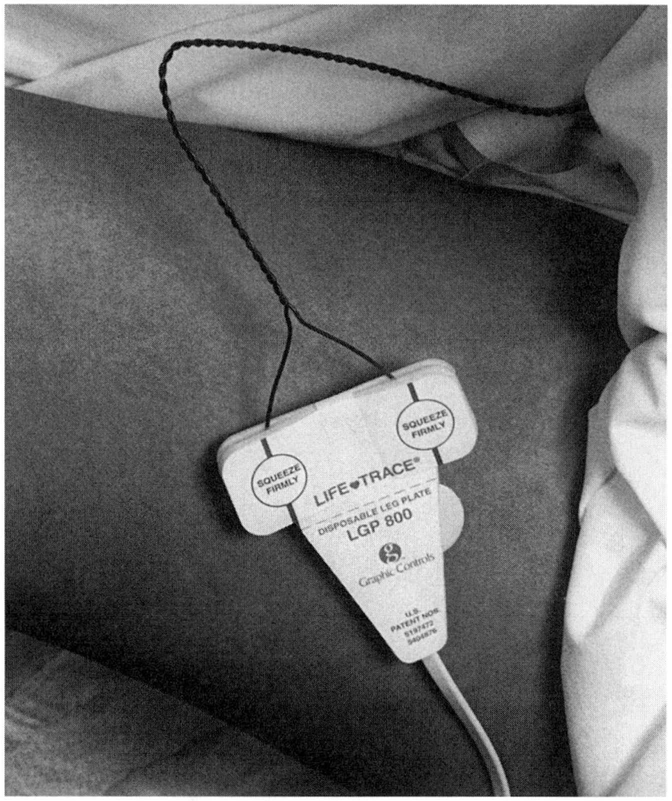

3.9 ***Disposable spiral electrode leg plate.*** (Photograph by Pam Barncastle, Castle Studio, Albuquerque, New Mexico).

DETERMINING THE FHR

Once the SE is in the fetal tissue, the fetal ECG and maternal ECG can be transmitted to the monitor for analysis. The monitor software identifies the tallest R waves on the QRS complexes. Because the spiral electrode transmits the fetal ECG, those R waves are usually the tallest. The time interval between each two R waves is determined and a beats per minute (bpm) rate is calculated. For example, if 1/2 second existed between two R waves, the bpm rate would be 120 bpm. A dot is printed at 120 bpm. Then, the next R to R interval is determined and a new bpm rate is printed. Connecting all these dots creates the FHR baseline, short-term variability (STV), and long-term variability (LTV). If a dysrhythmia occurs, sometimes the baseline cannot be seen.

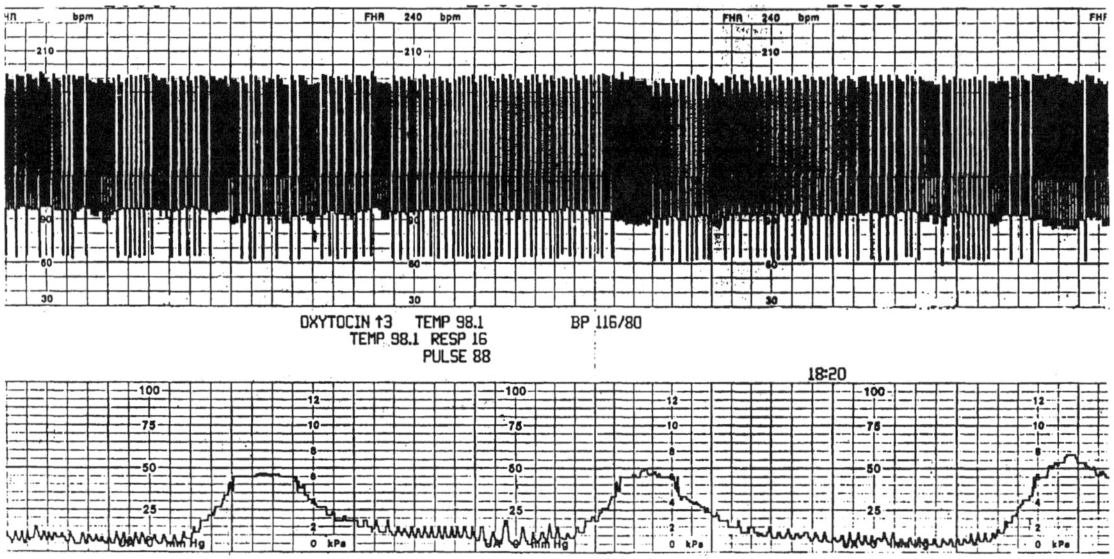

3.10 ***A series of fetal multifocal premature ventricular contractions (PVCs) creates lines that obscure the baseline.***

LOGIC, ECG ARTIFACT ELIMINATION SWITCH

In this case, to remove the up and down lines created by PVCs there may be a switch or button on the monitor which can be activated to delete these lines. Hewlett-Packard® calls this the "logic" button or switch. Corometrics® calls it the "ECG artifact elimination switch." Find this switch on the fetal monitor.

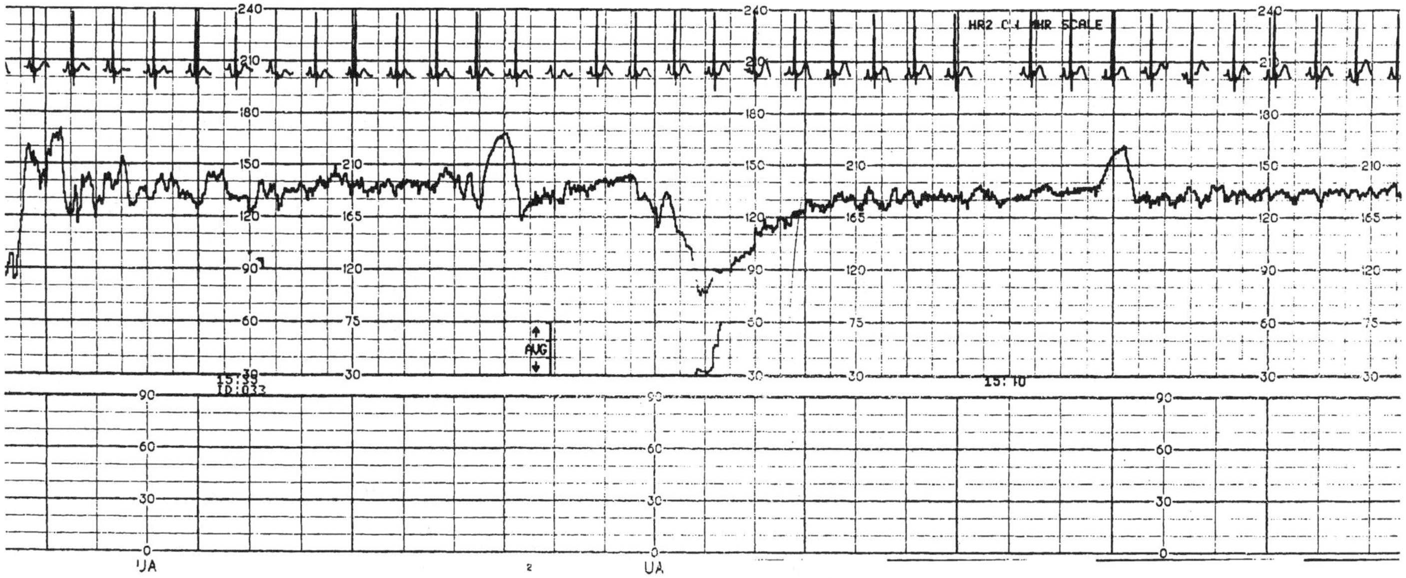

3.11 Spacelabs® monitors have an ECG plot feature.

ECG PLOT

Some machines have no logic button, but instead can print the fetal ECG for waveform analysis. These include Spacelabs® monitors, formerly called Advanced Medical Systems Monitors, and Oxford Sonicaid® monitors. The ECG plot can be turned on or off in the Space Labs monitors. A button is depressed to plot the FECG on Sonicaid fetal monitor paper.

Review your equipment with a skilled clinician. Identify:

- the spiral electrode
- the reference electrode
- the leg plate
- the "logic" button or ECG plot switch

TESTING THE LEG PLATE

Ask if your fetal monitor has the capacity to test the leg plate. To test the leg plate, the cable is plugged into the monitor, the power is turned on, and the end of the cable is pushed against two metal pins while the monitor test button is depressed. 200 bpm should appear on the screen of the Hewlett-Packard® monitors and 120 bpm appears when testing the Corometrics® leg plate. If these numbers do not appear, the cable may be faulty. Practice testing the leg plate.

NO NEED FOR ECG PASTE

There is no need to apply ECG paste to the leg plate unless the reference electrode is totally dry (in a dry pocket). Then the leg will be the site of the maternal ECG conducted into the fetal monitor. If the electrode is in a dry pocket and a Hewlett-Packard® monitor is used, a red wire is attached to a sticky electrode on the leg and inserted into the leg plate (see 3.12). This creates another site to transmit the maternal ECG. If the leg plate includes an active electrode to hold it in place, no ECG paste is needed.

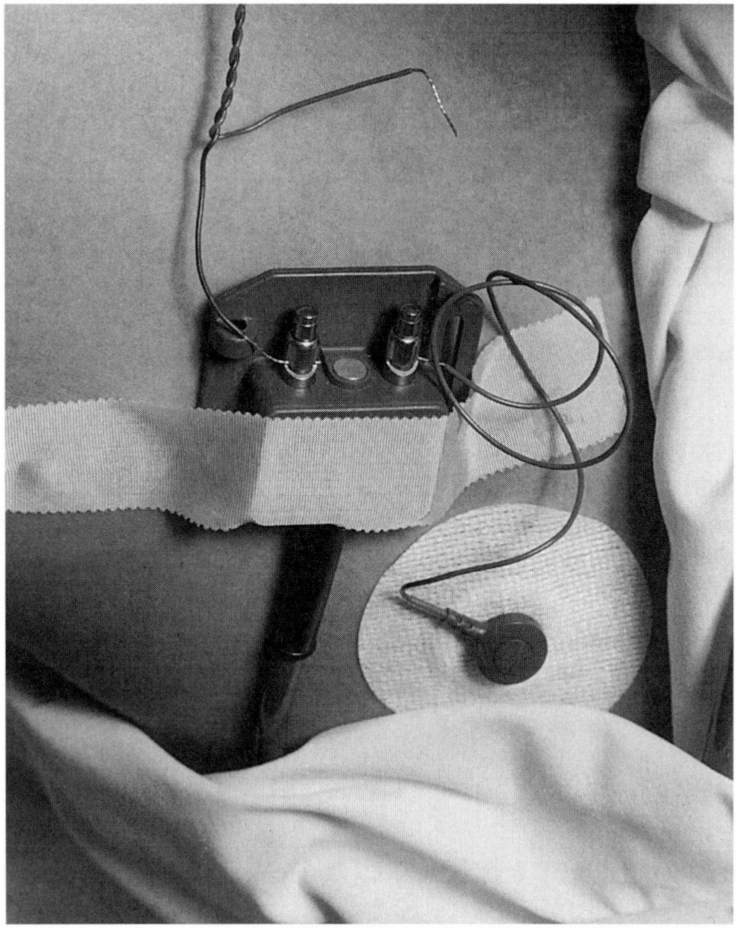

3.12 ***Single nonshielded lead with snap termination to conduct the maternal ECG when the reference electrode is in a dry pocket.*** (Photograph by Pam Barncastle, Castle Studio, Albuquerque, New Mexico).

Internal Monitoring of Uterine Contractions with an Intrauterine Pressure Catheter (IUPC)

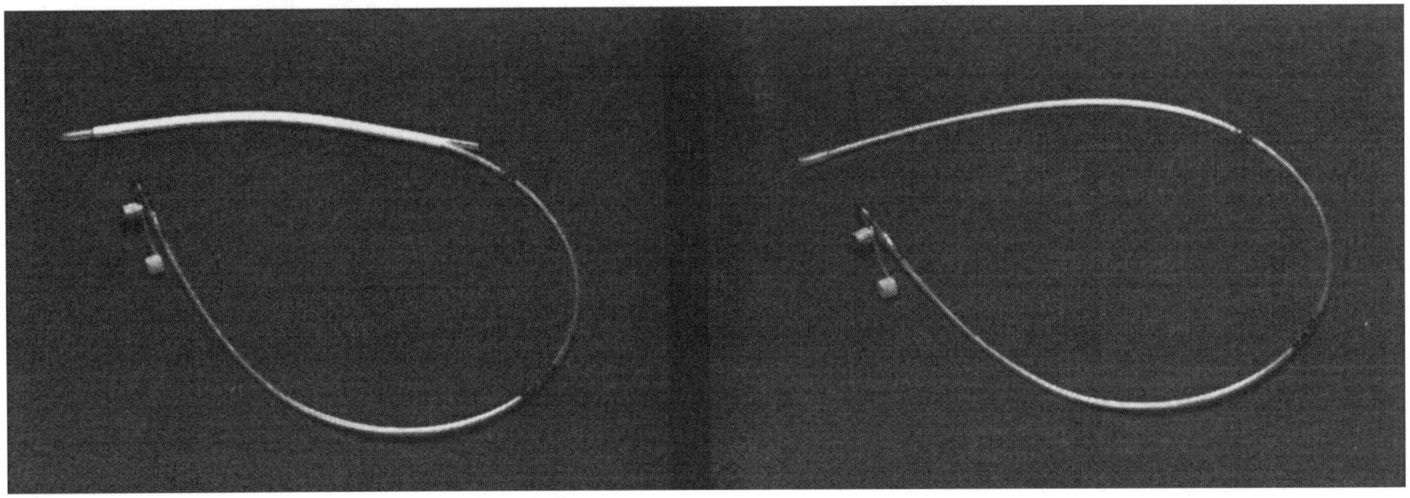

3.13 ***Koala™ intrauterine pressure catheter with and without insertion guide.*** (Photograph courtesy Clinical Innovations, Inc., Murray, Utah).

INTRAUTERINE PRESSURE CATHETER

The IUPC directly measures intrauterine pressure when properly placed in the amniotic space. The four components of pressure transmitted through the IUPC to the fetal monitor are:

- hydrostatic pressure
- elastic (myometrium tissue) recoil,
- contraction pressure and
- atmospheric pressure and/or cable "offset."

"Offset" means that you could add or subtract from the total intrauterine pressure 5 mm Hg due to the design of the transducer. To remove this "offset," zero the IUPC/cable system **prior** to insertion. Read the manufacturer's instructions prior to use.

For accurate measurement, it is vital that the IUPC is placed within the amniotic space. Placement of the IUPC outside the amniotic membranes (between the chorion and endometrial lining) can occur. Such placement may result in damped waveforms and one should not amnioinfuse into this space. One IUPC that helps identify proper placement is called the Koala™. It has a transparent lumen to visualize amniotic fluid "flashback" upon insertion to verify amniotic space placement. You can also look at the uterine activity waveform (see 3.14).

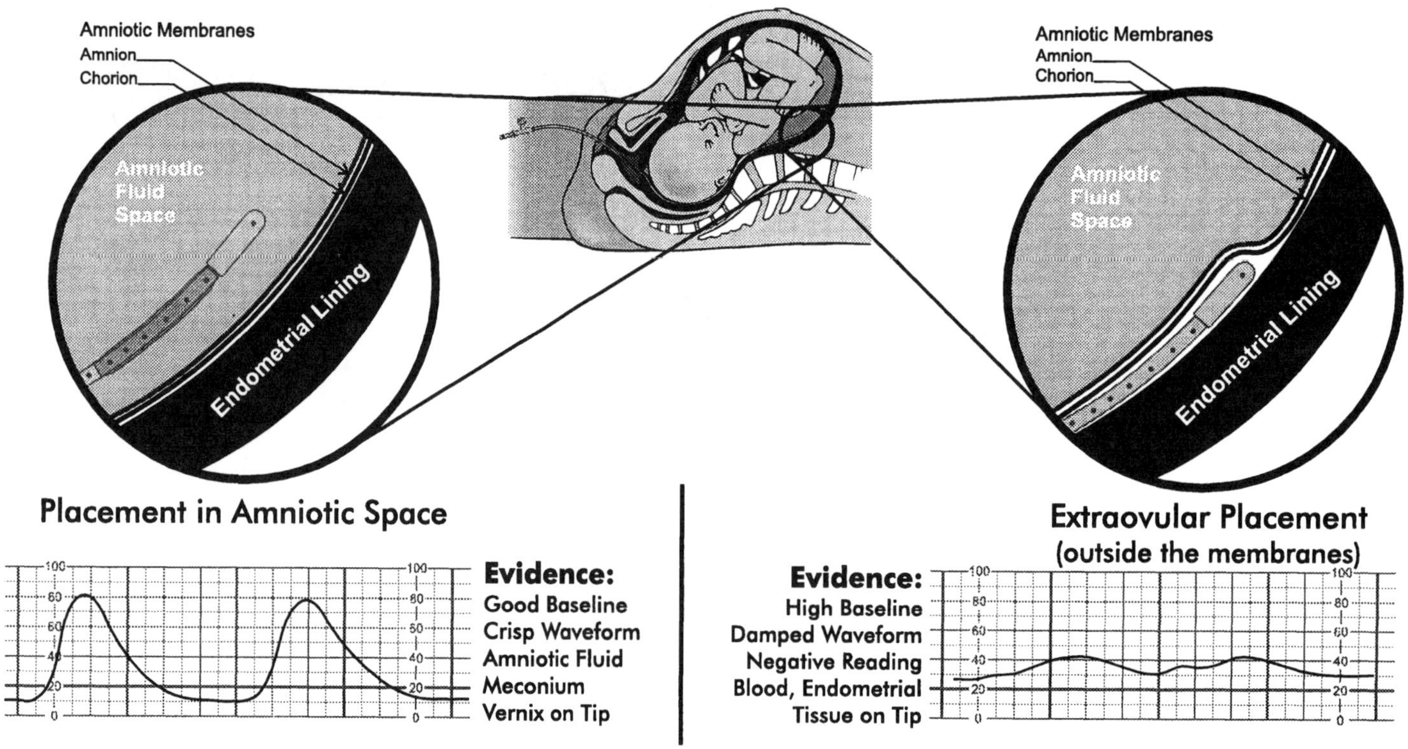

3.14 Accurate assessment occurs when the IUPC is placed within the amniotic space (Illustration courtesy of Clinical Innovations, Inc., Murray, Utah).

ZEROING THE SYSTEM

Learn about the IUPC used at your hospital. If you use a fluid-filled IUPC, be sure sterile water or sterile saline *without preservatives* is used to flush the catheter prior to insertion. Preservatives, such as benzyl alcohol, have been linked to intraventricular bleeds in preterm fetuses. Some sensor-tipped IUPCs should be "zeroed" before insertion, other IUPCs can be zeroed at any time. Zeroing is the process of "removing" atmospheric pressure and any electronic offset so that the recorded uterine activity only includes

- hydrostatic pressure
- elastic recoil (uterine wall resting tension) and the
- contraction pressure.

HYDROSTATIC PRESSURE

The pressure exerted by the weight of amniotic fluid above the IUPC sensing point is called hydrostatic pressure. Depending on the location of the IUPC sensor tip or pressure-sensitive transducer to the fluid, amniotic fluid may add to or decrease the pressure displayed. For example, if the IUPC is on the maternal left side and the woman lies on her right side, there will be less pressure recorded than when she lies on her left side (with the amniotic fluid above it). Recorded pressures may be affected by plus or minus 5 to 10 mm Hg due to position changes. Therefore, it is important to record position changes in order to know hydrostatic pressure effects.

ELASTIC RECOIL/RESTING TONE

Elastic recoil is also known as uterine wall (myometrium) resting tone. This is normal tension exerted by tissues in and around the uterus along with the uterine resting tension. Resting tone is often 7 to 15 mm Hg. The addition of hydrostatic pressure to the resting tone increases the uterine activity baseline reading. The *normal reading is between 5 and 25 mm Hg*. After the IUPC is inserted, it may be your hospital's policy to record baseline values on the woman's right side, left side, and in semi-Fowler's position in order to differentiate the effect of hydrostatic pressure on the uterine activity baseline. There should be at least one minute of rest between contractions. The time between contractions is called the interval.

PEAK IUP

The top of the uterine activity IUPC waveform is called the peak intrauterine pressure or peak IUP. When an IUPC is in place, contraction frequency, duration, strength (peak IUP), resting tone, and the interval between contractions is accurate. If the uterus should rupture, palpation of uterine tone is a more reliable indicator of uterine activity than the contraction tracing because contraction waveforms can continue although peak pressures tend to decrease.

IUPC RISKS

Risks associated with IUPC use include

- infection
- uterine perforation
- umbilical cord injury or entanglement
- placental injury such as abruption (more likely in extraovular placement)
- extraovular placement (between the uterine wall and amniotic sac).

If after IUPC insertion there is vaginal bleeding, a soft nontender uterus, with no uterine waveform recorded, suspect uterine perforation. If after insertion there is vaginal bleeding and uterine hyperstimulation, suspect placental abruption. Of course, perforation may be asymptomatic. Since membranes are ruptured to insert the IUPC, assess maternal temperature and pulse at least every 2 hours following rupture of the membranes. Record the color, amount, and odor of the amniotic fluid when you change the linen protector or chux. Notify the midwife or physician of any bleeding, abnormal FHR pattern, abnormal maternal vital signs or foul smelling amniotic fluid.

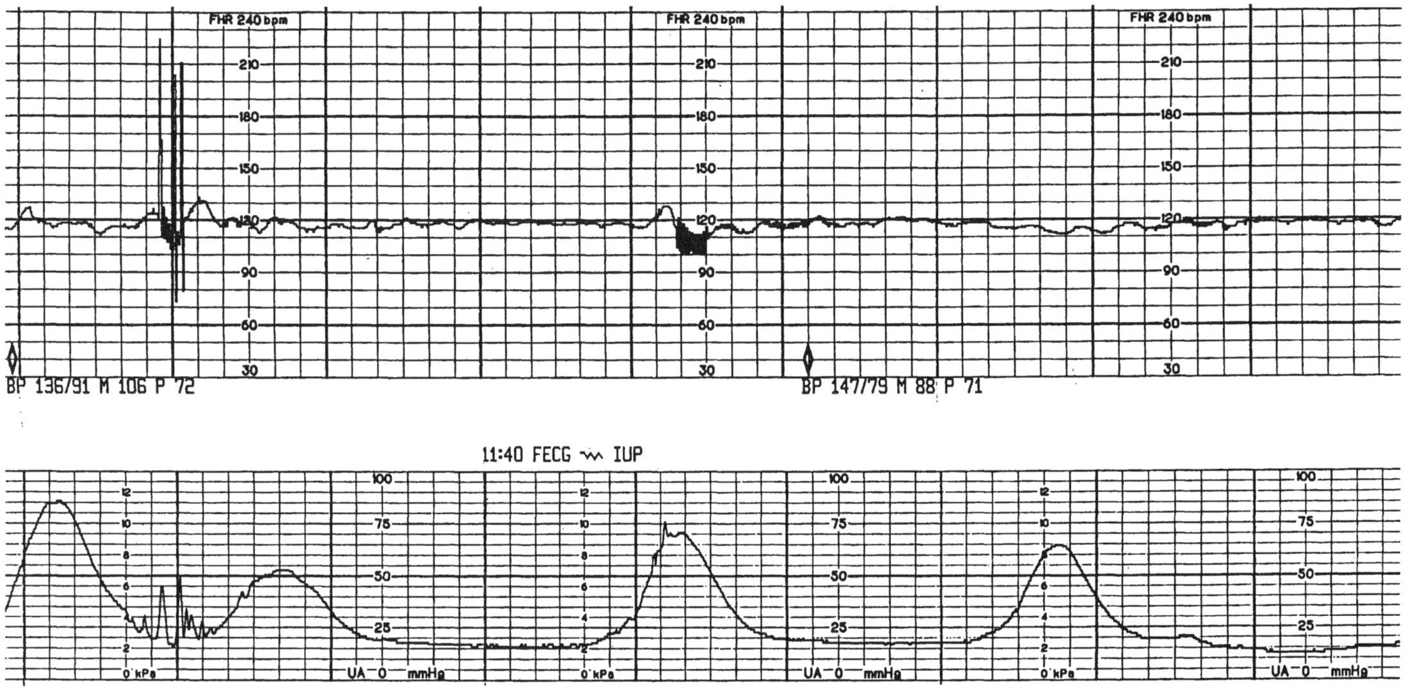

3.15 An intrauterine pressure catheter was used to record contractions with a peak pressure of approximately 53-85 mm Hg and a resting tone of 13-18 mm Hg.

SUMMARY

Summary

Autocorrelation has changed fetal monitoring with its improved analysis of the ultrasound signal. The printed rate is within 2.5 bpm of the true rate. If the fetal heart rate tracing looks good when the US (external monitor) is used, it's probably good when the spiral electrode (internal monitor) is used. Therefore, application of internal monitors should be considered after the risks and benefits have been weighed for the need for a continuous fetal heart signal and a pressure sensitive intrauterine device.

Testing of the tocotransducer and ultrasound transducer and proper transducer placement are critical to receiving accurate, interpretable data. Determine fetal position and the gestational age prior to transducer application. Confirm fetal life. Palpate fetal movement or auscultate with a fetoscope, especially if dysrhythmias are suspected.

The spiral electrode is used to transmit a direct fetal electrocardiogram (ECG) into the fetal monitor. When the fetus is dead, the maternal ECG will be conducted through the fetus, the spiral electrode and cable. It is important to convey the use of a spiral electrode to the newborn nurse so that this puncture site may be assessed during hospitalization.

The intrauterine pressure catheter should be zeroed properly (according to the manufacturer's instructions) to remove the electronic offset and/or atmospheric pressure. Hydrostatic pressure, elastic recoil, and contraction pressure make up the intrauterine pressure readings in mm Hg. Maximal normal resting tone is 25 mm Hg.

EXERCISES

Exercises

Examine these four tracings. Fill in the blanks under each one.

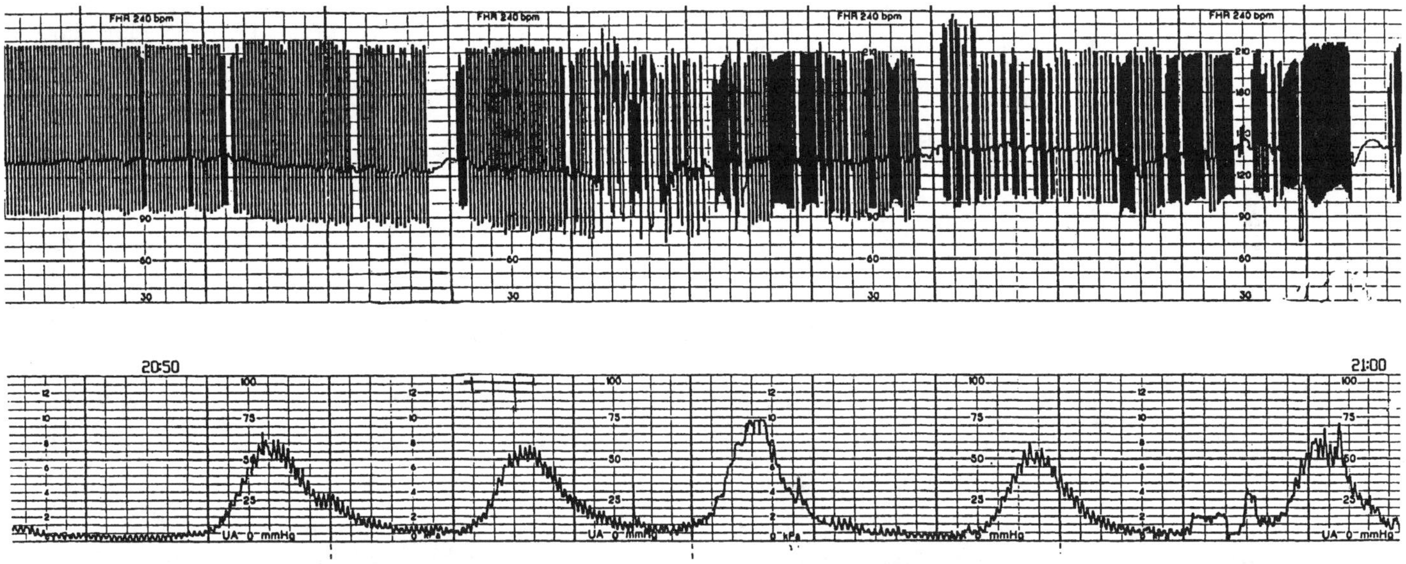

3.16 Recurrent fetal PACs. Tocotransducer in place. Apgar scores were 5 and 9 at 1 and 5 minutes.

1. Contraction frequency = _____ minutes
2. Contraction duration = _____ seconds

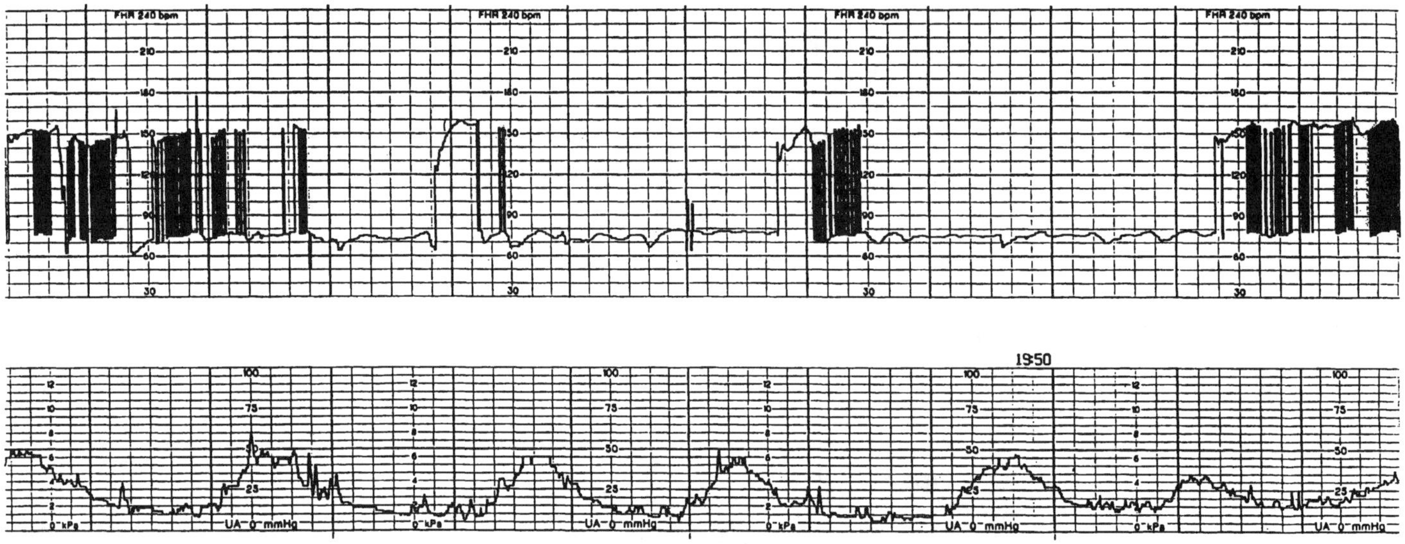

3.17 ***Dropped beats and second-degree heart block. Tocotransducer in place. Apgar scores were 5 and 9 at 1 and 5 minutes.***

3. Contraction frequency = _____ minutes

4. Contraction duration = _____ seconds

3.18 ***Unifocal PVCs. Tocotransducer in place. Apgar scores were 8 and 9 at 1 and 5 minutes.***

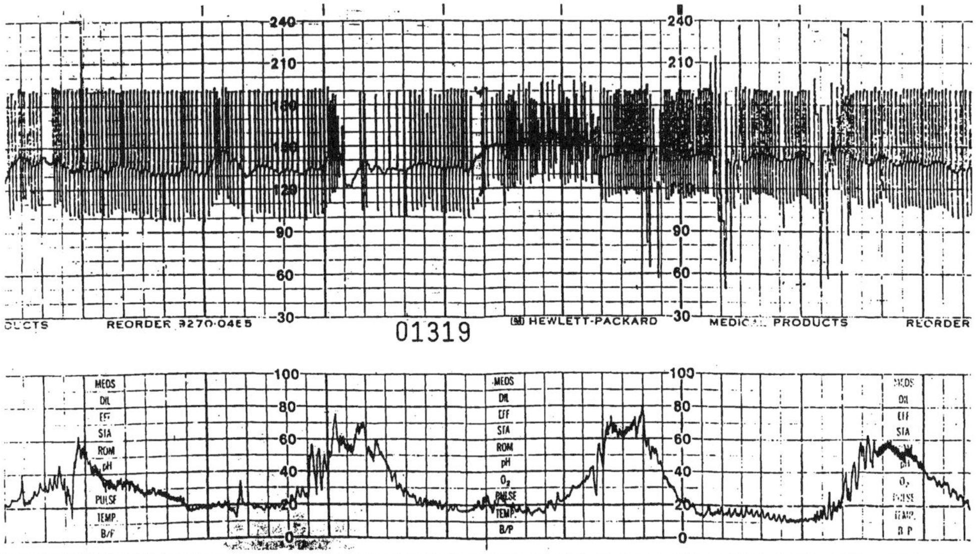

5. Contraction frequency = _____ minutes

6. Contraction duration = _____ seconds

7. Contraction peak IUP = _____ mm Hg

8. Contraction resting tone = _____ mm Hg

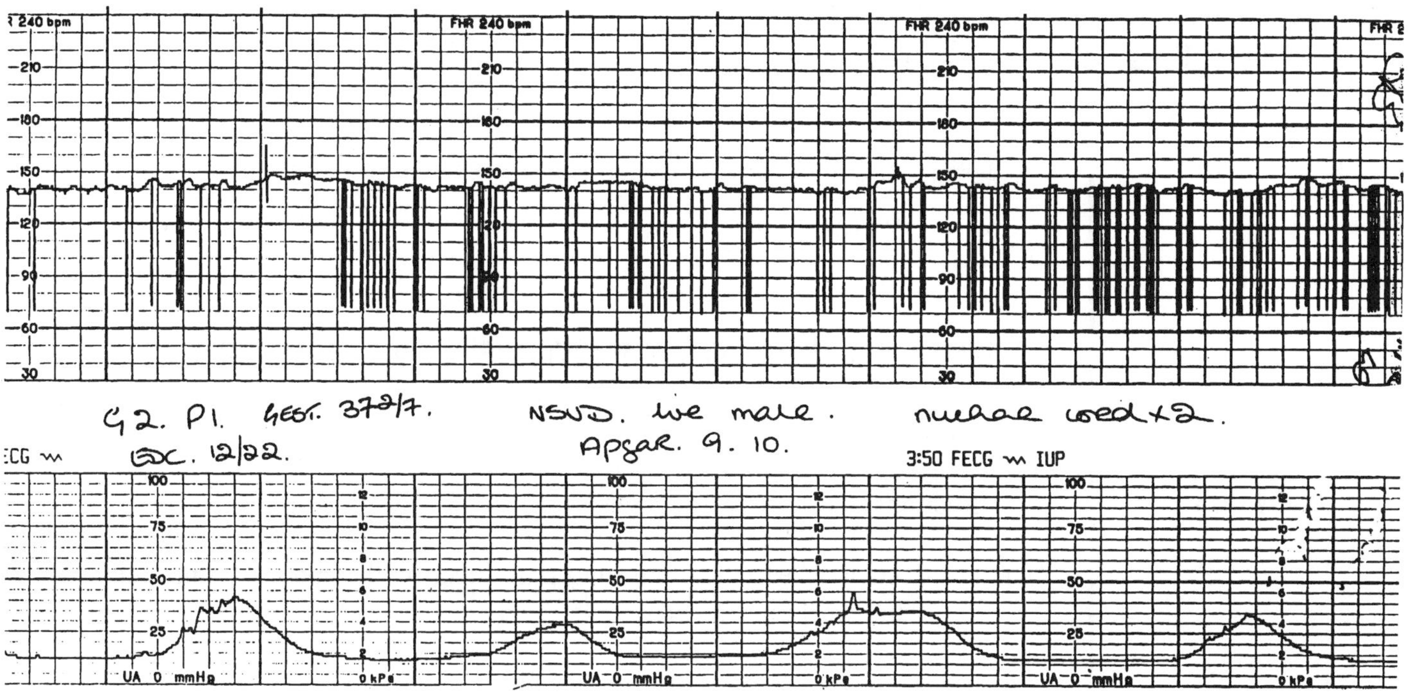

3.18 Dropped beats due to a second-degree heart block.

9. Contraction frequency = _____ minutes
10. Contraction duration = _____ seconds
11. Contraction peak IUP = _____ mm Hg
12. Contraction resting tone = _____ mm Hg

Answers on page 50.

ANSWERS TO EXERCISES

1. every 2 minutes
2. 70-90 seconds
3. every 2 minutes
4. 60-70 seconds
5. every 2-2 1/2 minutes
6. 80 seconds
7. cannot determine with a tocotransducer in place
8. cannot determine with a tocotransducer in place
9. every 2-2 1/2 minutes
10. 50-90 seconds
11. 30-40 mm Hg
12. 12-15 mm Hg

SECTION 3: EXTERNAL AND INTERNAL FETAL MONITORING

QUESTIONS

Directions: Circle T if the statement is true, F if it is false.

QUESTIONS

T F 1. Always keep the ultrasound transducer on the abdomen until the spiral electrode is in and working properly.

T F 2. Aquasonic gel helps transmit fetal heart sounds.

T F 3. The "logic" switch removes abnormal fetal heart rate lines due to premature atrial contractions and premature ventricular contractions.

T F 4. Zeroing removes the effect of hydrostatic pressure on the uterine activity printout.

T F 5. Normal resting tone of the uterus is 15-25 mm Hg.

T F 6. Autocorrelation creates a more reliable external tracing than peak detection.

T F 7. A spiral electrode and/or ultrasound transducer can detect the maternal heart rate.

T F 8. The ultrasound transducer detects the electrical energy of the heartbeat.

T F 9. Confirmation of fetal life can best be accomplished by utilizing a hand-held doppler if the ultrasound transducer failed to detect the fetal heart rate.

T F 10. Aquasonic gel is utilized on the spiral electrode leg plate when the reference electrode is in a dry pocket.

SECTION 4
Uterine Contractions

UTERINE PHYSIOLOGY

Uterine Physiology

The uterus is controlled by involuntary muscle fibers. Alpha receptors in the uterine muscle cells stimulate uterine contractions and beta receptors stimulate uterine relaxation. Norepinephrine and epinephrine stimulate both alpha and beta receptors. Prior to labor, progesterone stimulates the beta receptors and estrogen stimulates the alpha receptors. During pregnancy, progesterone and estrogen levels are balanced. Progesterone levels drop and estrogen becomes a dominant influence on the uterus prior to the onset of labor. The increase of estrogen and decrease of progesterone stimulates the formation of oxytocin receptors in the uterine muscle cells. The uterine cells begin to communicate by spreading their energy (action potential) through portals called gap junctions. This leads to synchronous uterine muscle cell contractions.

PACEMAKER

It is theorized that specialized cells exist in the fundus of the uterus that are responsible for initiating the electrical stimulus that precedes a contraction.

IMPULSE PATH

The normal contraction begins in the fundus and proceeds symmetrically downward toward the cervix. Asymmetry results when the uterine cells function independently and this leads to ineffective uterine contractions with minimal dilatation. Ketones in the urine during labor are often associated with ineffective uterine contractions. Therefore, it is important to provide adequate caloric intake either through hydration therapy, e.g., a controlled intravenous infusion of a dextrose-containing solution at 125-150 ml/hour, or by ingestion of glucose-containing liquids.

FEAR RESPONSE

Fear precedes the release of catecholamines (epinephrine, norepinephrine) which have an effect on uterine activity. Norepinephrine binds with alpha receptors and increases uterine resting tone and contraction frequency, duration, and strength. Epinephrine is secreted in small amounts and binds with beta receptors and decreases uterine activity. The overall uterine response to maternal fear is to increase activity, which is thought to produce ineffective contractions which may arrest labor progress. This is why many anxious women who think they are in labor are contracting so much more when they first arrive at the hospital and so much less after they calm down. By decreasing a woman's anxiety, contractions are more effective although less frequent.

FEAR ⇒ CATECHOLAMINES ⇒ INCREASED UTERINE ACTIVITY

The woman's childbirth preparation, coping skills, and support system determine educational and nursing care needs to minimize the effect of fear on uterine activity.

Contraction Concepts

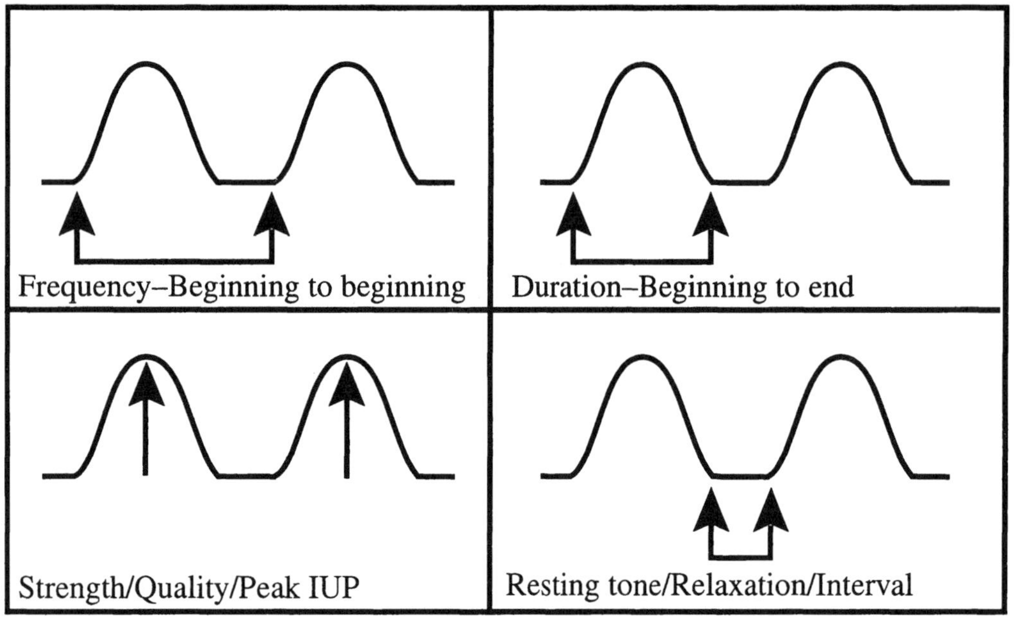

4.1 Contraction concepts.

PALPATION

A contraction occurs when the uterine muscle cells shorten. The uterus becomes more globular and tilts forward. You can feel this when your hand is on her fundus and the other hand is over the lower abdomen.

Palpation of resting tone is an important ongoing assessment. Contractions ideally should not be closer than 60 seconds apart. This resting period or interval facilitates optimal delivery of oxygen to and removal of carbon dioxide from the fetus.

DEFINITION OF TERMS

FREQUENCY

Contraction frequency is calculated from the beginning of one contraction to the beginning of the next contraction in minutes. It might be charted as "UCs q 4," meaning uterine contractions every 4 minutes.

DURATION

Contraction duration is timed from the beginning to the end of a contraction. It might be charted as UCs x 30-40 meaning contractions last 30-40 seconds.

INTERVAL

Interval is the time from the end of one contraction to the beginning of the next contraction. It should last 60 or more seconds so that the fetal oxygen reserves can be replenished. Resting tone is assessed during the interval. Interval duration is not documented.

HYPER-STIMULATION

When the interval is less than 1 minute and the frequency is closer than every 2 minutes, uterine hyperstimulation exists.

PEAK IUP

Peak intrauterine pressure (IUP) is usually above 35 mm Hg and may exceed 100 mm Hg during pushing. The peak is charted as "UCs ⇑ 80-90," meaning peak IUP ranges between 80 and 90 mm Hg.

INTENSITY

Intensity is measured as the difference between peak IUP and resting tone. Montevideo units are calculated by adding intensity of each contraction in a 10 minute period. Contraction intensity cannot be measured with a tocotransducer.

STRENGTH/ QUALITY

Strength or quality of contractions is judged at the contraction's peak. Push gently on the abdomen near the top of the uterus. Classify the strength as mild, moderate or strong.

Mild	⇒	abdomen easily indents to feel uterus, feels like pressing on your cheek
Moderate	⇒	abdomen firmer, some indentation occurs, feels like pressing on your nose
Strong	⇒	abdomen feels hard and cannot be indented, feels like pressing on your forehead

Strength with an intrauterine pressure catheter (IUPC) is the peak IUP on the uterine activity waveform. Documentation should include frequency, duration, peak IUP or strength, and relaxation or resting tone. For example, "UCs q 4-5 x 30-40, ⇑ 50-60, with resting tone 10-15."

RESTING TONE

Resting tone is the pressure exerted by uterine muscle cells and supportive tissues when they are at rest. It is measured accurately by an intrauterine pressure catheter in mm Hg. Resting tone between contractions should be 5 to 25 mm Hg, but is often closer to 8 to 12 mm Hg.

HYPERTONUS

A resting tone greater than 25 mm Hg is called **hypertonus**. Resting tone may be documented as "rest tone 10-15" meaning 10-15 mm Hg (when an intrauterine pressure catheter is in place) or "soft between contractions" when resting tone is palpated.

MONTEVIDEO UNITS

Montevideo Units (MVUs)

The original formula by Drs. Caldeyro-Barcia and Alvarez in 1952 was

MVUs = the *sum* of each contraction's *peak minus* the *resting tone* in a 10 minute period.

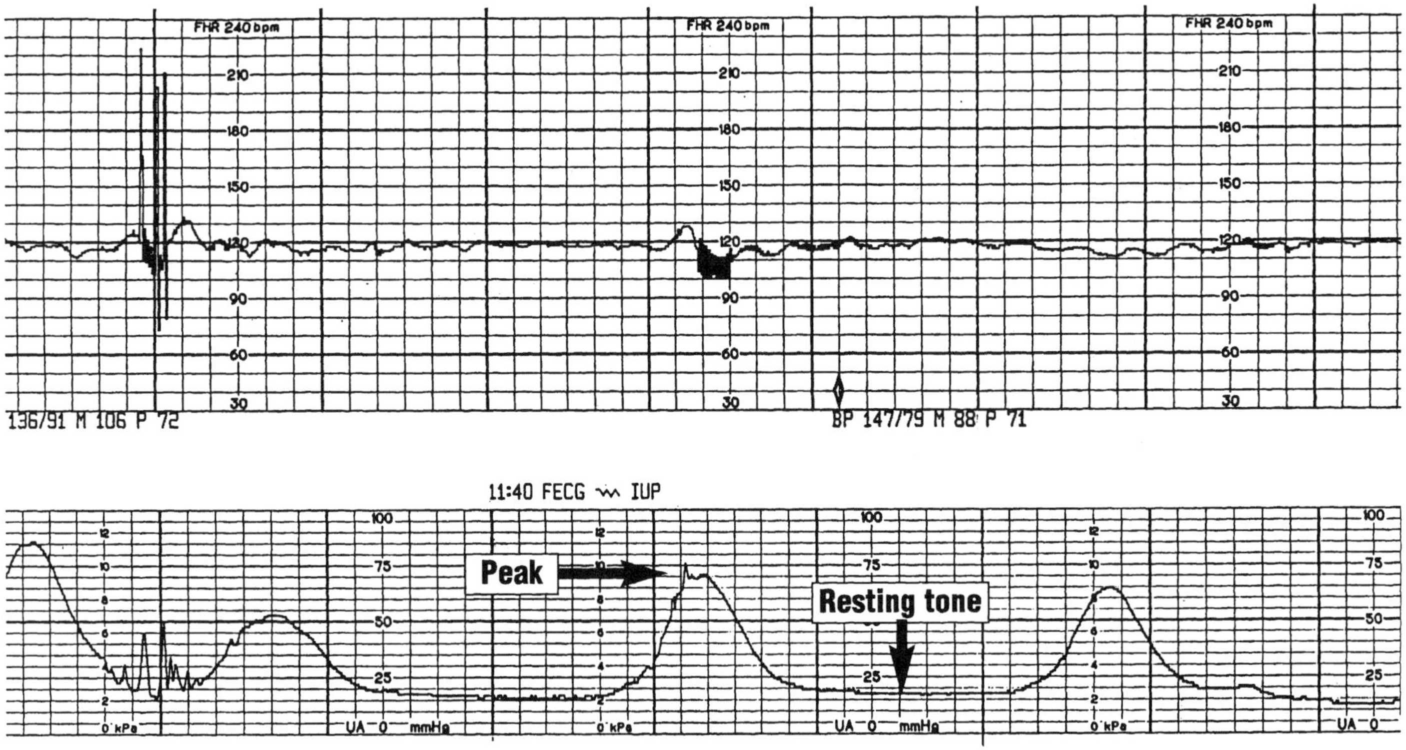

4.2 Contractions in 10 minutes.

There are 4 contractions with peak pressures of approximately 85, 55, 70, and 65 mm Hg. Resting tone averages 15 mm Hg. 85-15+55-15+70-15+65-15 = 70+40+55+50 or 215 Montevideo Units or MVUs.

ADEQUATE LABOR PROGRESS

Drs. Caldeyro-Barcia and Alvarez found that 150 to 250 MVUs were associated with adequate labor progress. Normal labors have ranged from 66 to 340 MVUs with an average of 100 in early labor, 200 by 10 cm dilatation, and 250 while pushing. MVUs are higher during ambulation (73 to 205) versus lying supine (80 to 176). Hypocontractile labor had lower MVUs (21 to 313), yet even overlapped values for normal labors. Therefore, MVUs should ***not*** be used to identify hypocontractility.

Maximize MVUs and labor progress, by using an upright position during labor and act to decrease maternal anxiety and increase maternal comfort.

Assessment of the maternal response to labor and palpation of contractions is more important in managing labor than calculation of MVUs. Often MVUs are calculated when pitocin® is infusing. MVUs between 150 and 250 suggest dilatation and descent should be progressing.

A third way to calculate MVUs is to add the mm Hg as you move from the base of each contraction to its peak. Adding all contractions in 10 minutes gives you the MVUs.

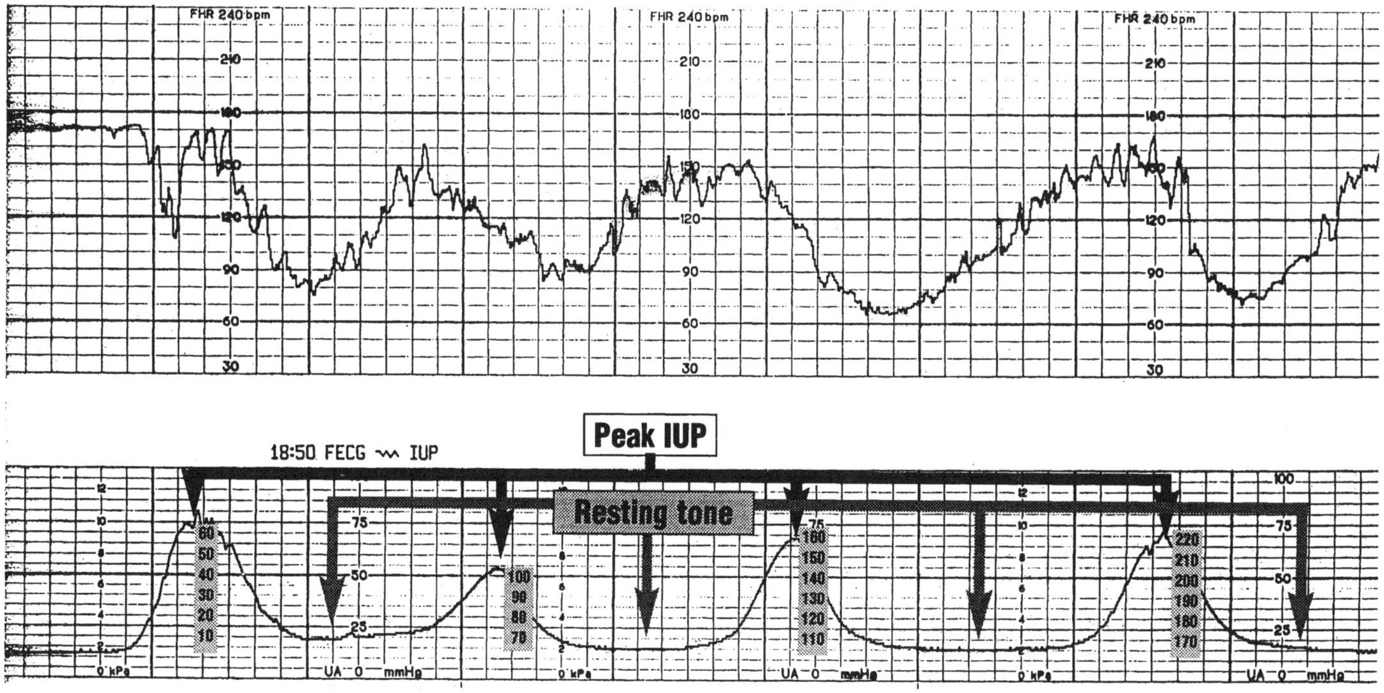

4.3 Calculate MVUs by adding the mm Hg under each contraction over a ten minute period.

EXERCISES

Exercises

Calculate the Montevideo Units

1. Peak pressures 50, 60, 70, 60 mm Hg
   Resting tone 10 mm Hg
   MVUs _____

2.	Peak pressures	50, 65	mm Hg
	Resting tone	5	mm Hg
	MVUs	_____	
3.	Peak pressures	100, 85, 75	mm Hg
	Resting tone	25	mm Hg
	MVUs	_____	

See the answers on page 71.

An alternative way to calculate MVUs is to calculate the average peak IUP in 10 minutes, subtract the average resting tone and multiply that number by the number of contractions. For example, if the peak pressures are 60, 75, and 95 mm Hg, their average peak is 60 + 75 + 90 ÷ 3 or 75. If the average resting tone is 15 mm Hg, 75 minus 15 is 60 mm Hg. 60 times 3 contractions in 10 minutes is 180 MVUs. With 180 MVUs you would expect adequate labor progress.

NORMAL CONTRACTION FEATURES

Normal Labor Features

- fundal dominance
- coordinated/symmetrical movement
- 2 - 5 contractions each 10 minutes
- 45 - 90 second duration
- 40 - 60 mm Hg early first stage peak IUP
- 70 - ≥100 mm Hg late first stage and second stage peak IUP

DYSTOCIA FEATURES

Abnormal Labor (Dystocia) Features

- no fundal dominance (discoordinate contractions)
- no cervical change or abnormally slow cervical change
- mixed "subnormal" and normal patterns that are ineffective for dilatation and effacement
- presenting part is not well applied to the cervix
- usually responds well to oxytocin augmentation, hydration, and/or narcotics

The frequency, duration, and or peak/strength of contractions may help identify abnormal uterine activity. You can also plot a labor curve to graphically assess labor progress.

LABOR CURVE

The purpose of plotting a labor curve is to visualize the progress of dilatation and descent. Graph paper is used to plot these values. The hospital's chart form may have a space for you to plot a labor curve.

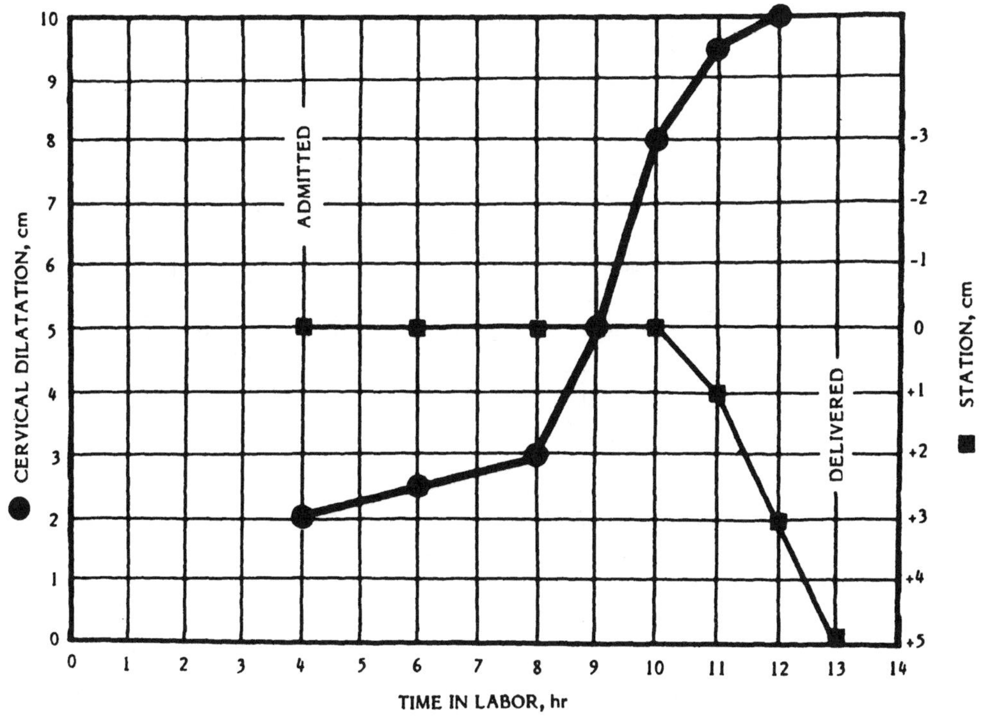

4.4 ***A sequence of observations of cervical dilatation and fetal station is entered on graph paper to display labor progress with the passage of time.*** (Cohen, W. R. and Friedman, E. A. (1983). Management of Labor. University Park Press).

If after 2 or more hours there is no progress in dilatation during active labor, an arrest of labor may exist. The woman should be evaluated by the midwife or physician. In addition, the midwife and/or physician should be called if:

- after 10 cm dilatation there is no descent for 1 or more hours of pushing. this is called an arrest of descent.
- there is a failure to dilate, perhaps the fetus is not well-applied to the cervix or contractions are weak and ineffective.
- there was some descent then failure to descend, perhaps pushing efforts were weak, an upright position might help, or the fetal or pelvic size limit descent.

BENEFITS OF TOCOTRANSDUCER USE

Benefits of the Tocotransducer (TOCO)

1. Provides a record of the contraction pattern and its relationship to the FHR
2. Noninvasive
3. Provides information on uterine contraction frequency, duration, and waveform configuration.
4. May be a closer representation of the *onset and duration* of contractions than reported by the woman or her coach.
5. Suggests fetal movement (spikes) and/or maternal breathing (rhythmic up and down fluctuations).

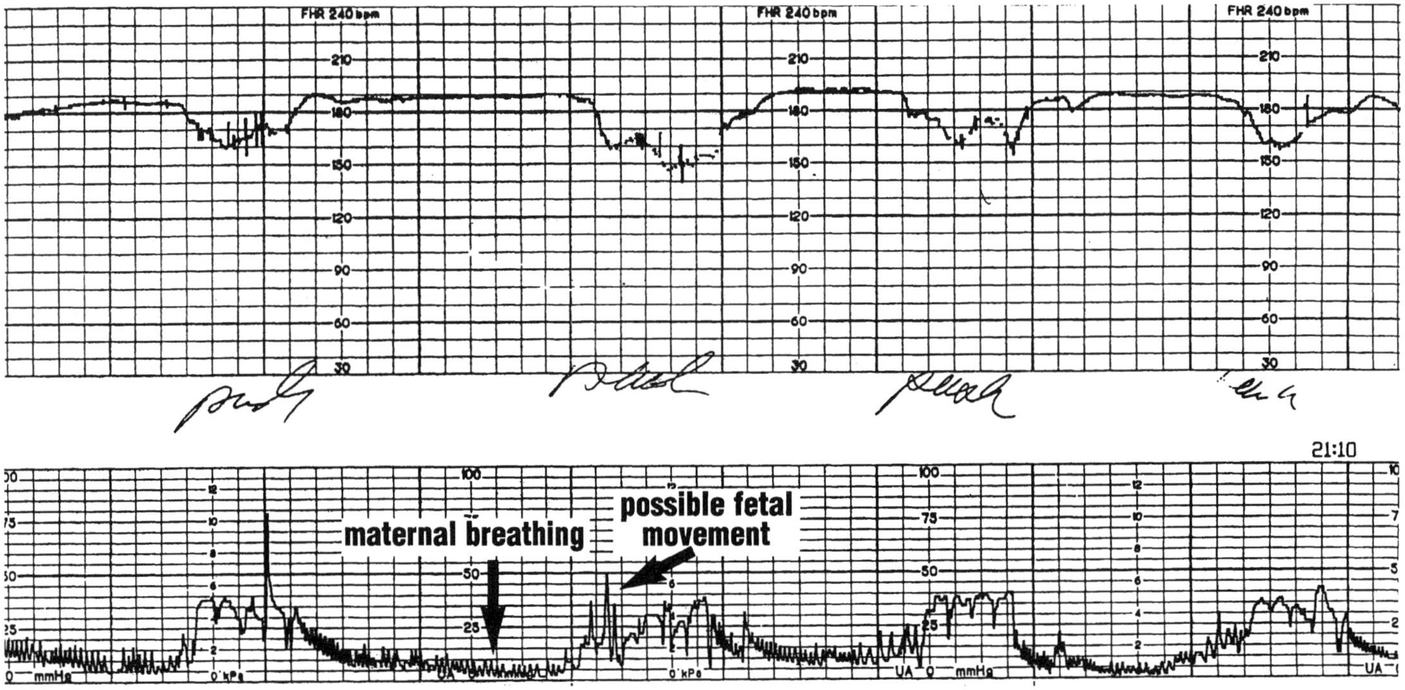

4.5 ***Pushing creates a picket fence appearance. Between and during contractions spikes suggest possible fetal movement. Fetal movement should be confirmed by palpation. The up and down small fluctuations between contractions suggest maternal breathing at a rate of approximately 28/minute. Hyperventilation may decrease oxygen delivery to the fetus. Coach the woman to slow down her breathing.***

- The TOCO should be placed above the woman's umbilicus in near-term to postterm pregnancies and at or below the umbilicus in preterm gestations.

EXTERNAL RECORDING OF UTERINE ACTIVITY: LIMITATIONS

Tocotransducer Limitations

- Incorrect positioning of the TOCO may lead to the inability to detect the contraction from beginning to end.
- Contractions in preterm pregnancies may be difficult to record because the electronic fetal monitor TOCO is not as sensitive as a home uterine monitor created specifically for preterm gestations.
- Subcutaneous tissue, especially in obese women, can interfere with the detection of contractions.

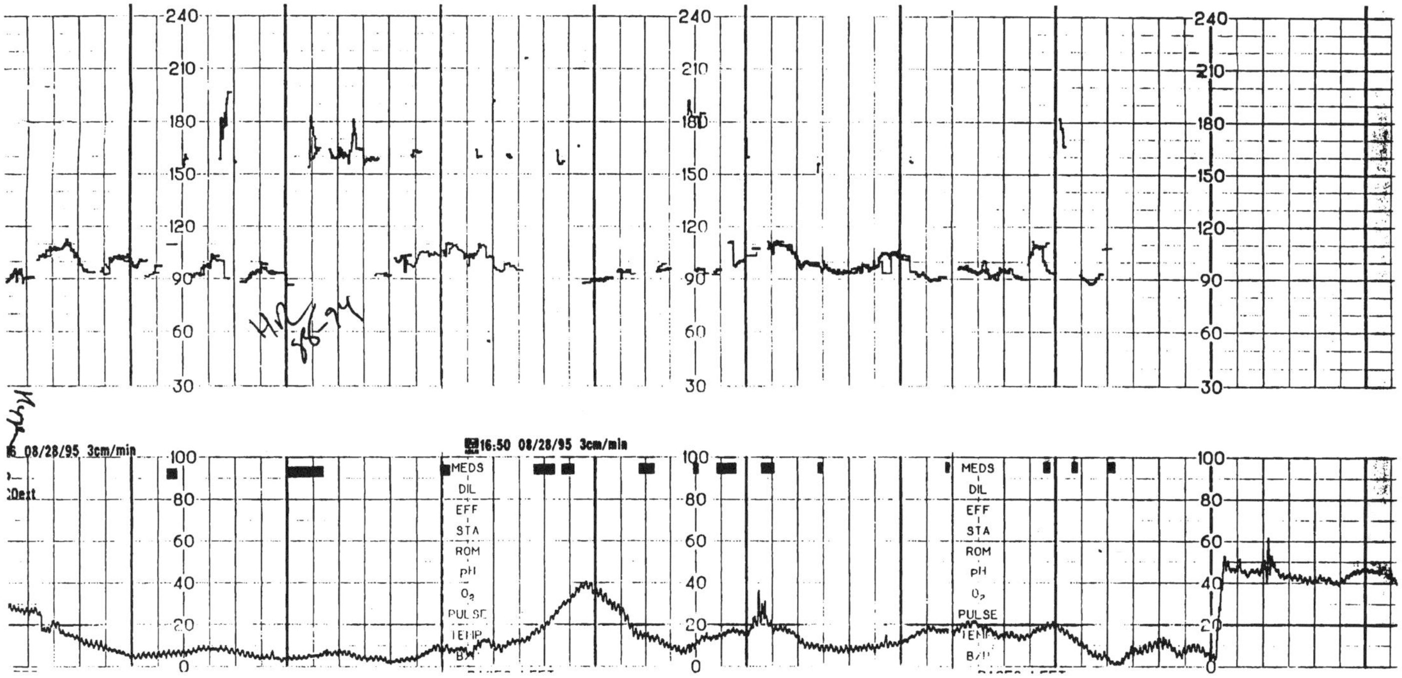

4.6 Maternal heart rate is printed (88-94 bpm). The black squares at the top of the uterine activity channel reflect maternal movement (since the maternal heart rate is also detected). The FHR or doubling of the maternal heart rate is intermittently recorded near 160 bpm. Contractions may or may not be too close together. Both the ultrasound transducer and TOCO need adjustments prior to making clinical decisions.

POSSIBLE IUPC INDICATIONS

Possible Indications for Intrauterine Pressure Monitoring (IUPC)

The use of an IUPC is based on a cost/benefit analysis. Risks of IUPC insertion include abruption, entanglement with the umbilical cord, lower segment uterine perforation, and infection. IUPCs may be used:

- to evaluate contractions during abnormal labor
- in case of a TOLAC (Trial of Labor After Cesarean) or a history of a uterine incision
- to monitor contractions accurately during oxytocin augmentation or induction
- to more closely examine the relationship between contractions and decelerations to possibly change the plan of care
- to evaluate the actual peak IUP and resting tone

UTERINE ACTIVITY VARIATIONS

Variations in Uterine Activity

The uterine activity pattern may vary. Examples of variations include

- coupling
- hyperstimulation
- hypertonus
- uterine reversal
- tetanic contractions, and
- low amplitude high frequency (LAHF) waves or uterine irritability.

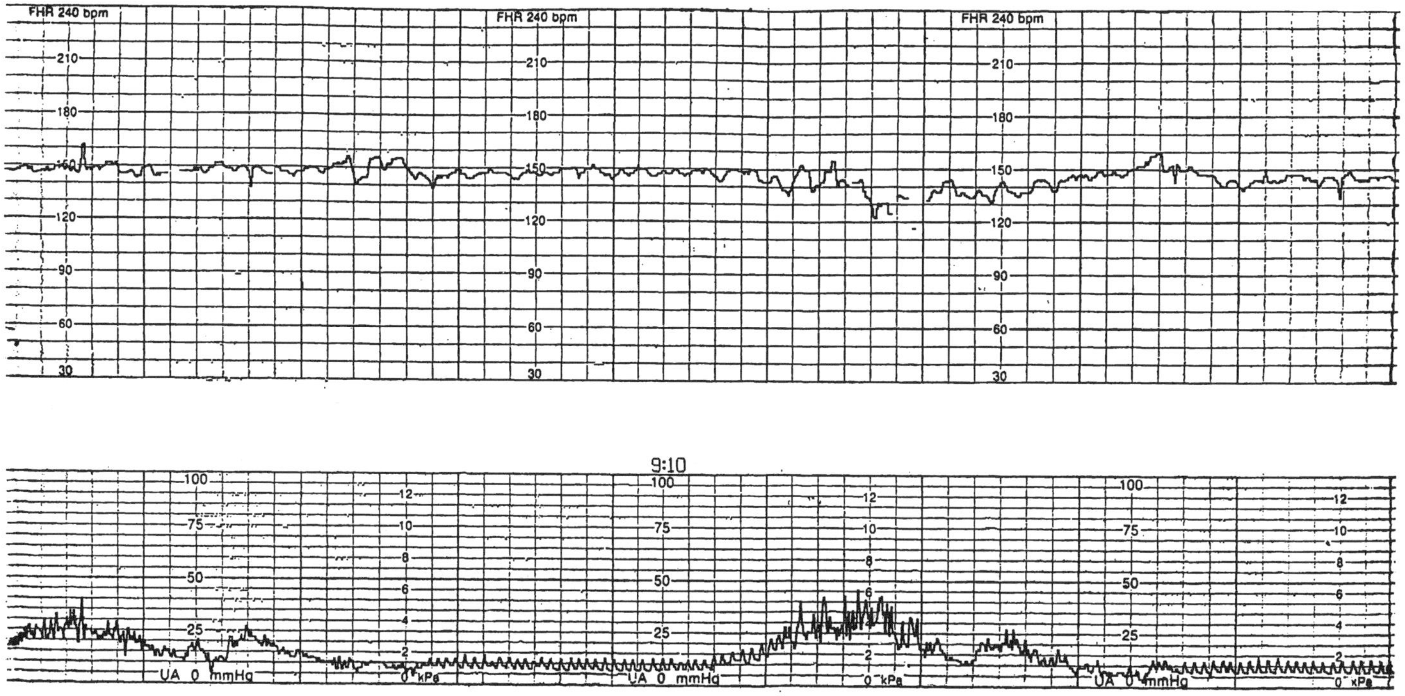

4.7 During coupling, the first contraction is always longer than the second.

COUPLING

Coupling

Coupling is often seen when the fetus is in an occiput posterior (looking up) position or OT (occiput transverse) position (looking sideways). To document coupling in this example, you might chart "UCs q 5 x 40-80, mild - mod with coupling." Of course, strength will be palpated. Or you could document "coupling q 5 x 40-80, mild - mod."

HYPER-STIMULATION

Hyperstimulation

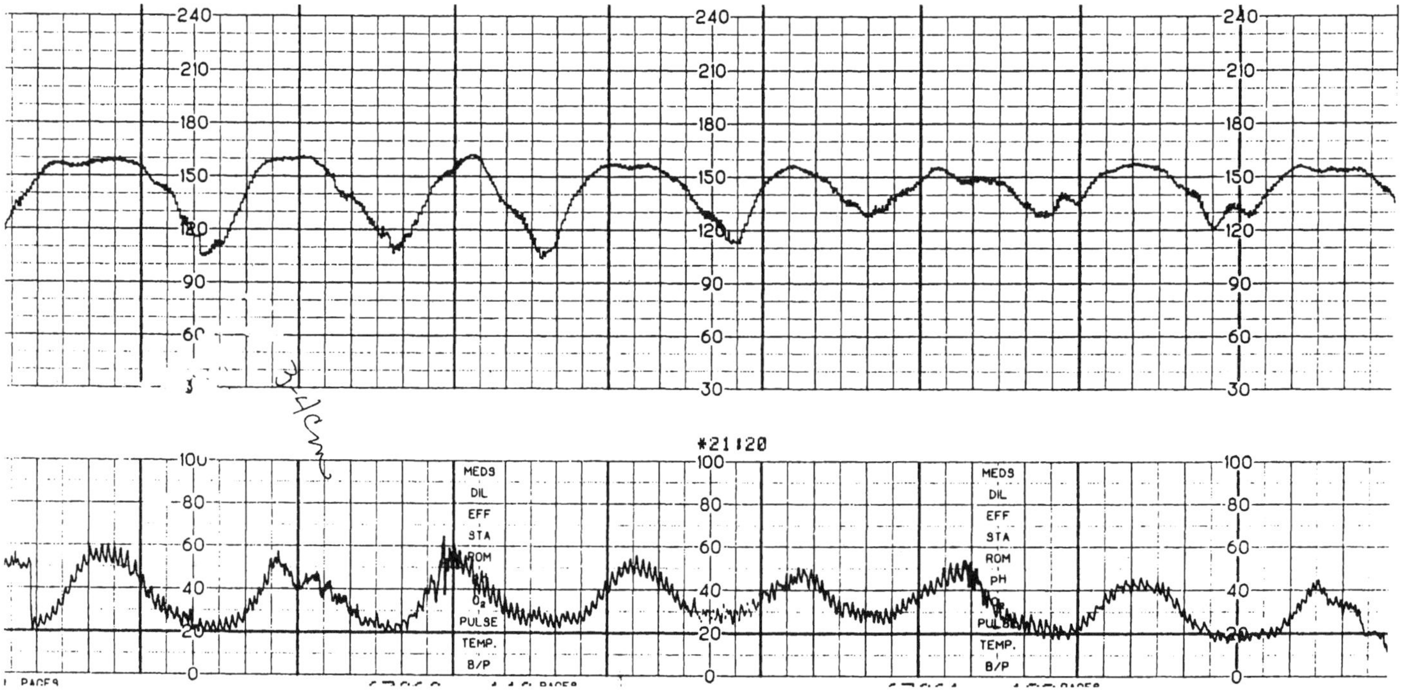

4.8 ***The frequency of contractions is approximately every minute with the interval only a few seconds between contractions. There are late decelerations with a baseline level of 155-160 bpm. This is a classic abruption pattern and a medical emergency.***

Hyperstimulation is often associated with pitocin® sensitivity or abruption. Pitocin® should be discontinued and is usually restarted at half of the dose once hyperstimulation ceases and an abruption is ruled out.

HYPERTONUS

Hypertonus

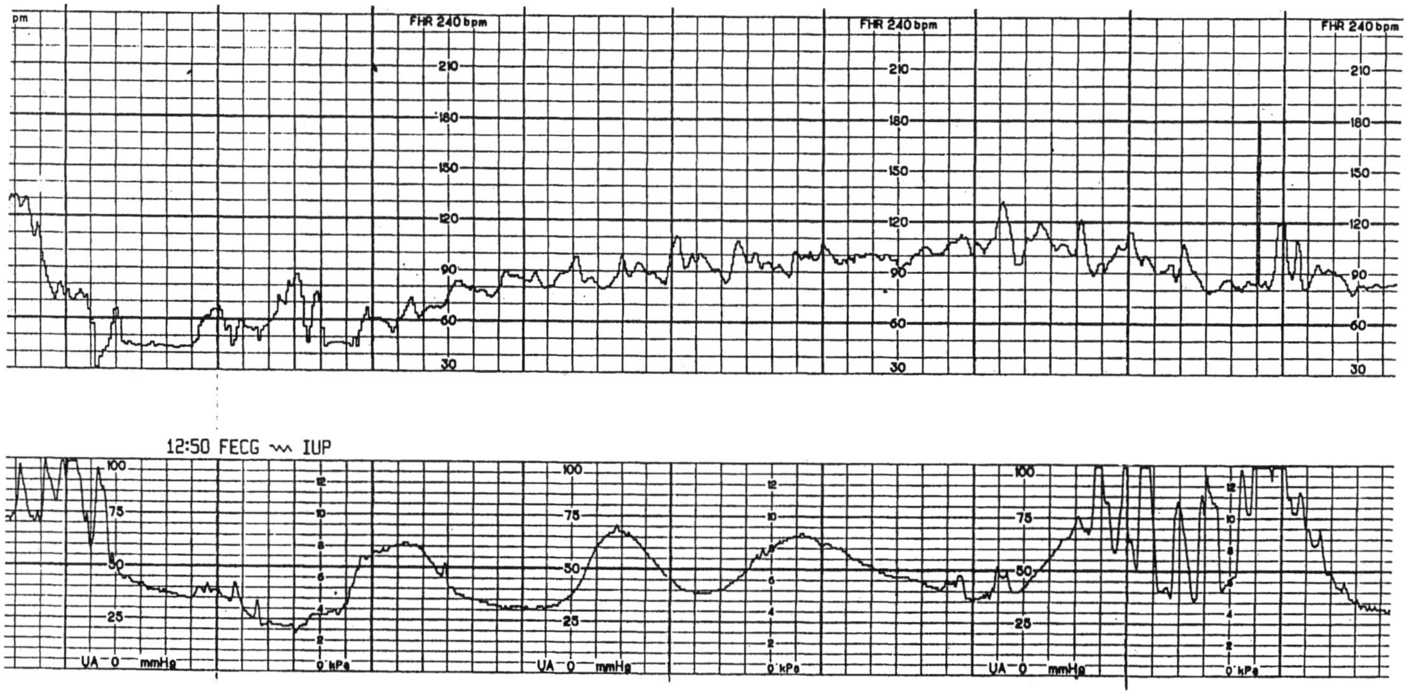

4.9 Uterine hypertonus often accompanies hyperstimulation. Hypertonus is a resting tone above 25 mm Hg.

In this example, the first and last contraction indicate maternal pushing. There is hyperstimulation and hypertonus. The fetus is bradycardic. If pitocin® is infusing, it should be discontinued immediately. The woman should be positioned on her side and encouraged to stop pushing. An intravenous bolus of lactated Ringer's solution should begin, oxygen should be administered at 8-10 liters per minute (LPM) by a simple face mask or 12 LPM by a partial rebreathing mask. A vaginal examination should be done to rule out umbilical cord prolapse and to assess dilatation, effacement and station. The midwife or physician should be promptly notified.

UTERINE REVERSAL

Uterine Reversal

If the TOCO is placed low on the abdomen or over the baby's buttocks and the fetus pulls away during the contraction, a negative versus positive pressure will be exerted. This will create a reversed image or uterine reversal pattern. If the woman is asleep, there is no need to adjust the TOCO as the tracing provides adequate information for decisions (see 4.10).

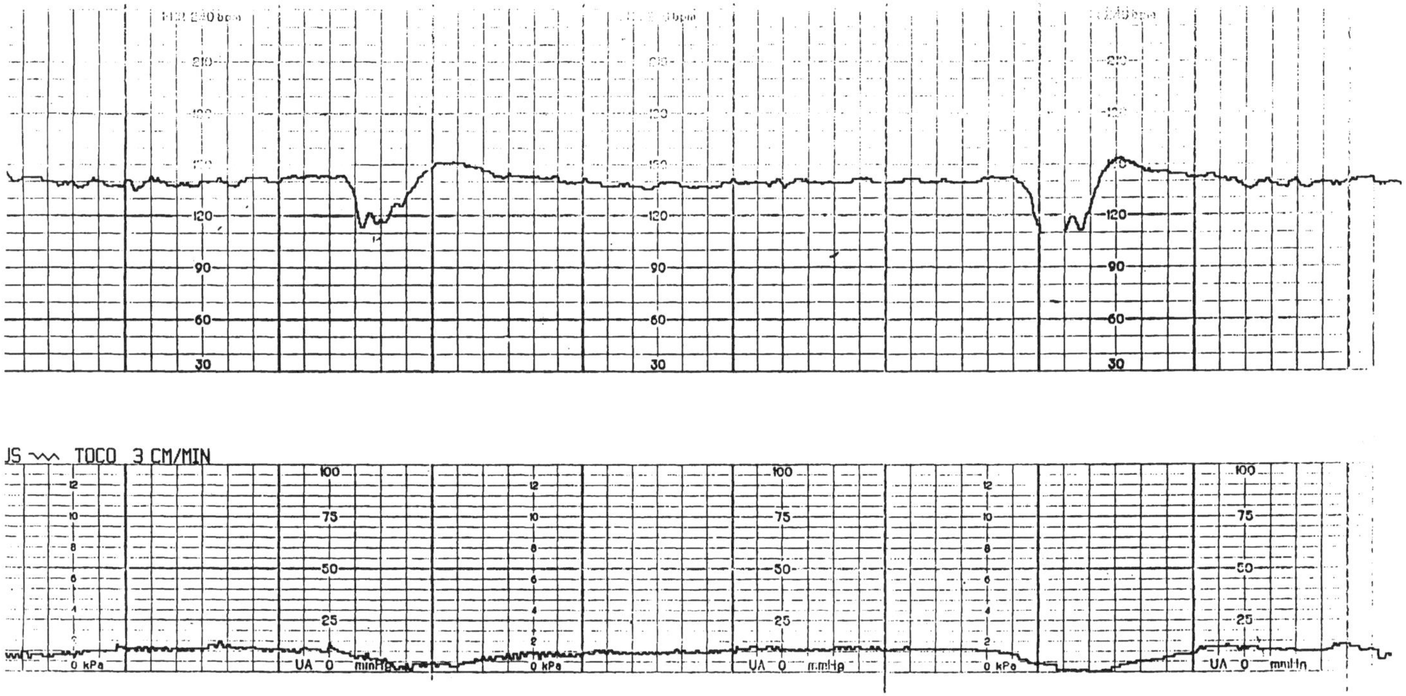

4.10 The FHR reflects variable decelerations with overshoots following the decelerations. The baseline is 136-140 bpm with minimal long-term variability. Contractions are reversed with a frequency of every 4½ minutes and a duration of approximately 70 seconds.

TETANIC CONTRACTIONS

Tetanic Contractions

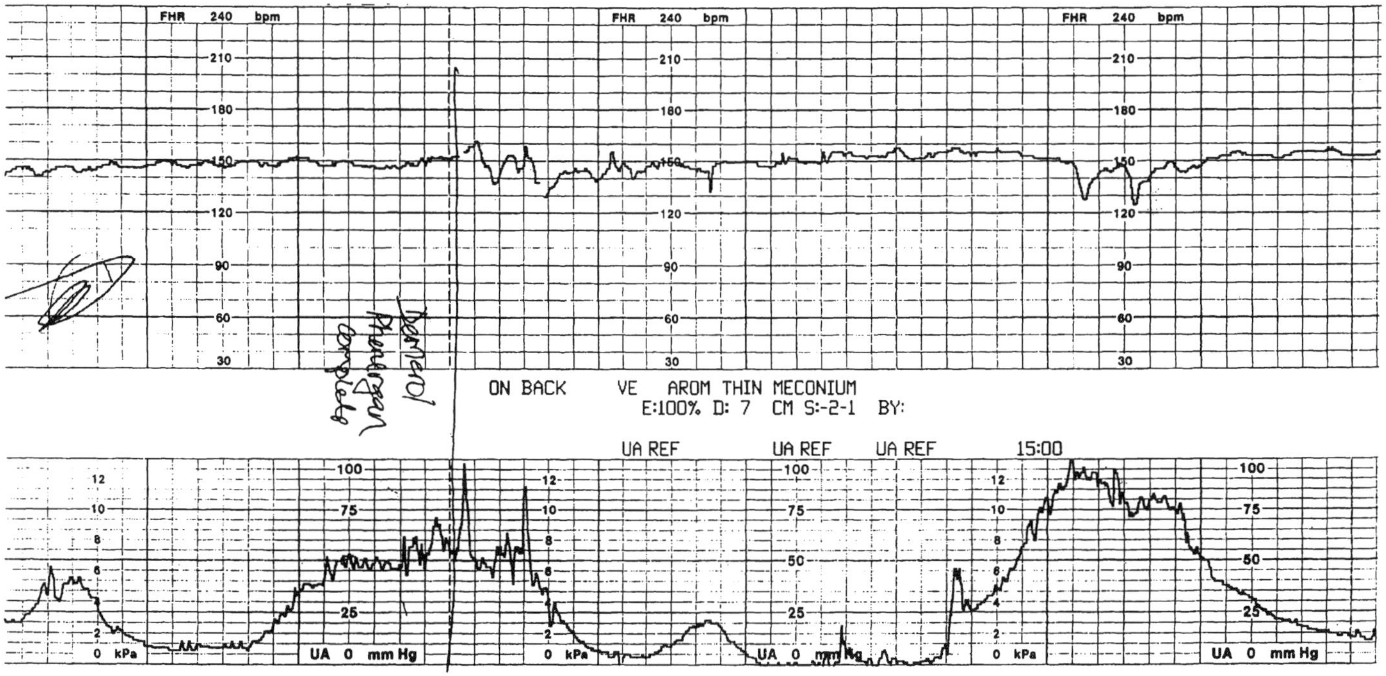

4.11 Tetanic contractions are strong and long (90 seconds x 90 mm Hg).

Tetanic contractions are long and strong, i.e., they usually last 90 seconds or more and are strong to palpation or reach or exceed 90 mm Hg. Tectonic contractions can normally occur. If they do, expect rapid labor progress. However, they can also occur as a response to cocaine. Cocaine causes the release of oxytocin from the posterior pituitary gland and has a direct effect on uterine cells.

UTERINE IRRITABILITY

Uterine Irritability

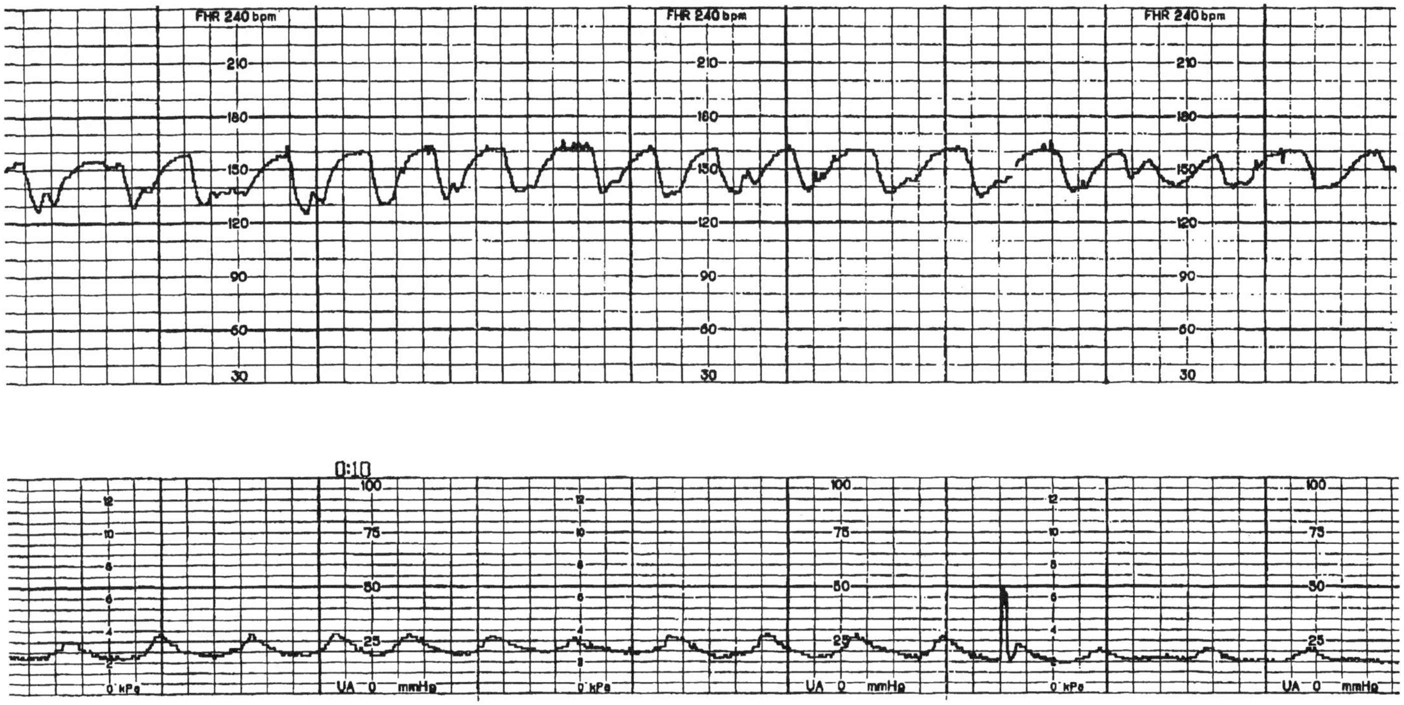

4.12 LAHF waves or uterine irritability. A series of accelerations are seen in the FHR pattern. The fetus eventually had a baseline of 120-130 bpm.

Low amplitude high frequency waves (LAHF waves), or uterine irritability, is often related to uterine prostaglandin release as a result of infection or lack of adequate uterine perfusion due to dehydration. If the woman is preterm, LAHF waves may occur in the 72 hours preceding the onset of preterm labor. Some women have LAHF waves when the placenta is abrupting.

EXERCISES

Exercises

For each example, describe the frequency, duration, strength, and relaxation or resting tone.

4.

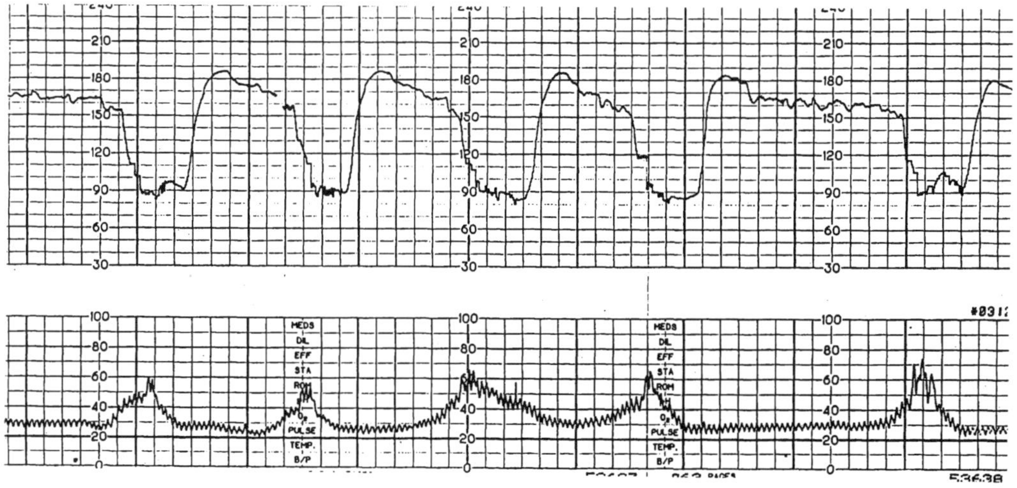

4.13 Variable decelerations with overshoots. Uterine activity pattern demonstrates maternal respirations.

Frequency ______________

Duration ______________

Strength ______________

Resting Tone ____________

5.

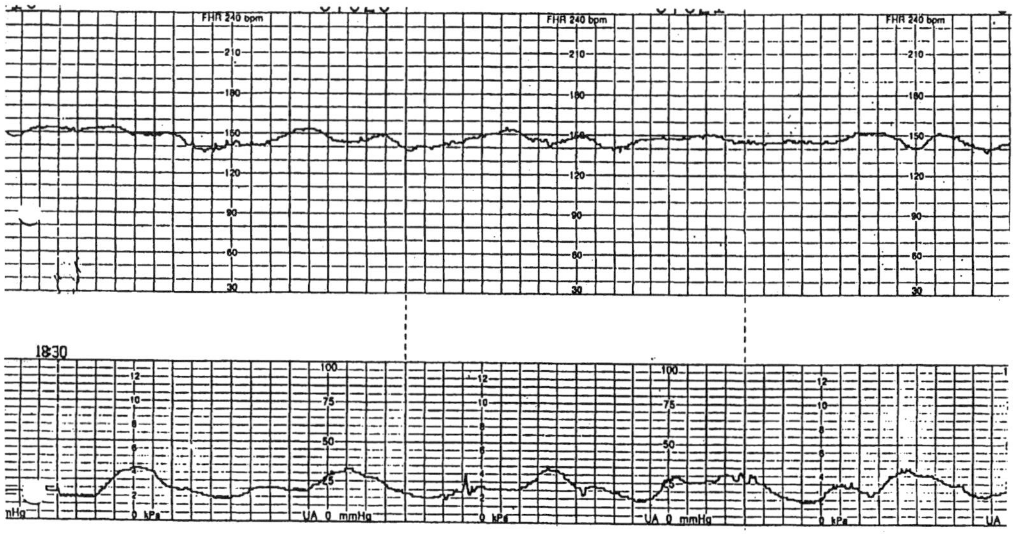

4.14 Abruption. Absent long-term variability.

Frequency ______________

Duration ______________

Strength ______________

Resting Tone ____________

6.

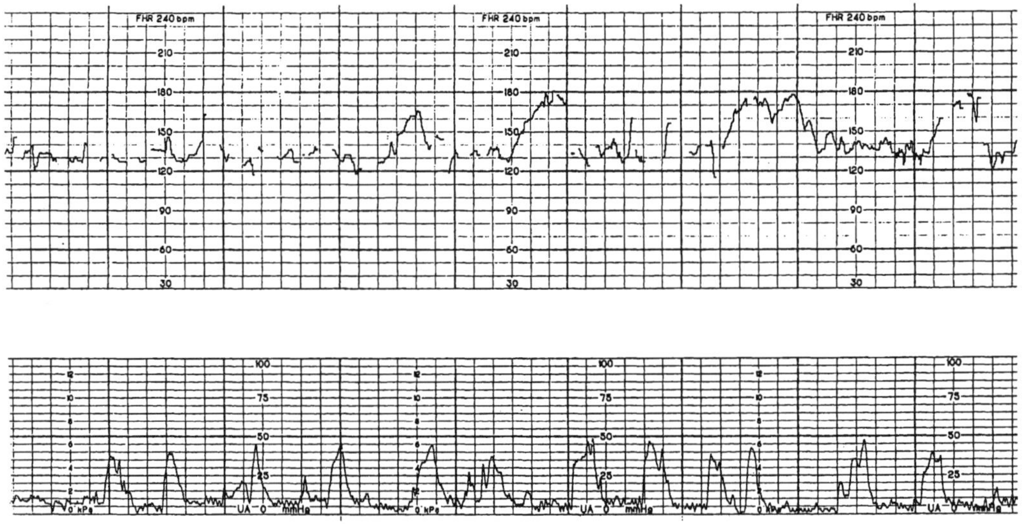

4.15 ***Ultrasound and tocotransducer used. Confirm uterine activity by palpation. Adjust toco as required.***

Frequency ____________

Duration ____________

Strength ____________

Resting Tone ____________

7.

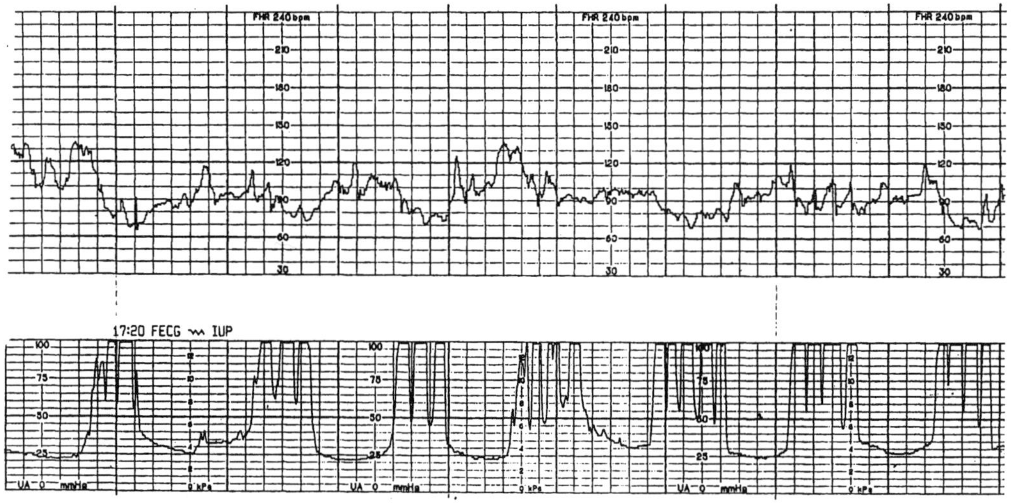

4.16 ***Pushing with second-stage or end-stage bradycardia. Uterine activity demonstrates patient pushing.***

Frequency ____________

Duration ____________

Strength ____________

Resting Tone ____________

8.

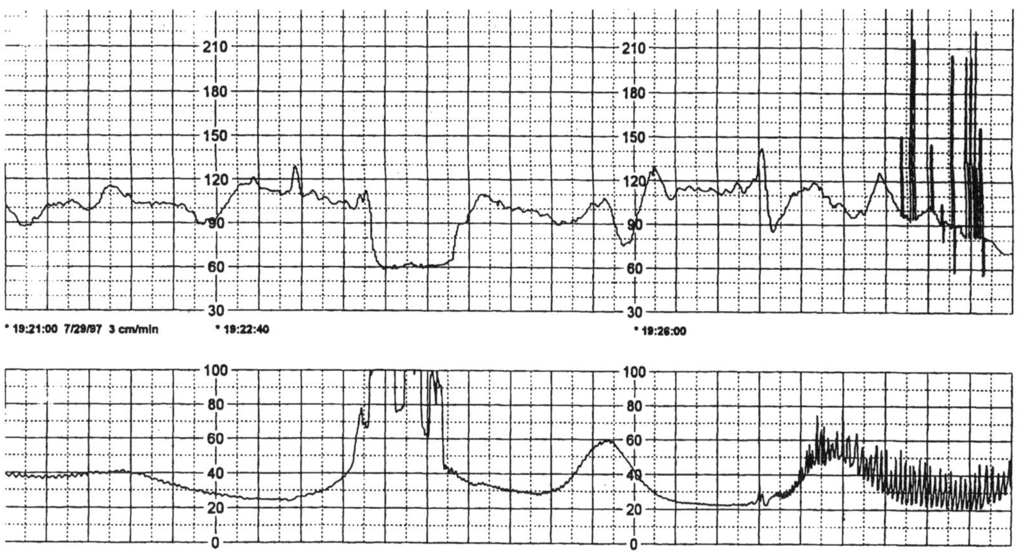

4.17 Computer printout of a fetal monitor tracing. Unstable FHR.

Frequency ____________

Duration ____________

Strength ____________

Resting Tone ____________

ANSWERS TO EXERCISES

1. 200 MVUs
2. 105 MVUs
3. 185 MVUs
4. q $1^1/_2$ -$2^1/_2$ minutes x 40-70 seconds, need to palpate strength and resting tone [q means every]
5. hyperstimulation, approximately q $1^1/_2$ minutes x 30-70 seconds, need to palpate strength. The placenta is abrupting. This is a medical emergency.
6. no uterine activity. Fetal or maternal movement spikes only.
7. hyperstimulation, occasional hypertonus, q $1^1/_2$ minutes x 50-70, strong (pushing), need to palpate resting tone and act to decrease uterine activity.
8. q $1^1/_2$ -2 minutes, 50-80, pushing then panting, palpate resting tone, act to facilitate delivery.

SUMMARY

Summary

Contraction frequency often increases when the woman is fearful and anxious. Frequency, duration, strength, and relaxation are documented when the uterus is palpated or a tocotransducer is used. Frequency, duration, peak intrauterine pressure, and resting tone are documented when an intrauterine pressure catheter is used.

Montevideo units (MVUs) are calculated by adding contraction intensities over a 10 minute period. Intensity is the contraction peak minus its resting tone. Intensity can only be measured when an intrauterine pressure catheter is in place. Greater than 150 MVUs has been associated with adequate labor progress.

Dystocia is associated with no or abnormally slow cervical change. Often, the presenting part is not well applied to the cervix. Oxytocin argumentation, hydration, and narcotics may improve uterine contraction effectiveness.

Contractions appear in sets (coupling) when the fetus is in a persistent occiput posterior or occiput transverse position. Hyperstimulation may be related to pitocin® hypersensitivity or abruption. Hypertonus is a resting tone above 25 mm Hg. Uterine reversal appears when the tocotransducer is not placed above the umbilicus at term or the abdomen moves away from it during a contraction. Tetanic contractions suggest rapid labor progress, imminent delivery, or are a response to cocaine. Uterine irritability or low amplitude high frequency waves suggest prostaglandin release due to infection, dehydration with a lack of uterine perfusion, or abruption.

SECTION 4: UTERINE CONTRACTIONS

QUESTIONS

Directions: Circle T if the statement is true, F if it is false.

QUESTIONS			
T	F	1.	Fear decreases uterine activity.
T	F	2.	The range of normal resting tone is 8 to 12 mm Hg.
T	F	3.	The interval is the time from the beginning of one contraction to the beginning of the next contraction.
T	F	4.	Intensity is synonymous with strength or quality of contractions.
T	F	5.	Calculation of Montevideo Units should be used to identify hypocontractility.
T	F	6.	Abnormal labor may include a fetal presenting part that is not well applied to the cervix.
T	F	7.	Tocotransducers provide accurate information on contraction frequency and duration.
T	F	8.	Contraction detection with a tocotransducer in a preterm gestation is as accurate as in a term gestation.
T	F	9.	An intrauterine pressure catheter is needed to evaluate peak intrauterine pressure.
T	F	10.	An occiput posterior position is related to uterine contraction coupling.

SECTION 5
The Baseline (BL)

SYSTEMATIC REVIEW

A systematic review of the fetal heart rate (FHR) includes the baseline, accelerations (accels), and decelerations (decels). A FHR pattern is a combination of BL, accels, and decels. There is actually no time limit for determining a BL rate. In fact, after a BL is observed, it will become obvious in one minute if it is flat, e.g., a persistent rate of 150 beats per minute (bpm).

In 1995 the National Institute of Child Health and Human Development (NICHD), in the National Institutes of Health held a research planning workshop on the topic of electronic FHR monitoring research guidelines. For the purpose of gathering data on the BL, the baseline was defined by the 17 perinatologists and one nurse as "the approximate mean (average) FHR rounded to increments of 5 bpm during a 10-minute segment, excluding:

- periodic or episodic changes (accels and decels)
- periods of marked FHR variability
- segments of the baseline that differ by more than 25 bpm."

In addition, this group believed that, "in any 10-minute recording, the baseline duration must be at least 2 minutes or the baseline for that period is undetermined." Since this definition is currently reserved for researchers and has not yet received widespread clinical acceptance, it may be easiest to determine the baseline as that part of the FHR pattern that is not an acceleration, deceleration, artifact, or arrhythmia.

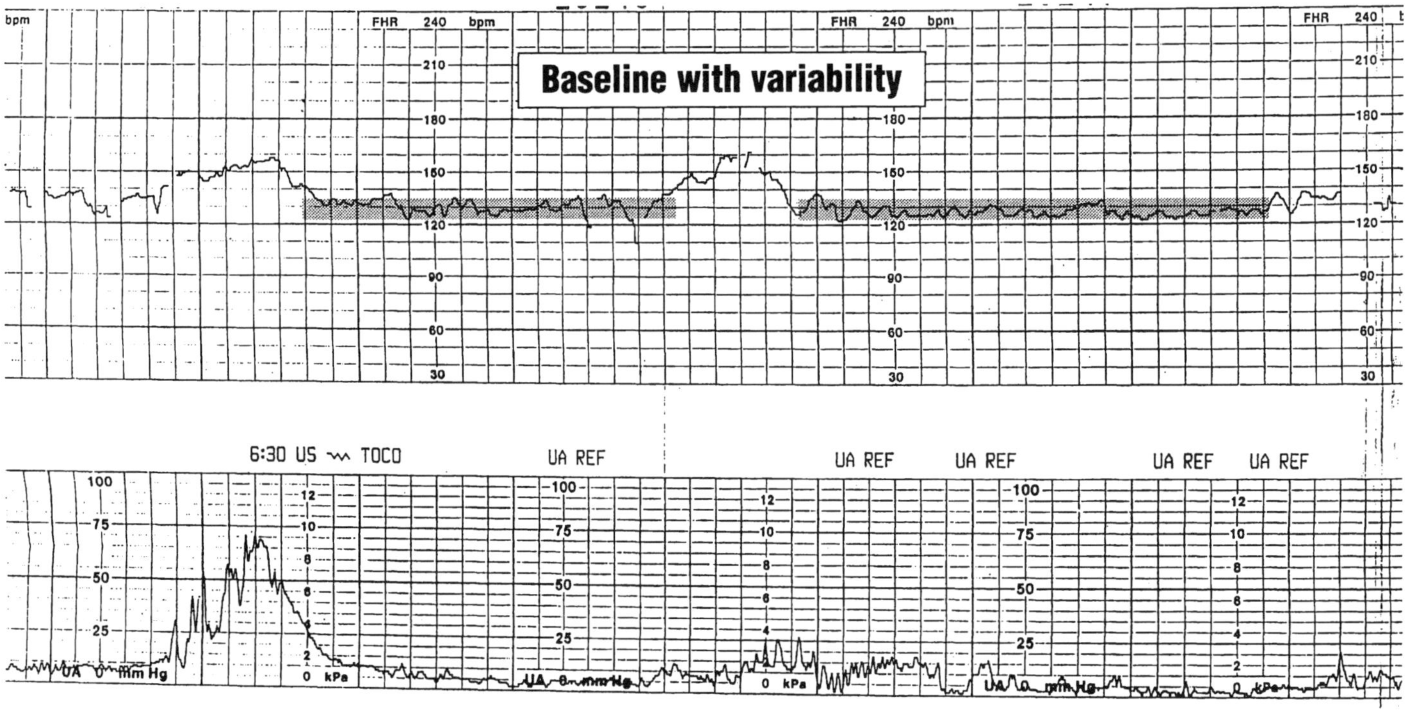

5.1 The FHR baseline is approximately 122-135 beats per minute in this illustration.

Scan the tracing above and you will see the baseline is fluctuating yet stable between 122 and 135 bpm. The baseline is the FHR created by the influence of the vagus and sympathetic nerves on the heart.

BASELINE PHYSIOLOGY

Baseline Physiology

The baseline is influenced by neural, hormonal, and pharmacologic factors.

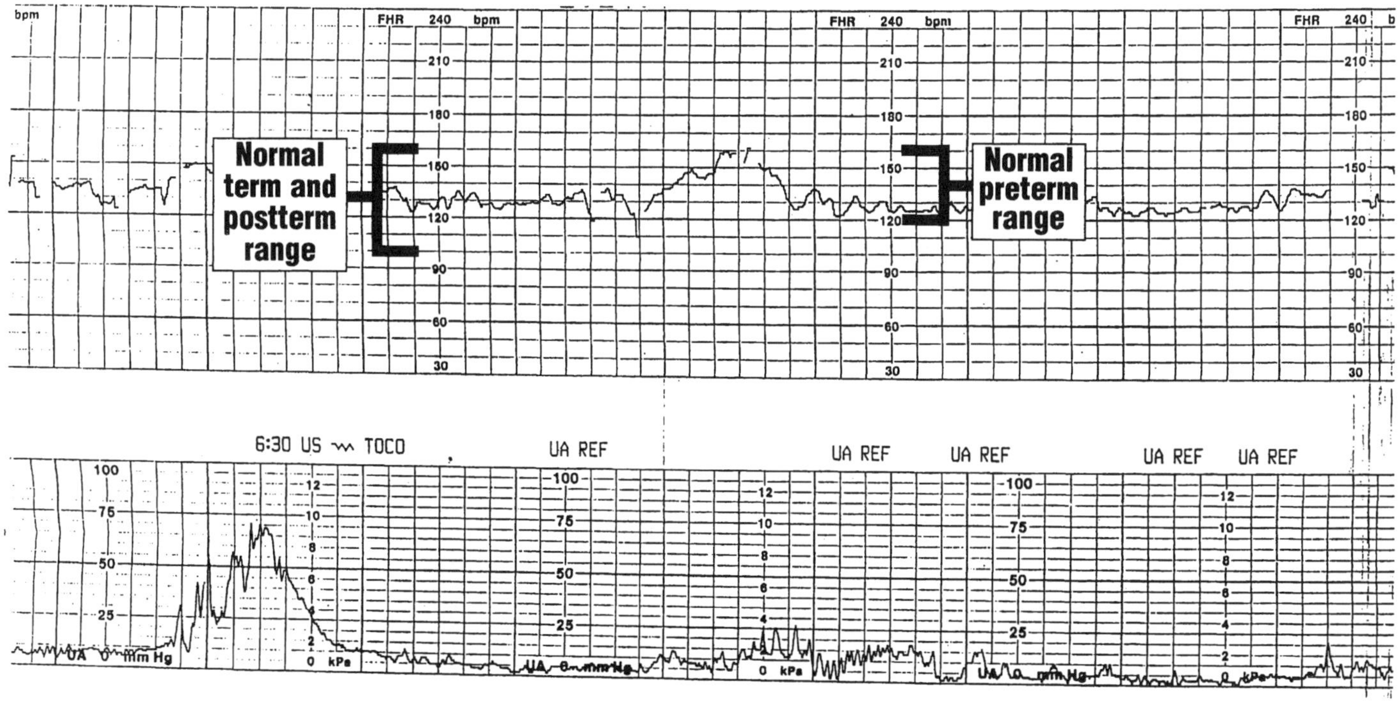

5.2 Illustration of baseline within the normal range for a term or postterm fetus.

The baseline is approximately 122-135 bpm. The normal baseline is between 100-160 bpm for term and postterm fetuses and 120-160 bpm for preterm fetuses. The baseline should stay at the same level from 35 weeks to delivery.

VARIABILITY

Variability

Variability is a baseline characteristic, not an acceleration or deceleration characteristic. Variability is present when the baseline is chaotic, irregular and fluctuating. Variability is absent when the baseline is regular, non-chaotic, and/or smooth. Variability was defined by the NICHD research planning workshop as "...fluctuations in the baseline FHR of two cycles per minutes or greater." One cycle looks like this:

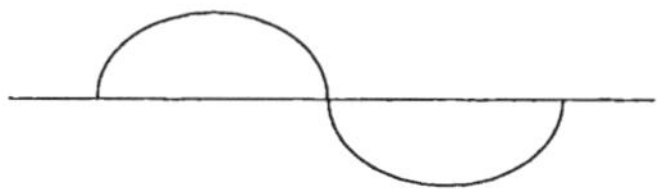

This NICHD definition of variability is essentially a definition of long-term variability. A series of cycles creates long-term variability. Section 6 discusses classifications of long-term variability.

Another characteristic of the baseline is short-term variability. Section 7 discusses short-term variability.

SIGNIFICANCE OF VARIABILITY

Variability should **not** be interpreted as reassuring unless accels are also present within the last 100 minutes of monitoring. Acute hypoxia abruptly increases variability. Causes of acute hypoxia include cord compression, uterine hyperstimulation, and maternal hypotension. The baseline range will be greater than 25 bpm with acute hypoxia.

Chronic hypoxia, with the accumulation of adenosine from the metabolism of adenosine triphosphate, decreases variability and the baseline flattens.

THE LOSS OF VARIABILITY/ FLAT BASELINE

The loss of variability may be caused by drugs such as narcotics. A flat baseline may be worse than a baseline with decelerations, particularly when the lack of variability is related to fetal metabolic acidosis. By obtaining a detailed history and reviewing clinical events, such as narcotic administration, the presence of maternal infection or meconium, and fetal movement, you can determine the most likely cause of absent variability.

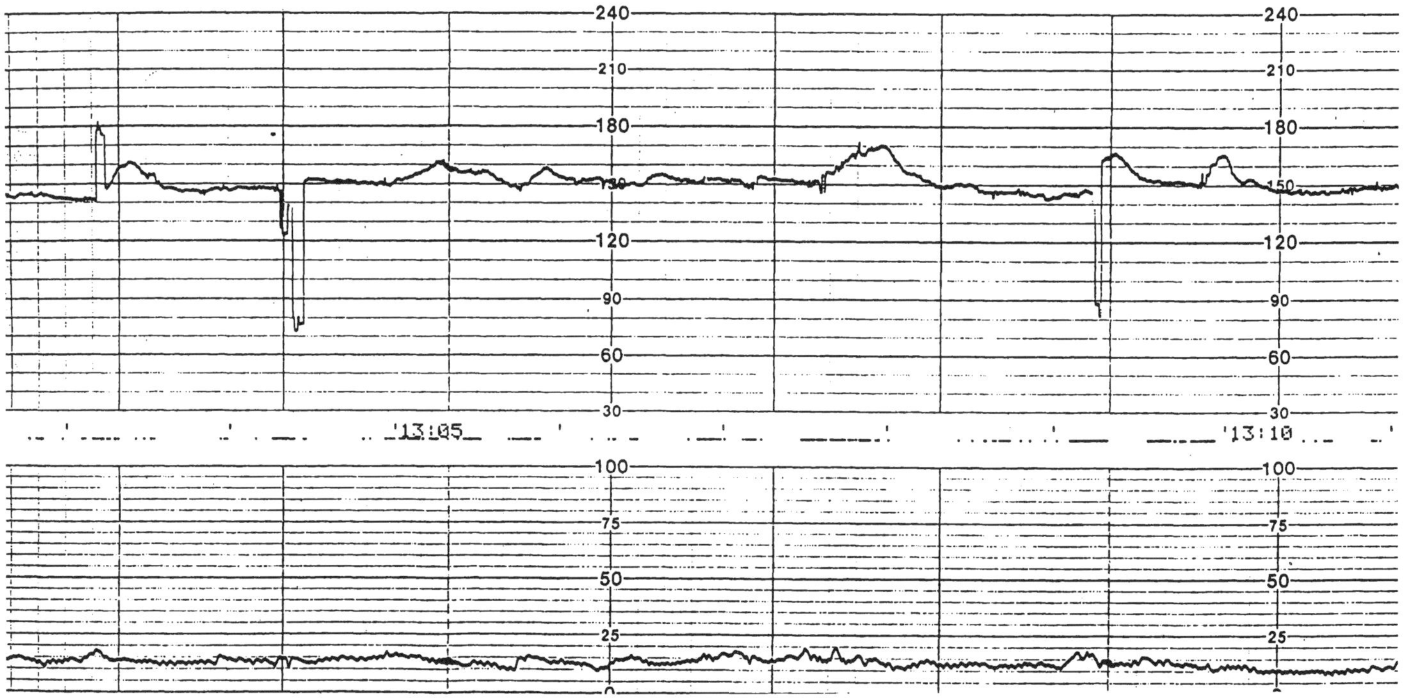

5.3 Baseline of 148-150 beats per minute with spontaneous accelerations to 160-170 bpm. Variability is most likely decreased due to Tegretol® and Prozac® to treat a panic disorder. Fetal movement is present. Apgars were at 7 and 9 at 1 and 5 minutes.

Persistent absent variability, or a flat baseline, may be due to direct myocardial depression as a result of metabolic acidosis. Over the course of two days and a prolonged labor, the fetus progressively deteriorated and was born asphyxiated (see 5.4 and 5.5).

The baseline may flatten, and/or rise over a period of minutes or hours, while accelerations disappear. At 1100, the baseline was 120-122 bpm (see 5.4). By noon, it was over 150 bpm with prolonged decelerations (see 5.5). The flattening and/or rising baseline is a response to hypoxia. By itself, a rising baseline is classified as compensatory. When you add one or more prolonged decelerations, the FHR pattern becomes nonreassuring. Hypoxic fetuses reduce their movement. Notify the midwife or physician when a rising baseline occurs. Assess fetal movement by palpation and/or ask the woman when her baby moved last.

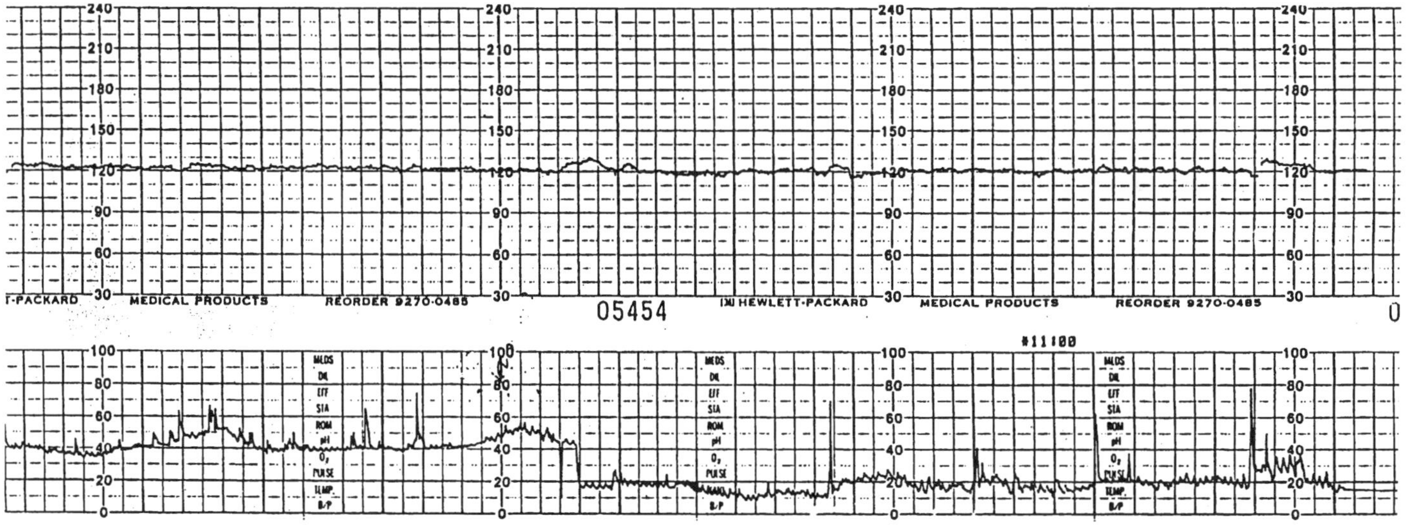

5.4 Initial baseline was 120-122 bpm.

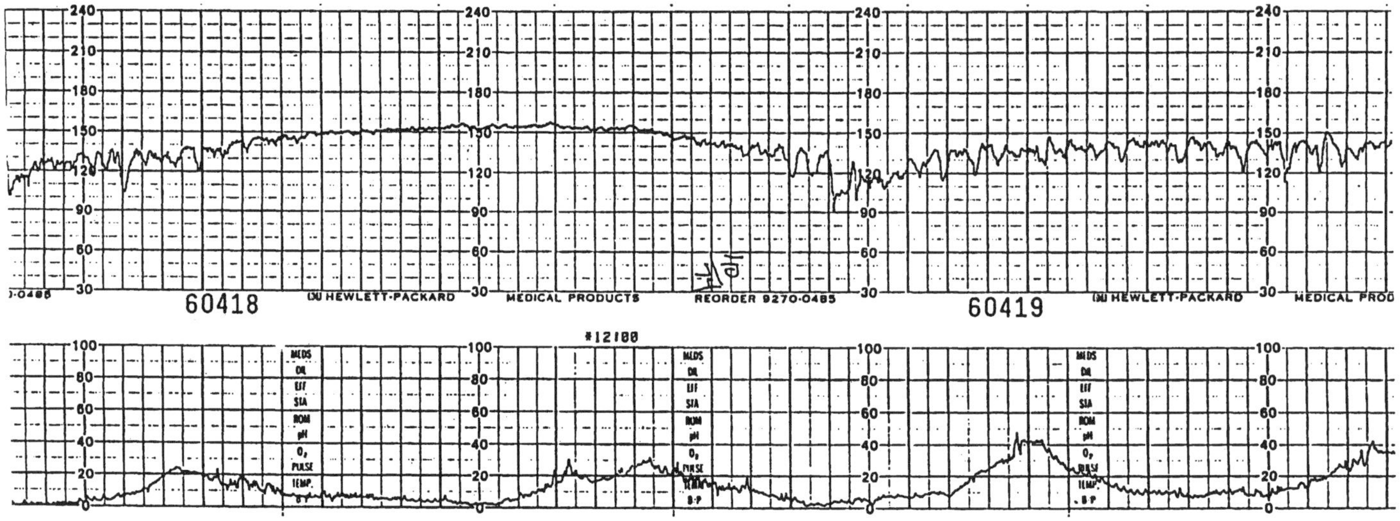

5.5 Rise in the baseline over 1 hour to 150-155 bpm.

TACHYCARDIA

When the baseline is consistently greater than 160 bpm, especially for 10 or more minutes, the fetus is tachycardic. This is abnormal and may be due to fetal hypoxia. To reassure yourself that this is not due to fetal oxygen deprivation, identify and document accelerations, fetal movement, and short-term variability.

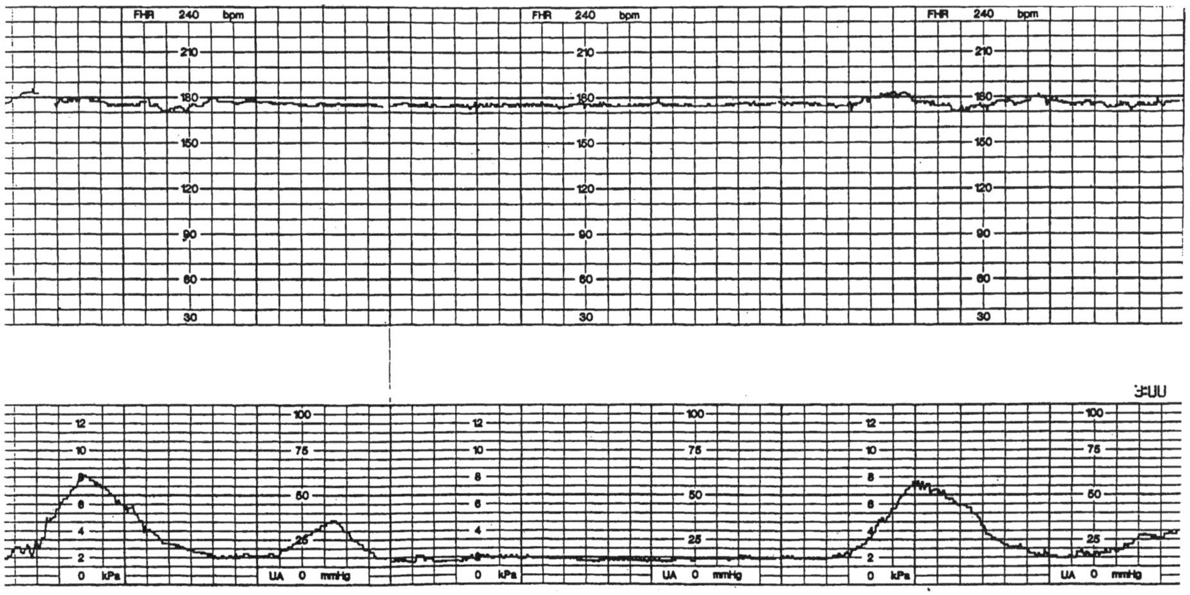

5.6 Tachycardia is defined by a FHR baseline greater than 160 bpm for 10 or more minutes. In this strip the baseline is 175 bpm.

BRADYCARDIA (TERM, POST TERM)

Some people would classify a baseline of 100 to 120 bpm as fetal bradycardia. However, this may be normal in a term or postterm fetus due to their mature vagal nerves. To reassure yourself that this is a normal rate and rhythm, identify and document accelerations, fetal movement, and short-term variability.

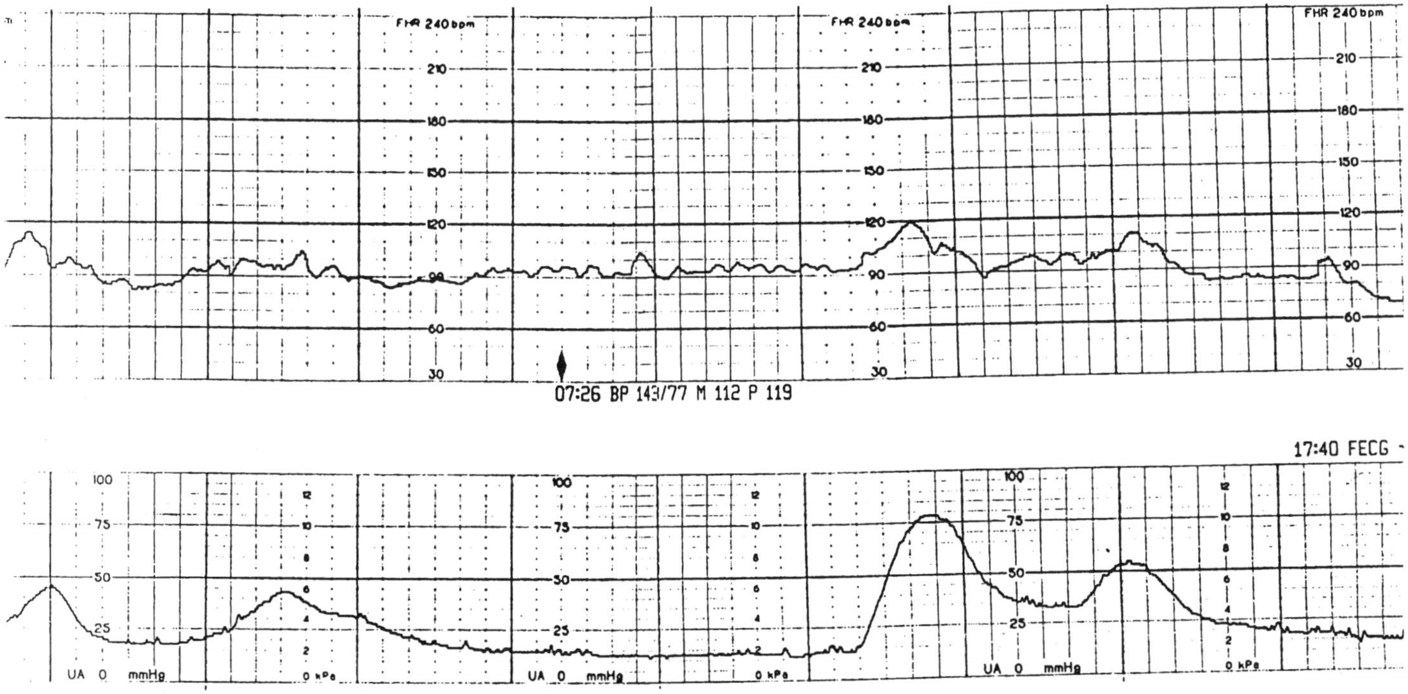

5.7 Bradycardia was a baseline less than 100 bpm in a term or postterm fetus. The baseline is 90-100 bpm. This baby was 39 weeks of gestation.

PRETERM BRADYCARDIA

A baseline less than 120 bpm is bradycardia if the fetus is preterm.

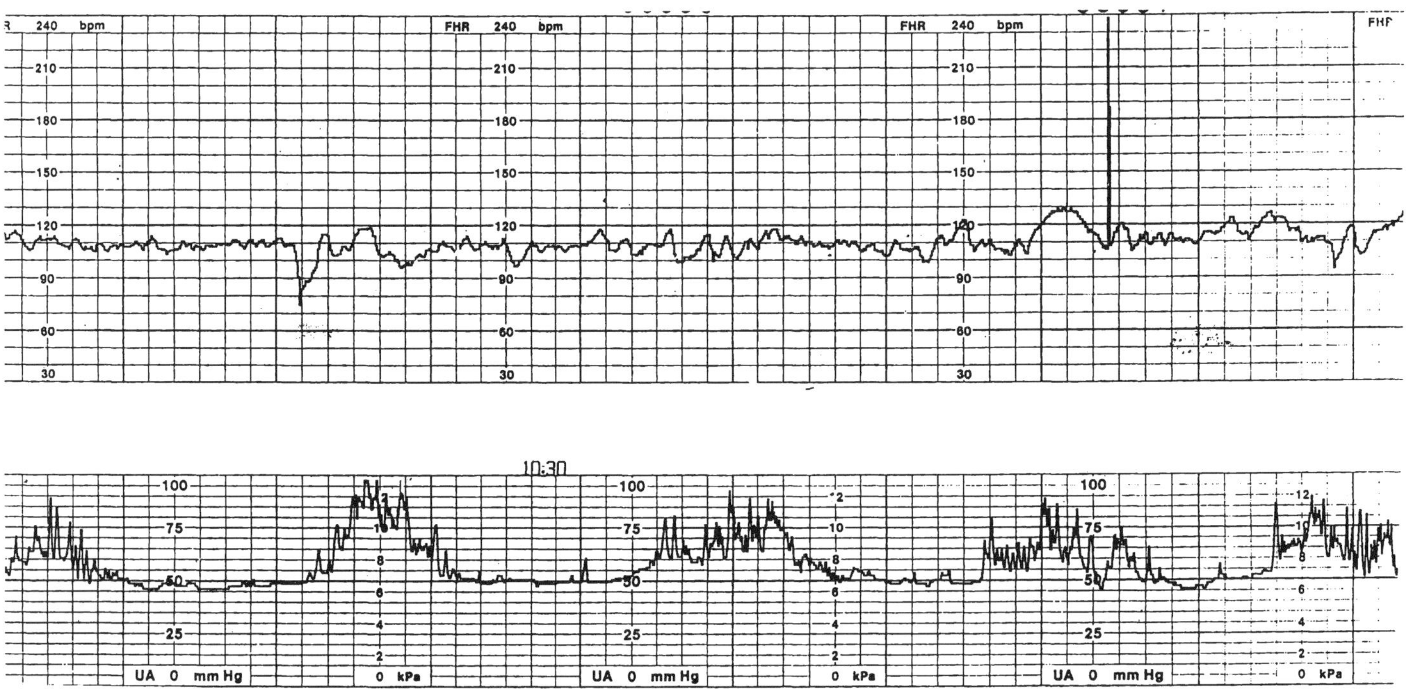

5.8 Preterm bradycardia. This baby was 37 weeks of gestation or near-term.

FALLING BASELINE

A falling baseline may occur abruptly or slowly. The fetus needs to be evaluated immediately. If there are no accelerations and a loss of variability or the baseline continues to falls, the pattern requires immediate medical attention.

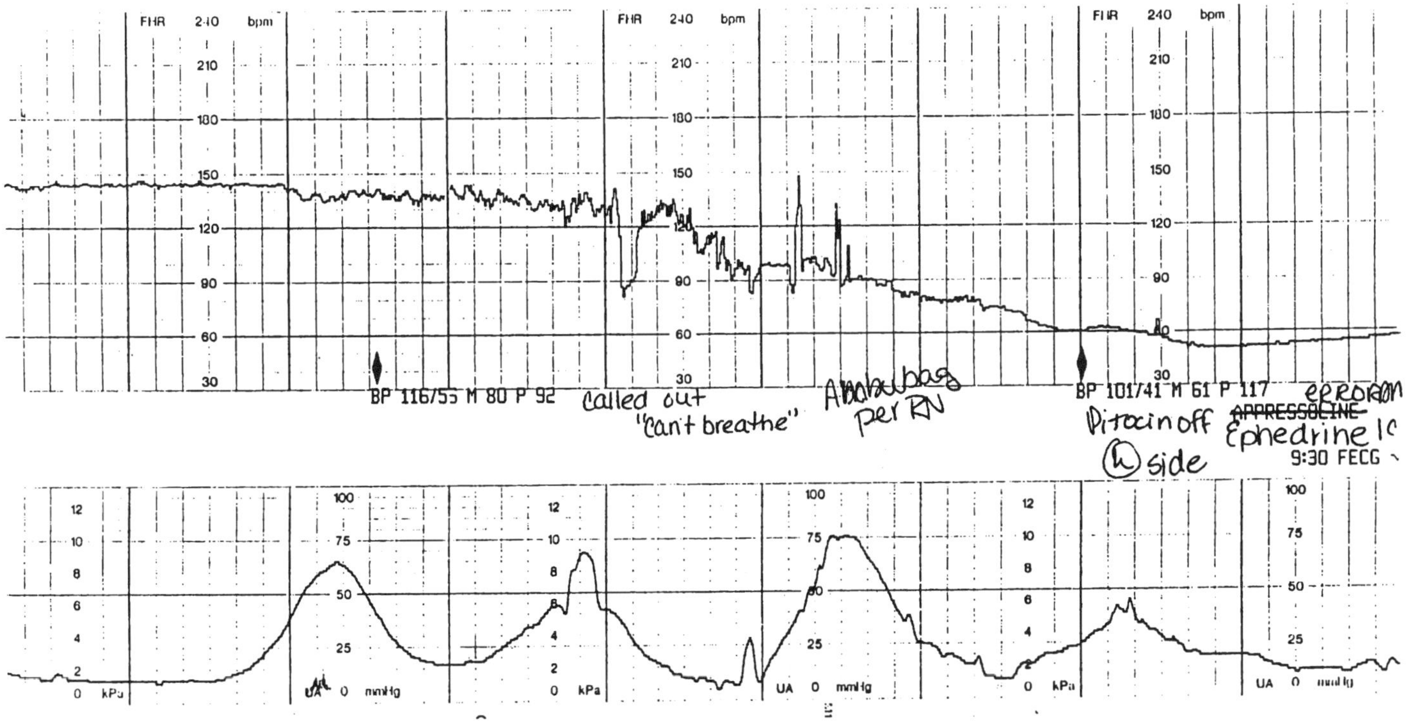

5.9 Falling baseline. This baby had Apgars of 0 at 1, 5, and 10 minutes. The cord artery pH was 6.4.

WANDERING BASELINE

A wandering baseline is a smooth meandering FHR with absent variability. It is unstable and ominous because it is usually associated with fetal asphyxia. Sometines the baseline rate will move between rates that are 40 or more bpm apart. It may never stabilize. Measures to enhance fetal oxygenation should be instituted immediately and delivery should be expedited, especially if congenital anomalies are ruled out by a previous ultrasound and metabolic acidosis is suspected.

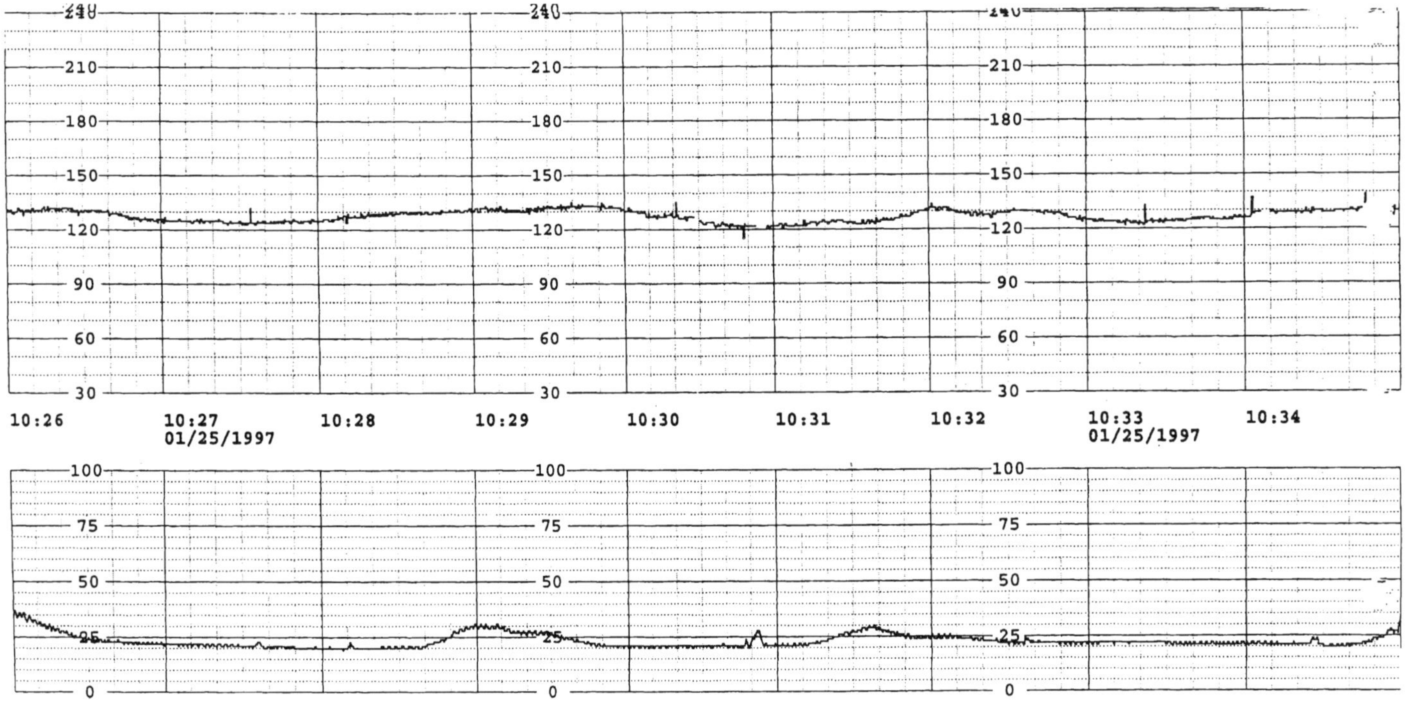

5.10 Wandering baseline.

AGONAL PATTERN

Agonal patterns are bradycardia usually related to cord compression, such as cord prolapse. The fetus is anoxic and unable to maintain its heart rate. The upward surge of the FHR is due to epinephrine and norepinephrine (catecholamines) from the fetal adrenal glands. In spite of this response, there is fetal decompensation with complete cardiovascular collapse. The FHR is ominous and demands immediate delivery and resuscitation. Document the rate, e.g., "60-100, 0 STV, 0 LTV." Do not write "agonal." Call the surgeon and neonatal resuscitation team stat. It is not appropriate to waste time or delay delivery with position changes or other measures to enhance oxygen delivery to the fetus unless the surgeon is not immediately available. Scalp stimulation is inappropriate as it is an assessment technique to stimulate the fetus when there is a baseline but no accelerations. Abdominal (external) manipulation has no effect on the fetus. Oxygen at 8 to 10 liters per minute via a simple tight fitting face mask or an intravenous bolus of lactated Ringer's solution may make little impact on fetal oxygenation. Discontinue oxytocics. A tocolytic, such as terbutaline®, may diminish uterine activity. Terbutaline® is contraindicated if there is a placental abruption.

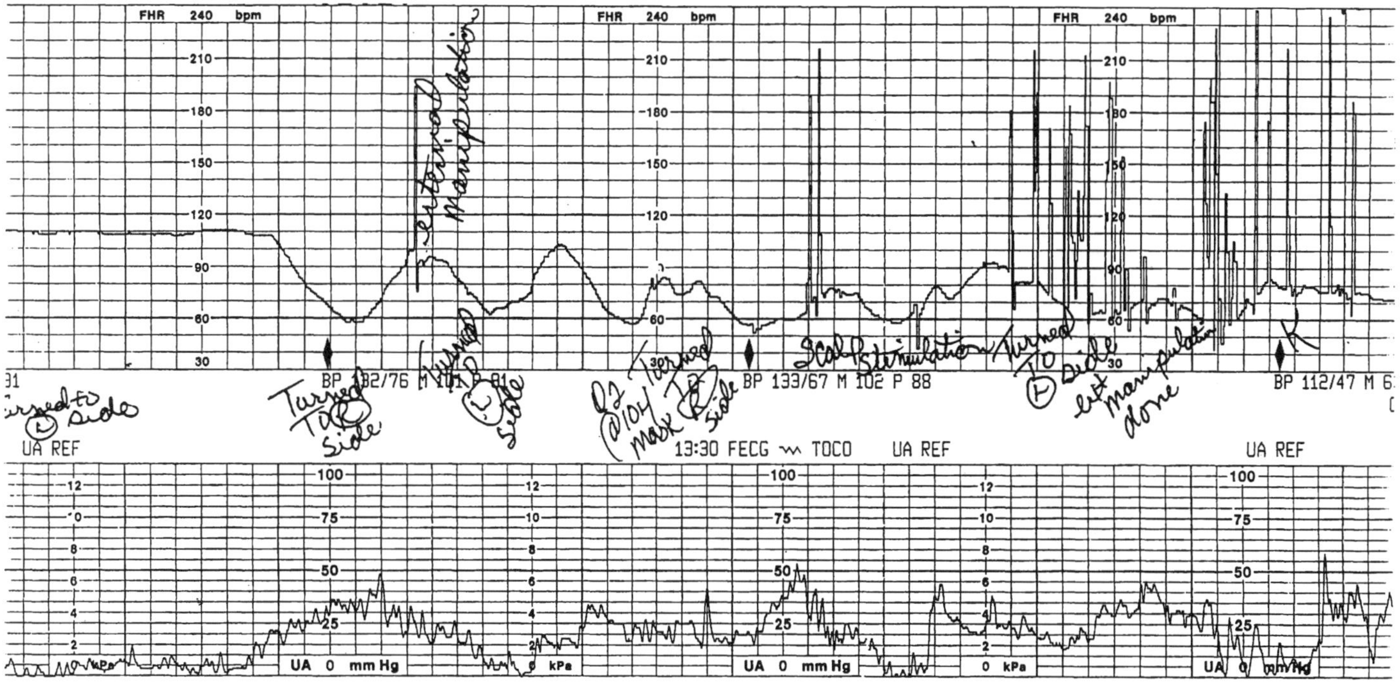

5.11 Agonal pattern.

DOCUMENTATION OF THE BASELINE

The baseline is documented as an average rate, e.g., 135 bpm, or as a range, e.g., 130s or 130-140 bpm. If the baseline is not exactly a 10 bpm range, do not generalize. Instead, be specific, e.g., 132-136. It is recommended to utilize the baseline range method in nursing notes as 5 percent of tracings are lost or are missing in actual lawsuits. From your note, the FHR pattern could be recreated. Thus, being specific creates a clearer image in the reader's mind of what you observed.

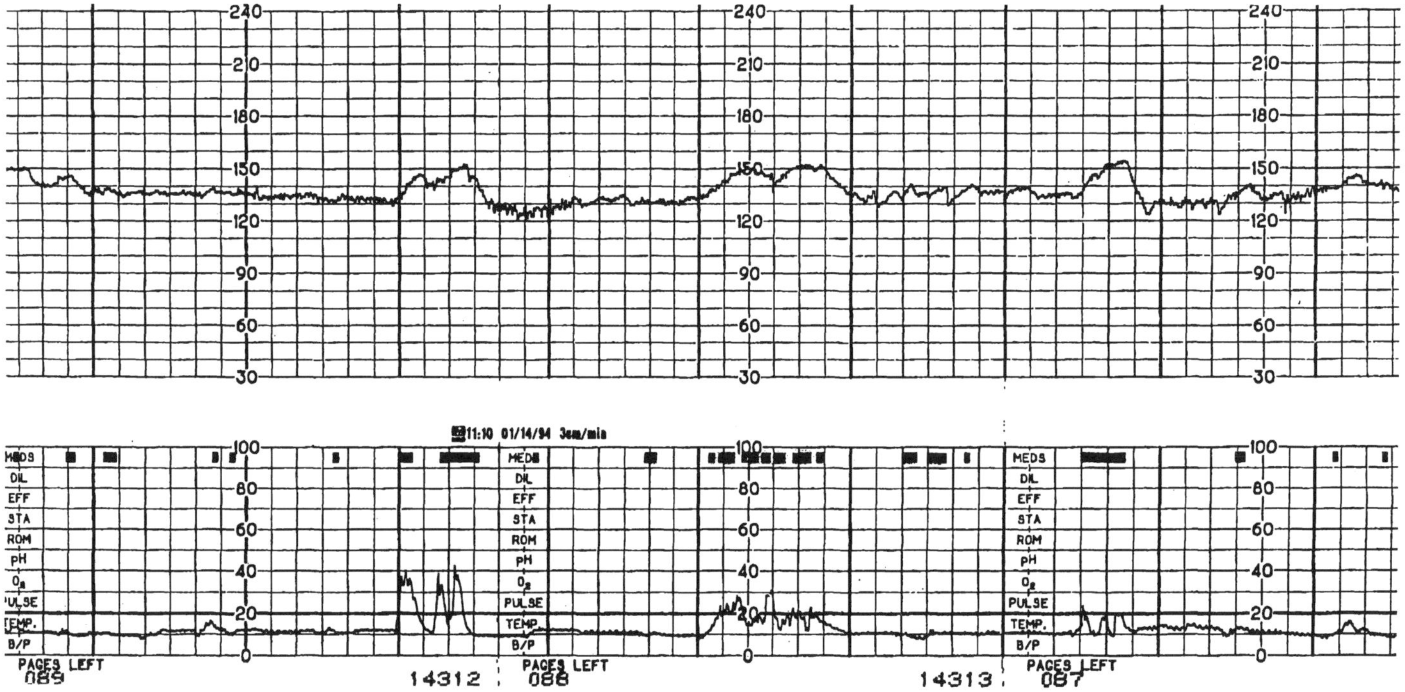

5.12 Baseline 130-140 bpm.

TERMINAL BRADYCARDIA

An ominous FHR demanding delivery and resuscitation is terminal bradycardia. Note the absence of variability. The FHR is less than 80 bpm. Document the rate, e.g., 60 bpm, 0 STV, 0 LTV. Do not write "terminal." Call the surgeon stat.

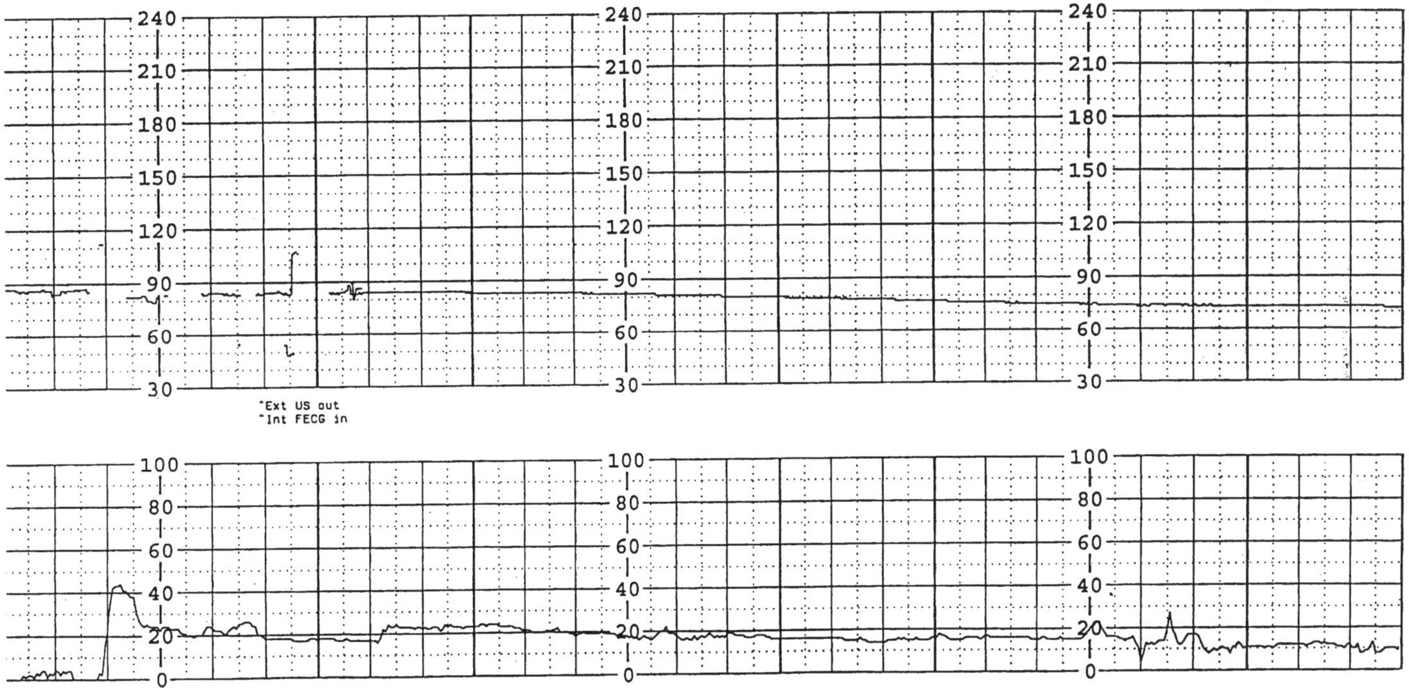

5.13 Terminal bradycardia in a primigravida woman at 40 weeks of gestation. Apgars 1, 3, and 6 at 1, 5, and 10 minutes.

Actions in Response to an Agonal Pattern and Terminal Bradycardia

- mobilize all available personnel
- prepare for cesarean section if vaginal delivery is not imminent
- prepare for neonatal resuscitation
- call stat:
  - "any available obstetrician" if the attending physician or surgeon is not in the hospital
  - anesthesia provider
  - neonatal resuscitation team, including a physician or neonatal nurse practitioner who can manage neonatal complications, including intubation and drug administration.

- act to improve fetal oxygenation, although this may not change the FHR pattern
- prepare the woman for delivery, which may include minimal preparations for a cesarean section, e.g., a foley catheter
- ask family members to wait in the waiting room
- if personnel are available, a member of the health care team should stay with the family and explain events
- deliver the fetus as soon as the team is mobilized.

END-STAGE BRADYCARDIA

End-stage or Second-stage Bradycardia

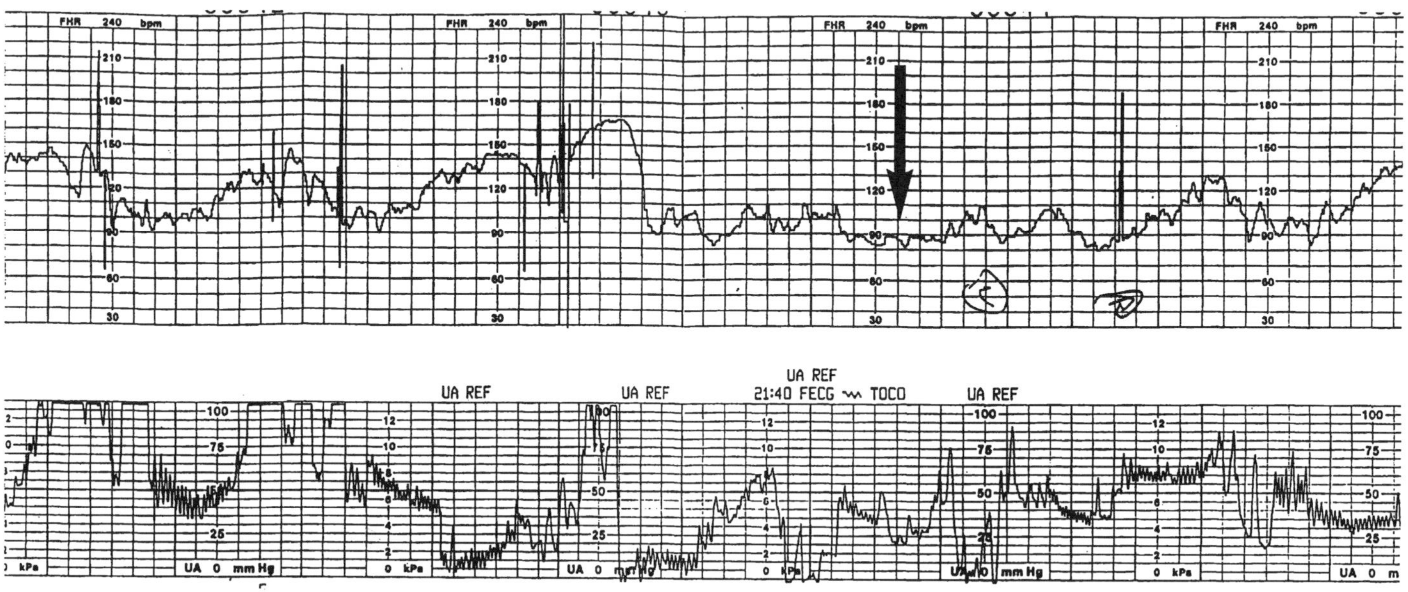

5.14 End-stage bradycardia.

End-stage bradycardia is a compensatory pattern that often precedes a vaginal birth. Usually during the minutes before birth when the head and cord are compressed the baseline drops to 80 bpm but long-term variability is average to moderate, accelerations occasionally appear. Variable decelerations or a prolonged deceleration often appear and short-term variability is present. As long as the FHR is greater than 80 bpm, supplemental oxygen is not needed. Document the bpm, e.g., "80-90 bpm." It is optional to write end-stage or second-stage bradycardia. Fetuses should be born with no more than a need for stimulus, e.g. dry them off, or you may need to provide brief blow-by oxygen for less than a minute.

SUMMARY

Summary

A systematic review of the fetal heart rate pattern includes assessment of the baseline, accelerations, and decelerations. The baseline may be assessed in one to two minutes, especially if it is flat. The baseline fluctuates due to vagal and sympathetic nerve influences. Variability, as a general concept, refers to the chaotic, irregular fluctuations in the baseline and consists of 2 or more cycles per minute. Acute hypoxia creates a baseline range greater than 25 bpm (marked or saltatory long-term variability). The loss of variability may be due to narcotics or other central nervous system (CNS) depressant drugs. Variability is only reassuring if accelerations are present within 100 minutes of monitoring. Persistent absent variability may be due to metabolic acidosis.

Alterations in the baseline, such as a rising baseline, suggests a compensatory response to hypoxia. Tachycardia is a baseline greater than 160 bpm for 10 or more minutes. A falling baseline suggests fetal decompensation. Bradycardia in a term or postterm fetus is a rate less than 100 bpm for 10 or more minutes. Bradycardia in a preterm fetus is a rate less than 120 bpm for 10 or more minutes. Terminal bradycardia is ominous. It is an FHR which suggests a high risk for asphyxia and death. Once a fetus has terminal bradycardia, they never spontaneously recover. Therefore, the goal is to deliver and resuscitate.

A wandering baseline is usually related to fetal asphyxia and rarely related to a congenital defect.

An agonal pattern is fetal bradycardia that lacks variability, but has upward and downward swings in the fetal heart rate. It is ominous and a predeath pattern. The FHR pushes up at times from a flat 60 to 70 bpm rate due to a surge of fetal catecholamines. Agonal patterns are often related to cord compression, e.g., due to cord prolapse. The immediate goal is to deliver and resuscitate.

End-stage or second-stage bradycardia is common prior to vaginal delivery due to head and cord compression. Since variability and accelerations persist, one can expect a good outcome.

SECTION 5: THE BASELINE

QUESTIONS

Directions: Circle T if the statement is true, F if it is false.

QUESTIONS

T	F	1.	A systematic review of the fetal heart rate includes the baseline, accelerations, and decelerations.
T	F	2.	The baseline has cycles.
T	F	3.	A baseline is determined over a 20 minute period.
T	F	4.	The baseline is influenced by neural, nutritional, hormonal and pharmacologic factors.
T	F	5.	Baseline changes can occur abruptly or over minutes.
T	F	6.	Preterm infants have a normal heart rate range between 100 and 160 beats per minute.
T	F	7.	Variability is a baseline characteristic.
T	F	8.	A rising or falling baseline may indicate hypoxia.
T	F	9.	An asphyxiated fetus' baseline has variability.
T	F	10.	A wandering baseline requires actions to improve fetal oxygenation and expedite delivery.

SECTION 6
Long-Term Variability (LTV)

In Section 5 you identified the fetal heart rate (FHR) baseline. In this section you will learn to identify long-term variability (LTV). LTV is a baseline characteristic and is not evaluated in a deceleration or acceleration.

SINE WAVE, OSCILLATION, CYCLE

As each consecutive FHR is determined and printed, the baseline may appear to rise and fall creating small undulations or waves around an average rate. This is long-term variability (LTV). One wave is also called a sine wave, oscillation, or cycle. Most oxygenated fetuses have 2 to 8 cycles per minute (cpm). You should first determine the cycle amplitude within a FHR baseline prior to categorizing LTV.

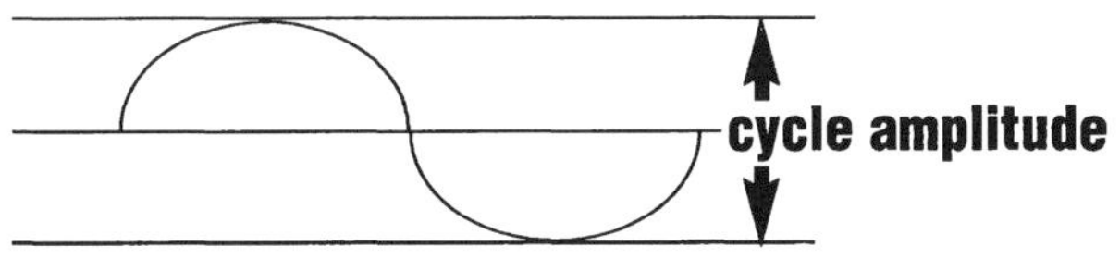

1 cycle or sine wave

Documentation of Cycles

BANDWIDTH

AMPLITUDE/ RANGE

Although LTV is observed as cycles per minute, it is not documented as such. Instead, LTV is classified and documented based on the bpm range between the top and bottom of the majority of cycles. This range is called the *bandwidth*. It is usually similar to the baseline range especially when the baseline is stable. The bandwidth is also called the *amplitude* of the baseline.

CLASSIFICATION OF LTV BASED ON AMPLITUDE

Over the years, several systems have been developed to document LTV observations for the time period you have assessed. In fact, LTV may fluctuate between a narrow bandwidth, e.g., 3 bpm, to a wider bandwidth, e.g., 25 bpm or more. Therefore, it is common to document more than one category of LTV. Determine the top of most of the cycles, the bottom of most of the cycles, and then calculate the bpm between these two levels.

Five categories of LTV are listed with their bandwidth range.

LTV Category	Bandwidth Range
absent	0 - 1 bpm or < 1 1/2 cpm
minimal or decreased	3 - 5 bpm
average	6 - 10 bpm
moderate	11 - 25 bpm
marked, saltatory, or increased	> 25 bpm

LTV in and of itself, has no predictive value concerning fetal well-being. The absence of LTV may suggest fetal compromise. You must also identify accelerations and short-term variability (STV). Your facility may not use all 5 categories for documenting LTV. Refer to your documentation record to verify the categories used.

To judge the quality of your documentation ask, "Could I draw the pattern from what I charted?" Accuracy in charting LTV helps recreate the tracing should it be lost.

ABSENT LTV

Absent LTV

Most babies have average to moderate LTV. Absent LTV is less than one and a half cycles per minute or a baseline with a range of 0 to 2 bpm (flat or nearly flate). Absent LTV is more likely related to a depressant drug such as narcotics. It can also occur during fetal quiet sleep (quiescent fetal state) which lasts an average of approximately 20 minutes in near-term or term fetuses. However, it may last up to approximately 100 minutes.

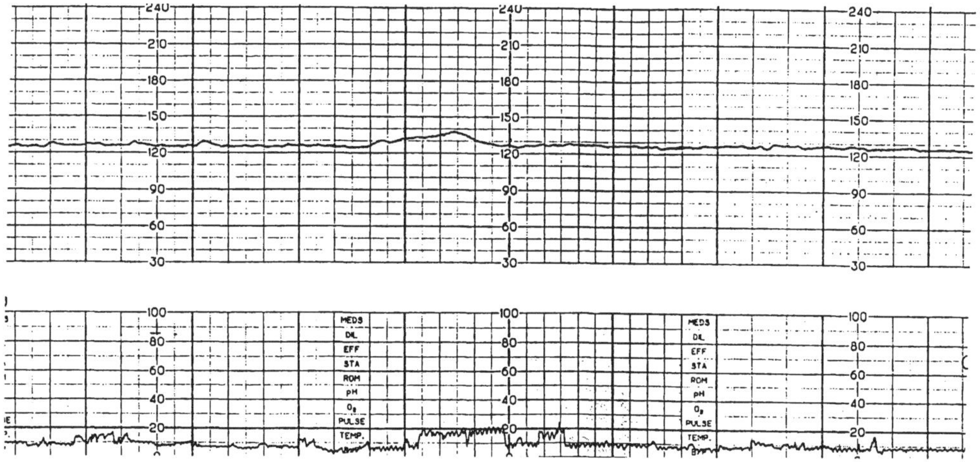

6.1 Illustration of long-term variability that is absent to minimal. Magnesium sulfate (6 gm bolus) may be associated with the loss of LTV. However a well baby will still accelerate.

CAUSES OF ABSENT LTV

Cause(s)/Physiology of Absent LTV

- machine artifact: test button is stuck in the "in" position
- fetal 1F quiescent state
- drugs, e.g., narcotics, cigarettes, and cocaine
- hypoxia
- severe fetal anemia, e.g., as a result of a fetal viral infection
- arrhythmia such as supraventricular tachycardia or complete heart block
- fetal brain death or decerebration
- congenital brain anomaly, e.g., anencephaly or heart anomaly
- cardiovascular lesions or chromosomal aberration, often accompanied by bradycardia and variable decels
- cerebral ischemia.

Absent LTV is also a late sign of deterioration of the intrauterine growth restricted fetus. *Bradycardia and absent LTV, not related to an arrhythmia, suggests impending intrauterine death, e.g., terminal bradycardia.*

ACTIONS WHEN LTV IS ABSENT

Actions When LTV is Absent

Absent LTV is nonreassuring until the etiology is determined. Actions to determine the significance of absent LTV include obtaining a fetal movement history, assessing fetal movement by palpation or real-time ultrasound, and review of the tracing to determine if there have been any accelerations in the last 60 to 100 minutes. Rule out machine malfunction, check to make sure the test button is not in the "in" position. Obtain a maternal drug use history.

WANDERING BASELINE WITH ABSENT LTV

One cycle per minute is abnormal and reflects absent LTV. Absent LTV in the non-narcotized fetus is usually indicative of fetal metabolic acidosis, asphyxia, or neurologic damage. A wandering baseline (with absent LTV) should be reported immediately! It is abnormal.

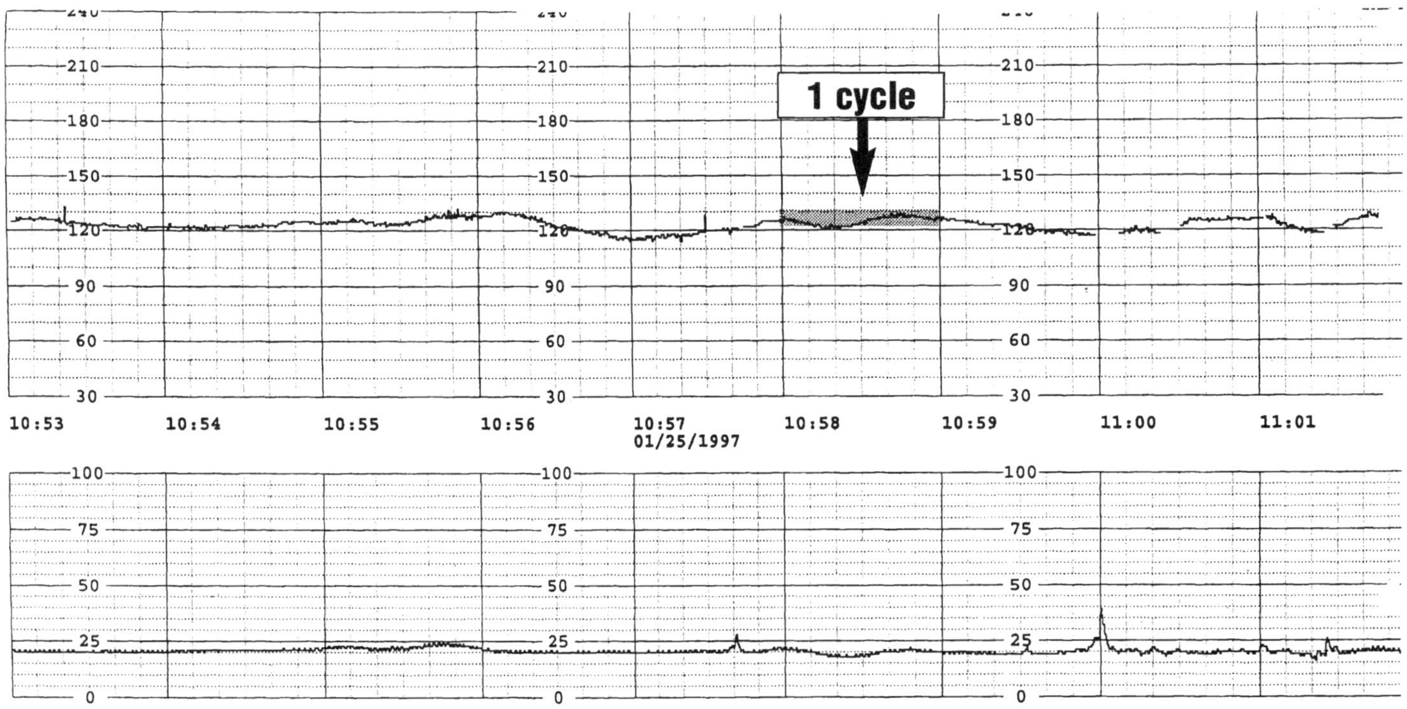

6.2 A wandering baseline with less that 2 cycles per minute or absent long-term variability.

MINIMAL LTV

Minimal LTV

Minimal LTV (3 to 5 beats per minutes bandwidth) may occur when the fetus is in a quiet sleep state or has a narcotic "on board." Minimal LTV may also represent a lack of oxygen or hypoxia. To differentiate hypoxia from a quiet sleep state or medication administration, examine the fetal heart rate tracing 60 minutes prior to the "minimal" LTV. Do you see accelerations? Review the nurses' notes for drug administration. Determine the probable cause of minimal LTV.

Causes(s)/Physiology of Minimal LTV (3-5 bpm)

Alternative Label: decreased LTV

Minimal LTV may be present when the fetus has:

- a temperature elevation (tachycardia will be present too)
- hypovolemia, hypoxia, or acidosis (tachycardia may be present too)
- a central nervous system depressant "on board"
- moved into a quiescent (1F) state

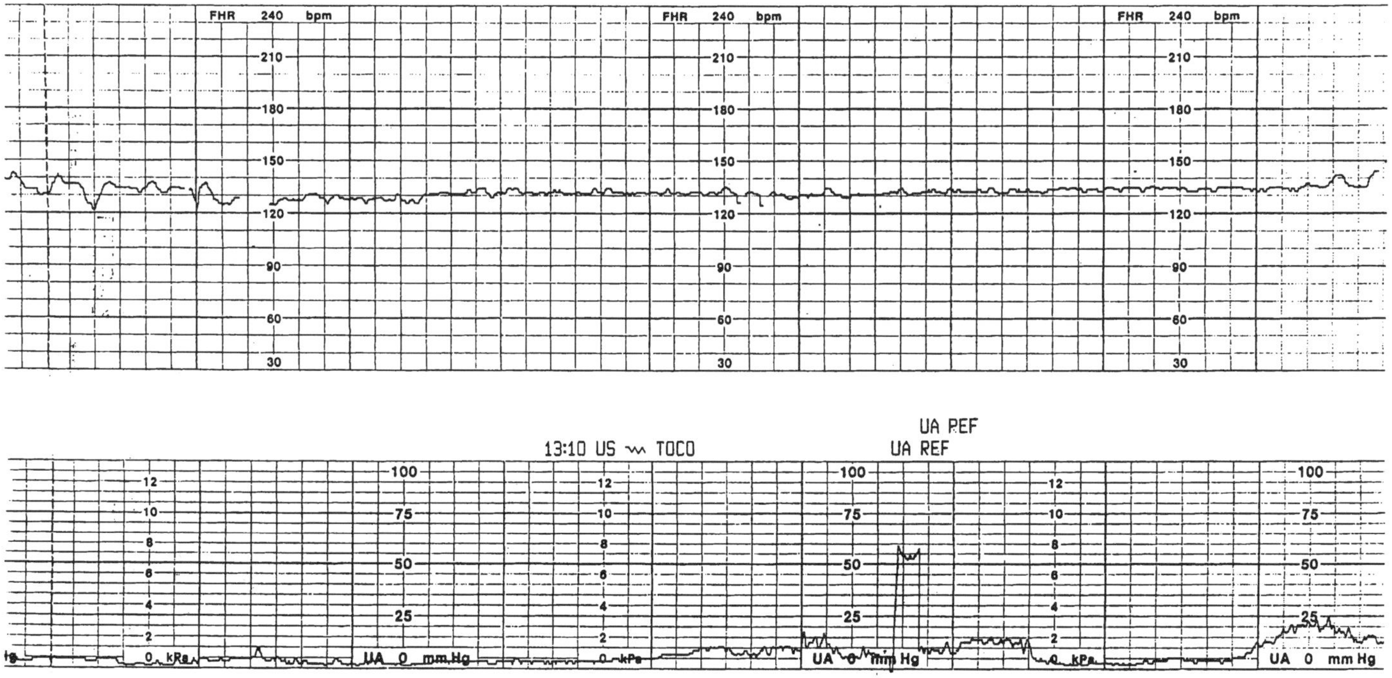

6.3 Minimal long-term variability.

AVERAGE LTV

Average LTV

Average LTV usually is a normal finding and represents integrity of the sympathetic and parasympathetic (vagus) nervous systems. There is adequate oxygen delivery to the brainstem. There should also be spontaneous accelerations and fetal movement. A pathological sinusoidal pattern may have average LTV but there will be decreased to no fetal movements and no accelerations.

Cause(s)/Physiology of Average LTV (6-10 bpm):

- neural integrity when accompanied by accelerations and fetal movement

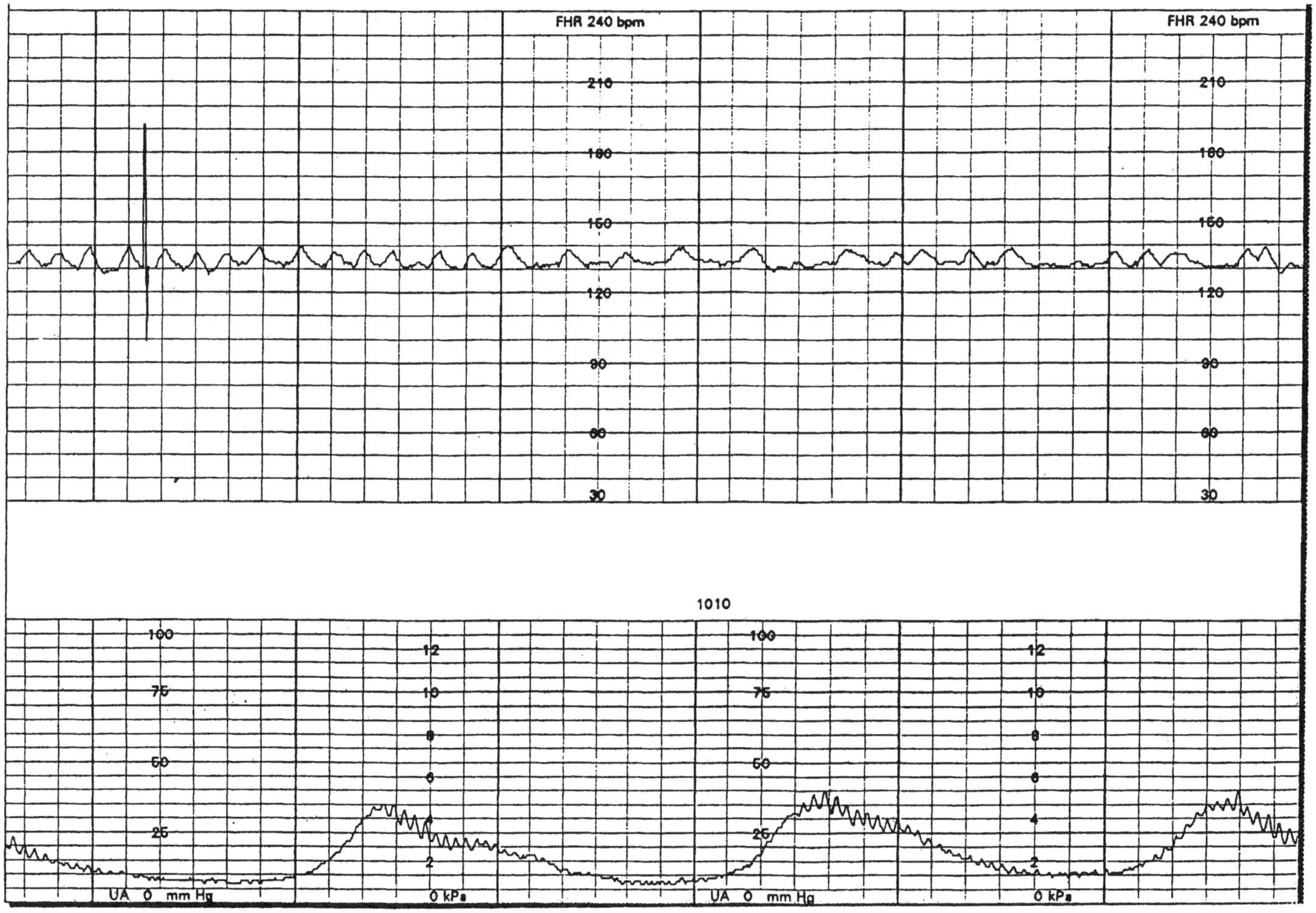

6.4 Average long-term variability.

MODERATE LTV

Moderate LTV is normal. Moderate LTV is seen when there is fetal movement and accelerations. However, it may be a response to ephedrine administration, vacuum extractor application, or a slight decrease in oxygenation.

Cause(s)/Physiology of Moderate LTV (11-25 bpm):

- active awake state of fetus (2F or 4F fetal behavioral state)
- application of the vacuum extractor (may also see marked LTV)
- maternal ephedrine to correct hypotension (may also see marked LTV)

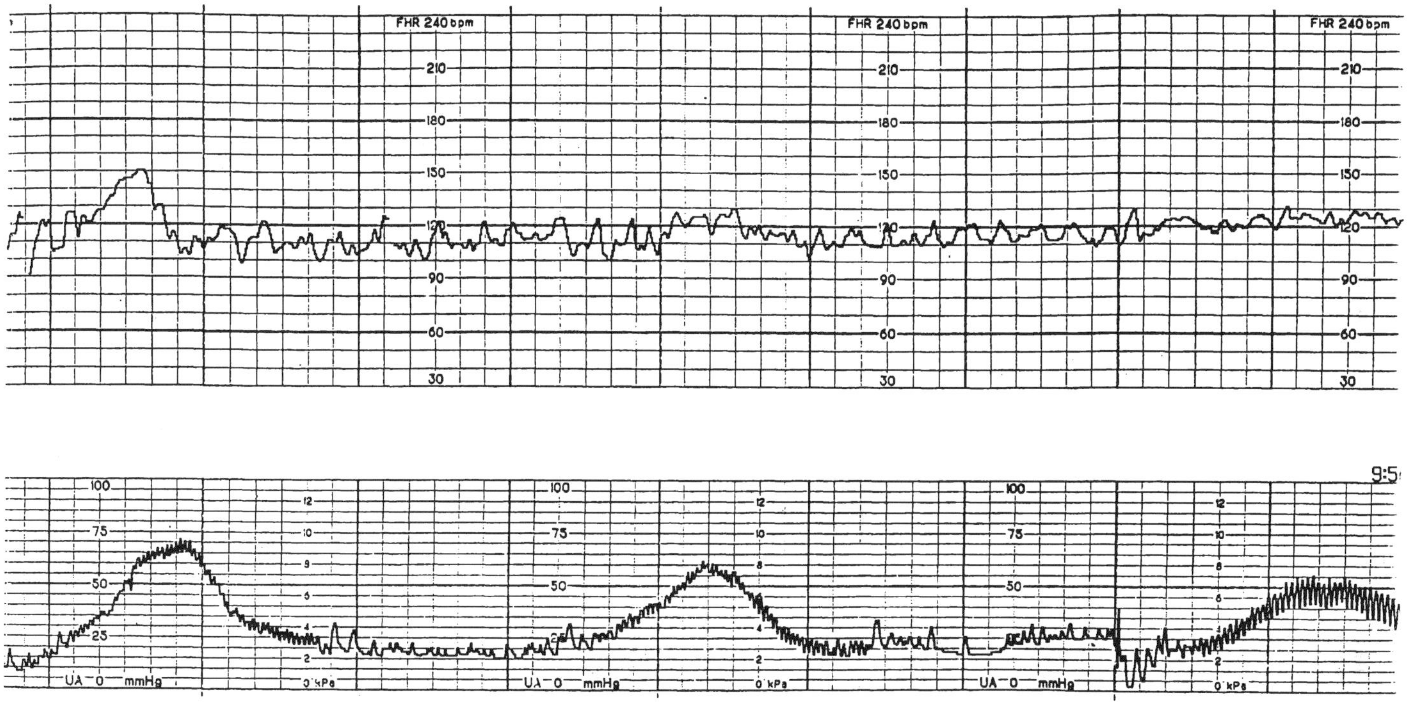

6.5 Moderate long-term variability following a spontaneous acceleration.

Some clinicians have suggested that 6 to 25 bpm is moderate FHR variability. This is one way to collapse two categories into one. However, if the baseline range is not near 25 bpm, and the strip is lost, the tracing will be difficult to recreate.

MARKED OR SALTATORY LTV

Marked LTV, also called a saltatory pattern, usually suggests an acute fetal compensatory response to a hypoxic event such as umbilical cord compression, uterine hyperstimulation, or maternal hypotension. A saltatory pattern is a chaotic, jumping baseline with a cycle bandwidth of more than 25 bpm. It may be preceded by a variable or prolonged deceleration. It may also follow maternal hypotension and ephedrine administration. Actions to improve fetal oxygenation are taken, such as a maternal position change, an intravenous bolus with a non-glucose solution such as Lactated Ringer's, and even hyperoxygenation with a face mask. If a simple mask is used, set the oxygen flow to 8 to 10 liters per minute. If a partial rebreathing mask is used, set the flow at 12 liters per minute to prevent carbon dioxide from entering the oxygen reservoir.

The benefits of maternal oxygen administration include:

- increased fetal brain oxygen
- improved fetal circulation
- increased fetal PaO_2
- increased fetal SaO_2
- increased fetal tissue O_2
- increased fetal breathing movements
- increased fetal body movements
- accelerations reappear
- variability improves
- late decelerations decreased or cease
- fewer neonatal resuscitations.

Oxygen should be in the fetus by the 10th minute after its initiation. If the FHR pattern does not improve by the 20th minute, oxygen delivery may be impeded. The midwife or physician may need to consider expediting delivery. Therefore, it is important to let them know within 10 minutes of beginning interventions.

Marked LTV

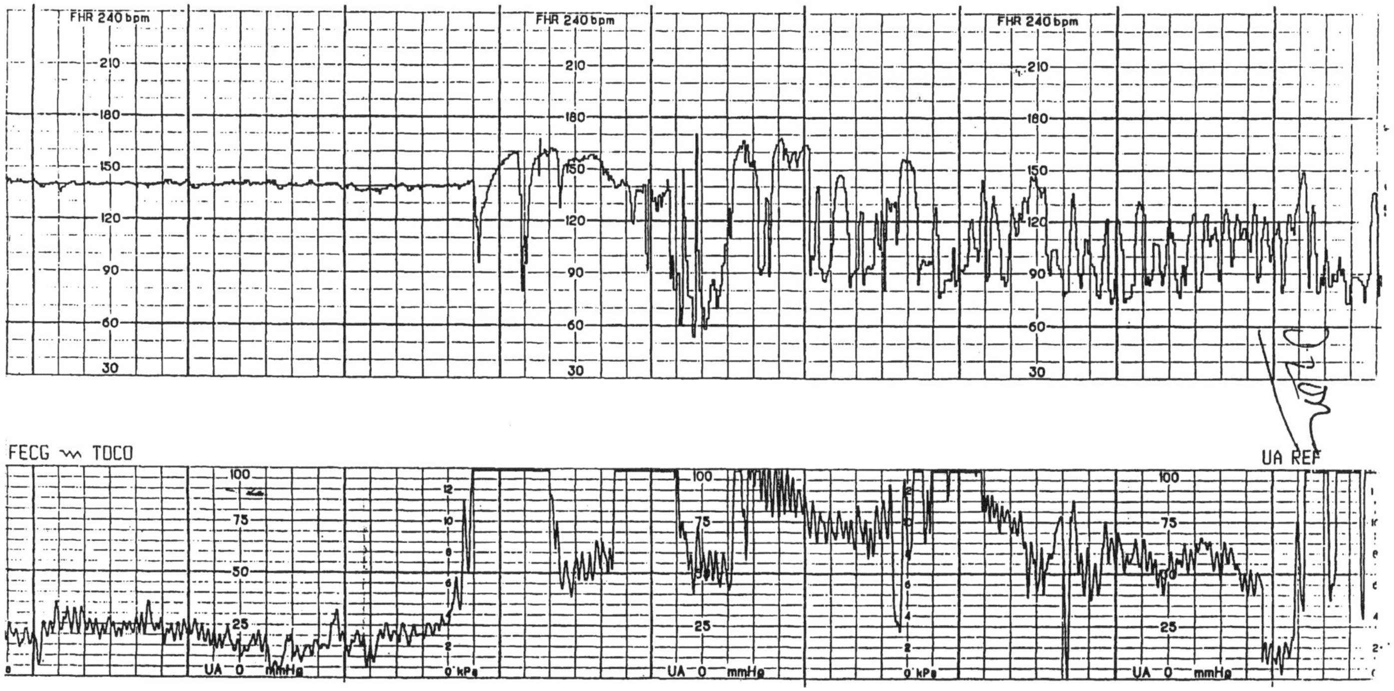

6.6 In this strip the long-term variability (LTV) changed from minimal to marked close to the time of delivery due to cord compression and acute hypoxia.

Cause(s)/Physiology of Marked LTV:

- if noted when an ultrasound transducer is used, may be caused by a fetal dysrhythmia such as premature ventricular contractions
- rare in preterm fetuses
- high incidence in postterm fetuses, possibly due to neurologic maturation
- usually a compensatory response to a hypoxic event, e.g., umbilical cord compression or uterine hyperstimulation
- may follow ephedrine administration for hypotension
- may be observed during the second stage of labor, especially with use of the vacuum extractor.

PATHOLOGIC SINUSOIDAL PATTERN

A series of sine waves creates a *sinusoidal pattern or sinusoidal baseline*. Sinusoidal patterns may represent a *pathological* process such as fetal hypoxia, acidosis, or asphyxia.

Cause(s)/Physiology of a Pathologic Sinusoidal Pattern:

- Rh disease (erythroblastosis fetalis) with hemolysis/anemia
- hypoxia, metabolic acidosis, and/or asphyxia
- possible cord compression, hypoxia, and/or infection
- preeclampsia, abruption, or amnionitis, probably related to hypoxia
- fetal hypovolemia

Some clinicians feel a sinusoidal pattern differs from variability because they believe the pattern is smooth with regular frequency and amplitude. Yet, even smooth, regular cycles are a baseline characteristic. Indeed, a sinosoidal pattern is a specific type of baseline.

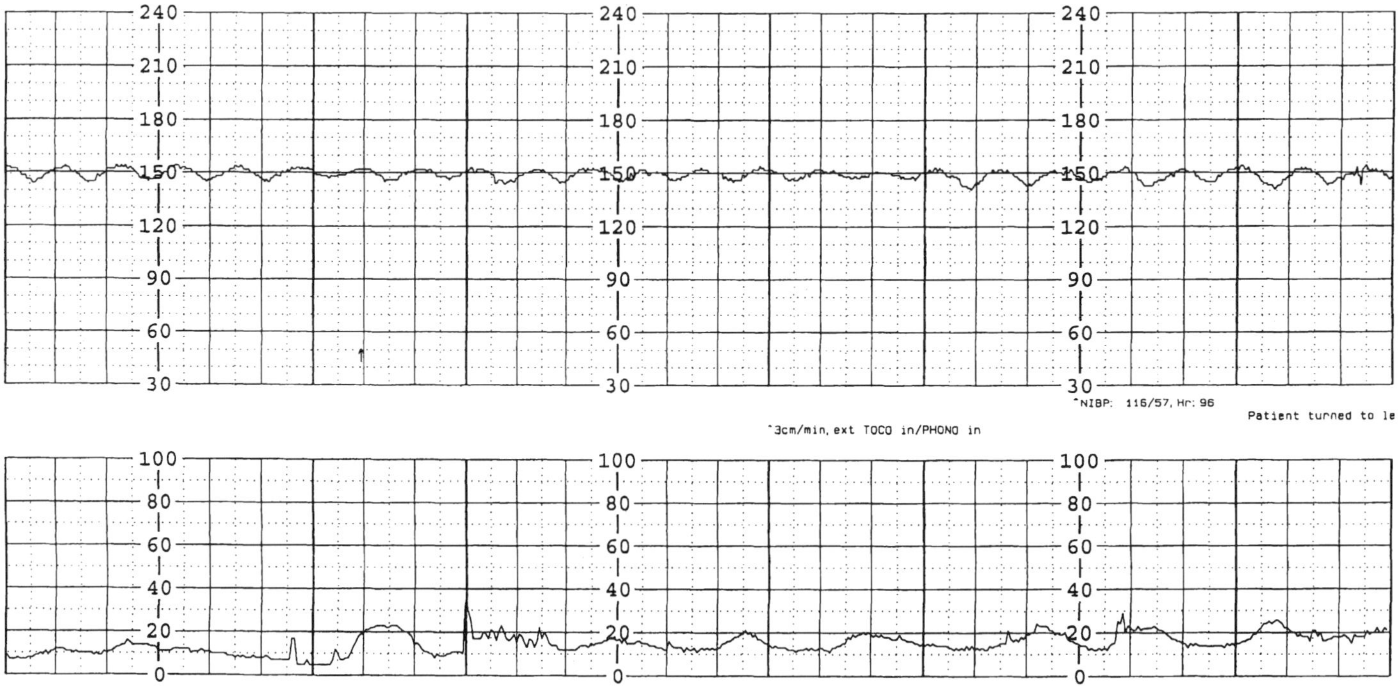

6.7 Pathological sinusoidal pattern. Count the number of cycles in each minute.

Did you see 2½ cycles in the first minute, 2½ cycles in the second minute, and 2 cycles in the third minute? Sinusoidal patterns or sinusoidal baselines have 1½ to 5 cycles each minute. Pathologic sinusoidal patterns never have accelerations, however they may have decelerations. Sometimes, a sinusoidal baseline looks as if the lower portion of each cycle is hanging lower than the upper portion height. But, it is still called a sinusoidal pattern.

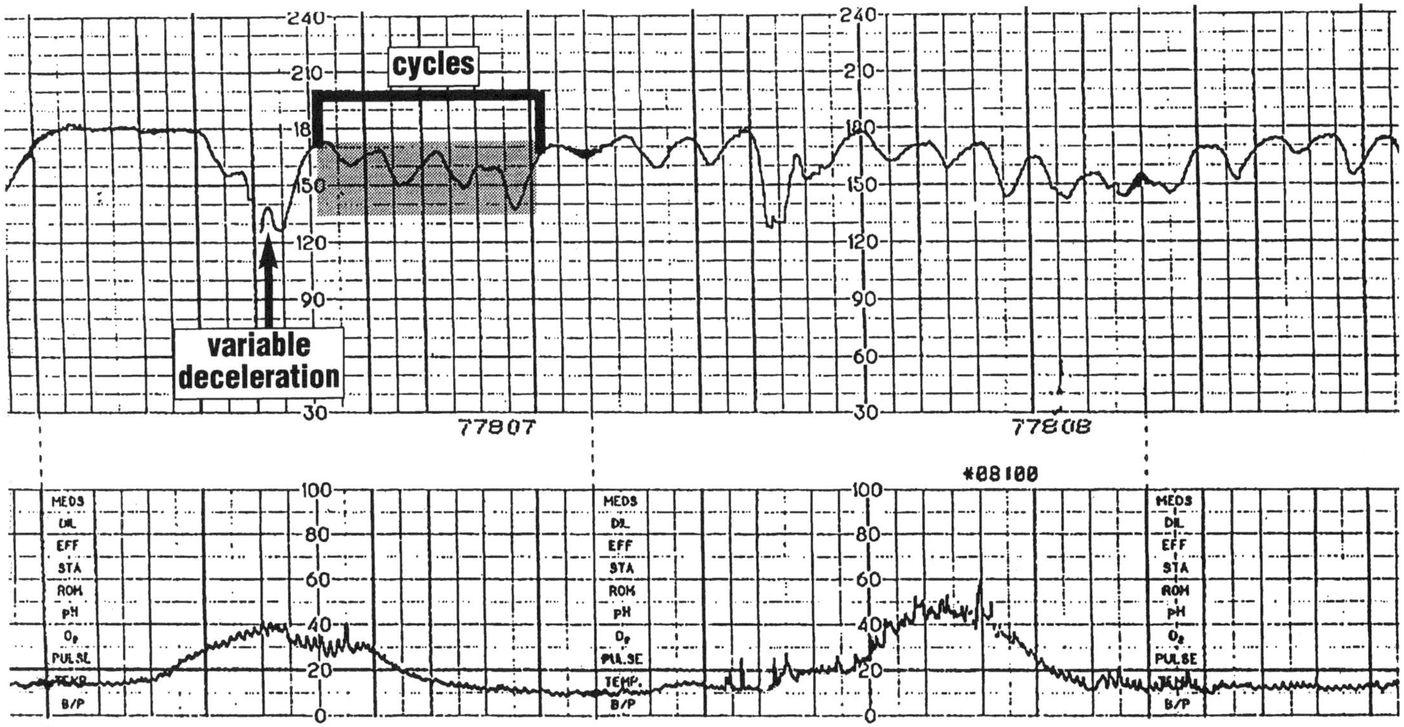

6.8 Sinusoidal pattern with "V" shaped lower portion of cycles. Hemoglobin was 6 gm/dl and the hematocrit was 18% at 33½ weeks of gestation. Bleeding from placenta previa occurred. Variable decelerations are also present.

ACTIONS REQUIRED

When you see a sinusoidal pattern, it is important to

- assess fetal movement now and in the recent past
- review the entire tracing, there should be an acceleration within 100 minutes of monitoring
- assess maternal blood type. Rh negative? possibility of erythroblastosis fetalis?
- communicate your assessments to the midwife and/or physician.

BENIGN SINUSOIDAL PATTERN

Benign sinusoidal patterns are preceded and followed by FHR accelerations. Benign sinusoidal patterns also have 1½ to 5 cpm but decelerations are usually absent and accelerations are present before or after the sinusoidal baseline. Fetal movement may be present spontaneously or in response to acoustic stimulation or scalp stimulation. These patterns were called *psuedosinusoidal* in the past. These fetuses are not hypoxic, acidotic, or asphyxiated. They may be relaxed and making breathing, mouthing, or sucking movements, or simply reflecting the cardiac/brainstem response to narcotics.

To differentiate between a pathologic and a benign sinusoidal pattern:

- obtain a fetal movement history (fetus may respond to acoustic stimulation)
- assess fetal movement by palpation or a real-time ultrasound
- identify accelerations present before the benign sinusoidal baseline began
- identify the change in the FHR pattern after narcotics administration
- relax! This is a benign pattern that requires no intervention.

Document this pattern's baseline rate, LTV, STV, and acceleration(s). You need not to write "benign sinusoidal."

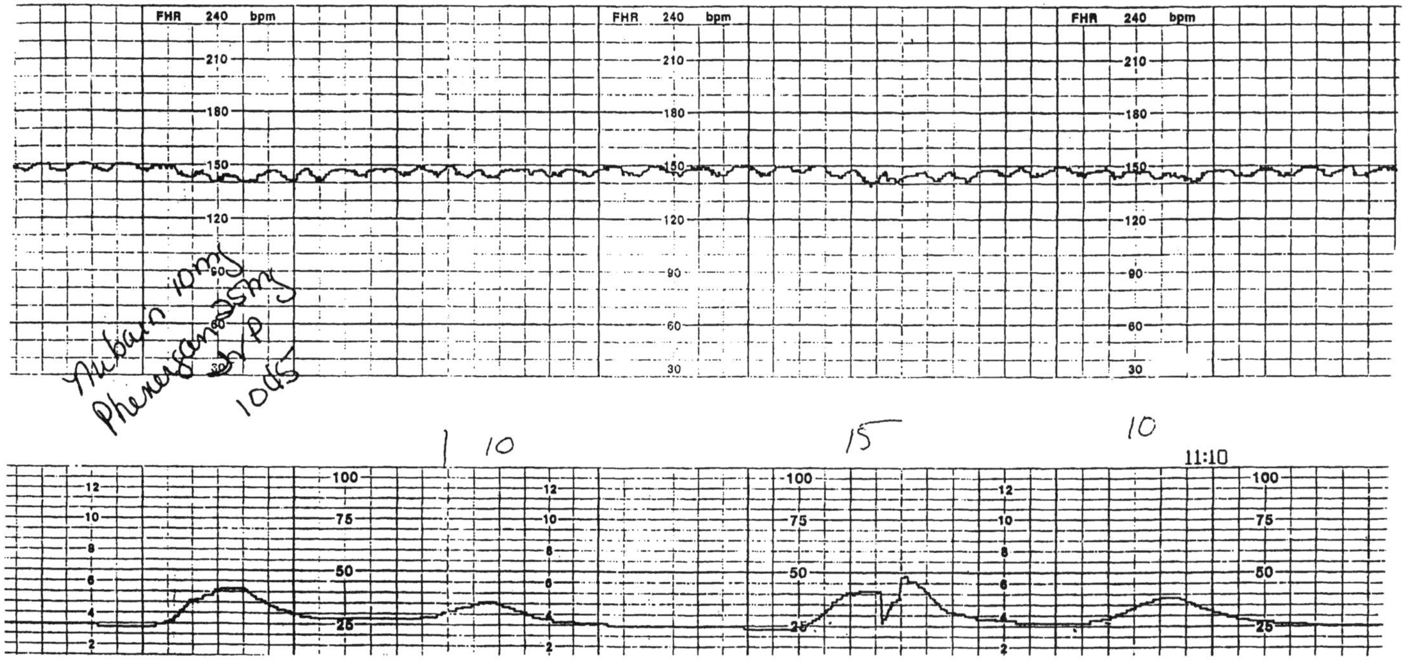

6.9 Benign sinusoidal pattern following Nubain® administration.

EXERCISES

Exercises

1. On the fetal monitor paper, draw 4 cycles per minute with average LTV.

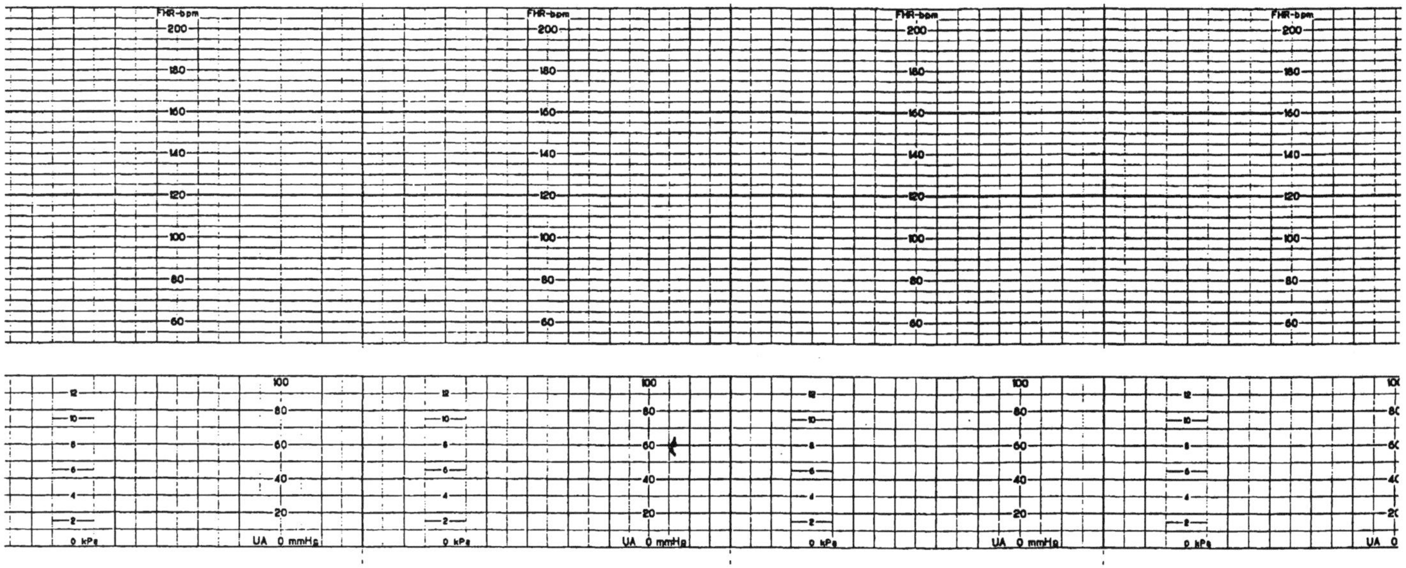

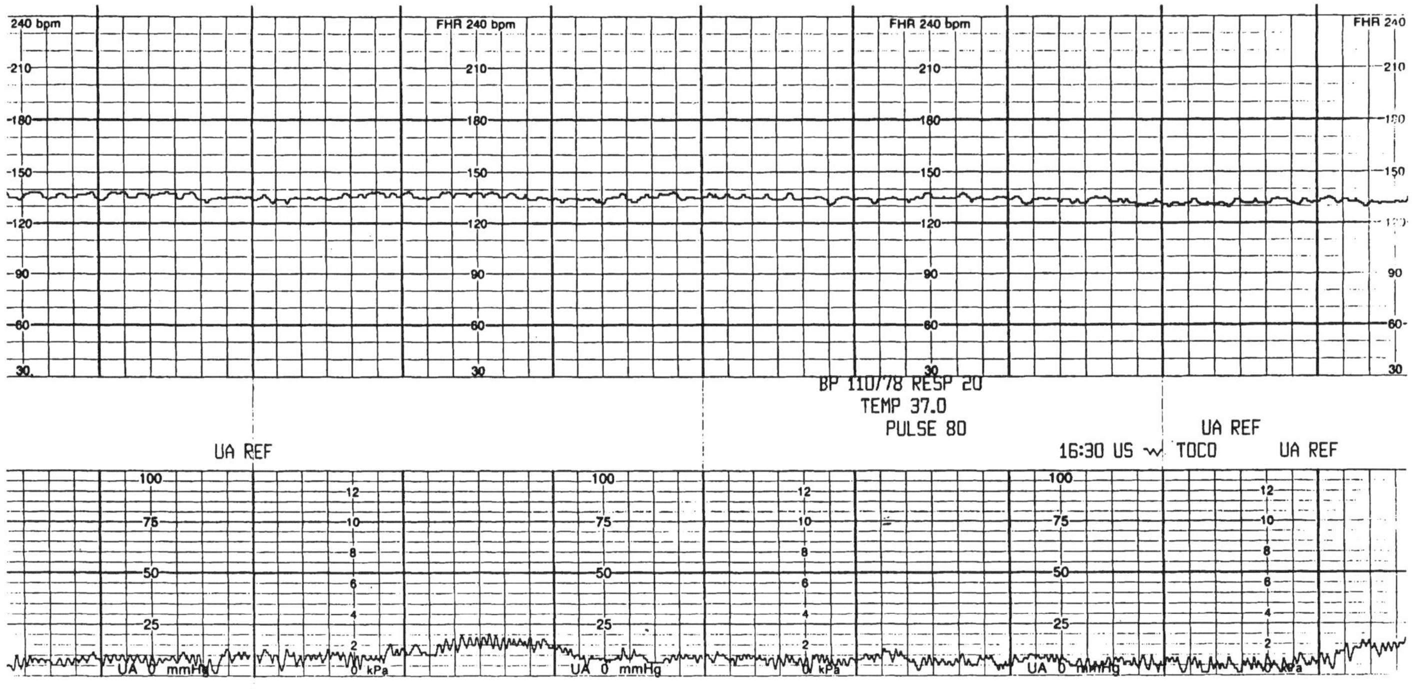

2. Classify LTV using a 5 category system.

   LTV is _______ to ________.

3. If there is only 1 cycle per minute, how would you classify LTV?

4. Match the type of LTV with its cause

1. absent LTV	A. quiescent fetal state _______________ (1 response)
2. minimal LTV	B. narcotics _______________ (2 responses)
3. average LTV	C. compensation for an acute hypoxic event _______________ (1 response)
4. moderate LTV	D. neural integrity _______________ (3 responses)
5. marked LTV	

5. LTV is categorized and recorded based on
   A. baseline bandwidth
   B. sine waves
   C. oscillations
   D. cycles per minute

6. A pathologic sinusoidal pattern can be obtained from a fetus with the following:
   A. narcotics "on board"
   B. hypoxia or acidosis
   C. sucking or mouthing

7. Which best describes categories for documentation of LTV?
   A. present or absent
   B. minimal, marked, moderate, increased, decreased
   C. absent, minimal, average, moderate, marked
   D. cpm, bpm

ANSWERS TO EXERCISES

1. show your instructor
2. minimal to average
3. absent LTV
4. A = 1, B = 1 & 2, C = 5, D = 2, 3, 4
5. A
6. B
7. C

SUMMARY

Summary

Long-term variability is a baseline characteristic with cycles and a bandwidth or amplitude. Cycles are also called sine waves. A special type of baseline is a sinusoidal baseline, also called a sinusoidal pattern. LTV can be classified using as many as 5 categories: absent, minimal, average, moderate, and marked. Depending on your facility, you may be asked to use less than 5 categories. The key question is, can you draw the baseline from your documentation description? Documenting more than one category, e.g., av to mod LTV, is acceptable because baselines fluctuate over time. **Absent and minimal LTV may be related to hypoxia. Marked LTV suggests fetal hypoxia**, usually from cord compression. Actions should be taken to improve fetal oxygenation. A return to minimal to moderate LTV with accelerations suggests interventions were successful.

SECTION 6: LONG-TERM VARIABILITY

QUESTIONS

QUESTIONS

Directions: Circle T if the statement is true, F if it is false.

T F 1. Long-term variability has two components: sine waves and amplitude in beats per minutes.

T F 2. "Absent long-term variability" is documented if there are less than $1\frac{1}{2}$ cycles per minute.

T F 3. Persistent absent long-term variability with spontaneous accelerations and fetal movement suggests fetal asphyxia.

T F 4. A wandering baseline is the same as long-term variability.

T F 5. A pathologic sinusoidal pattern has long-term variability.

T F 6. To use long-term variability categories in documentation you must first identify the bandwidth of the baseline.

T F 7. Absent, minimal, and marked long-term variability require further assessments and possible actions to improve fetal oxygenation.

T F 8. Fetal sleep and awake cycles are accompanied by changes in long-term variability.

T F 9. "Present long-term variability" is clear terminology that enhances visualization of the tracing if the tracing is lost.

T F 10. Long-term variability is created by the effect of sympathetic and vagus nerves on the fetal heart.

SECTION 7
Short-term Variability (STV)

Short-term variability is reflected by consecutive changes in the beats per minute (bpm) rate. Section 6 explained long-term variability cycles. Each cycle is the combination of consecutive printed rates. These consecutive rates might appear on the lighted display of the fetal monitor as 118, 119, 121, 118, 120, 122, 124, 121, etc. The changes from one bpm rate to the next bpm rate rarely exceeds 8 bpm, e.g., 120 to 129 bpm. This, however, is rare. Usually the rates differ by 1 to 3 bpm. As each consecutive rate is printed on the moving fetal monitor paper, the baseline may appear bumpy, nonlinear, and/or chaotic. The bumpy look is called short-term variability. STV is a baseline characteristic. STV does not include accelerations or decelerations. STV is usually recorded as present or absent. Rarely it is intermittent, with several minutes of STV and then several with absent STV.

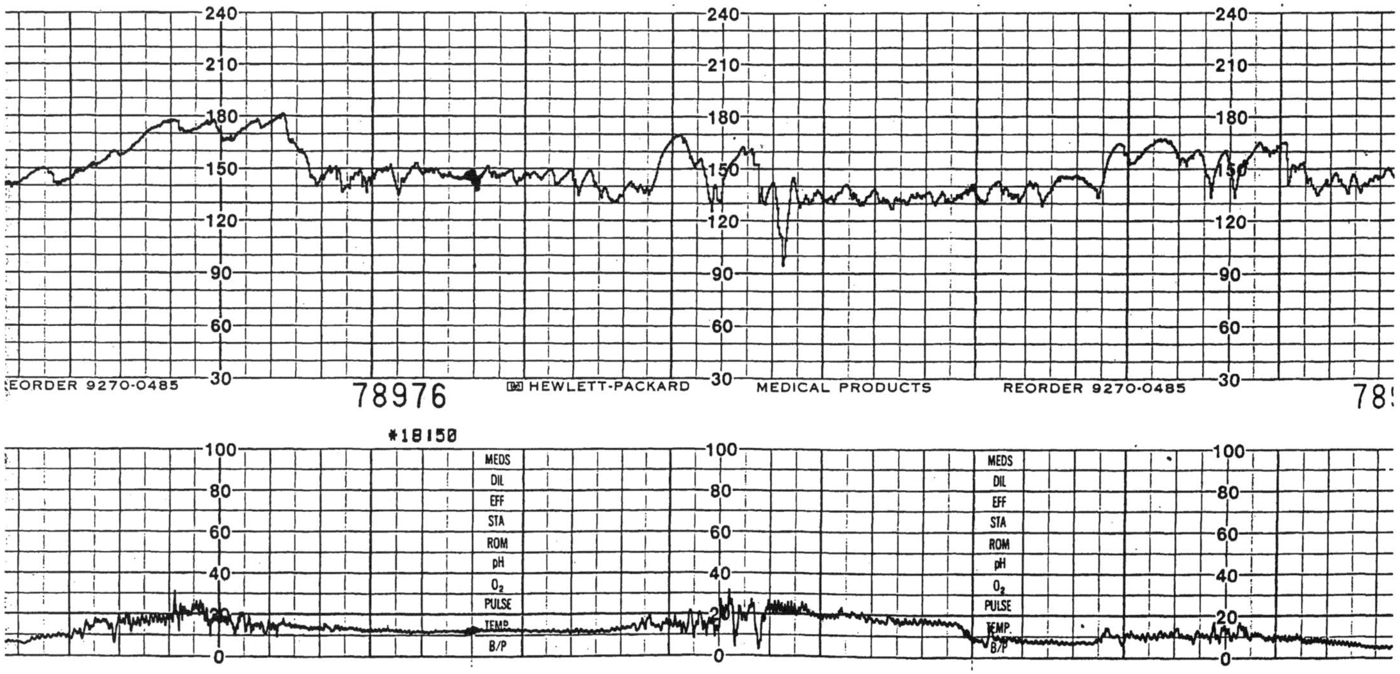

7.1 ***STV is present, as are spontaneous accelerations to 162 to 180 bpm x 15-100 seconds. The baseline has a normal shift from 140-150 to 130-140 bpm. Long-term variability is average to moderate.***

PHYSIOLOGY OF STV

STV IS PRESENT AND ABSENT

BEAT-TO-BEAT VARIABILITY (BTBV) IS RELATED TO SHORT-TERM VARIABILITY BUT IS NOT SHORT-TERM VARIABILITY

Physiology of Short-term Variability

The vagus nerve is the 10th cranial nerve. It splits into two branches. The *right* vagal branch innervates the *sinoatrial (SA) node*. The *left* vagal branch innervates the *atrioventricular (AV) node*. The SA node is the heart's pacemaker, creating time fluctuations between heartbeats. **When the brainstem, vagus and SA node are oxygenated, STV will be present.** When there is metabolic acidosis, asphyxia, or neurologic damage, STV will be absent. Parasympatholytic drugs, such as scopolamine and atropine, decrease the variation between R to R (systole to systole) intervals and decrease STV.

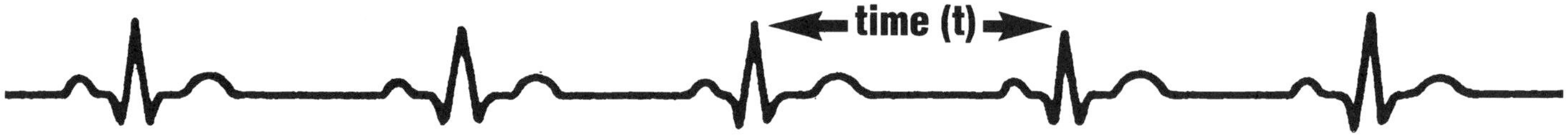

7.2 ***If t= 0.5 seconds, the rate = 120 bpm. The beat-to-beat (time) interval will determine the bpm rate displayed and printed on the paper.*** (Reproduced and modified with permission of Prentice-Hall, Inc. from Walraven, G. (1986). Basic Arrhythmias, p. 27).

The time interval between heartbeats or systole is measured 100% accurately when the fetal electrocardiogram (ECG) enters the fetal monitor via a spiral electrode in the fetus' buttocks or scalp. Changes in the R to R intervals varies the bpm rate and creates STV. If the R to R interval decreases, the bpm rate increases. When the R to R interval is unchanged, the baseline will appear flat and smooth, like a rate calculated by a pacemaker. *The fluctuation in the time interval between consecutive heart beats is called beat-to-beat variability (BTBV).* BTBV is measured by the fetal monitor in milliseconds (msec). *BTBV determines STV.* BTBV is determined by the fetal monitor's computer. BTBV is the interval between heartbeats and is not visible. STV is visible as a bumpy or rough appearance of the baseline. The presence of STV is reassuring. If BTBV is absent, STV will be absent. Absent STV is nonreassuring and requires interventions to improve oxygenation if the absence of STV is not related to a drug with depressant effects.

DOCUMENTATION OF STV

The Association of Women's Health, Obstetric, and Neonatal Nurses (AWHONN) supports the use of a two-category system for charting STV: present or absent. Present STV is recorded as STV +. Absent STV is recorded as O STV, STV O, or STV –.

Look at the next two tracings.

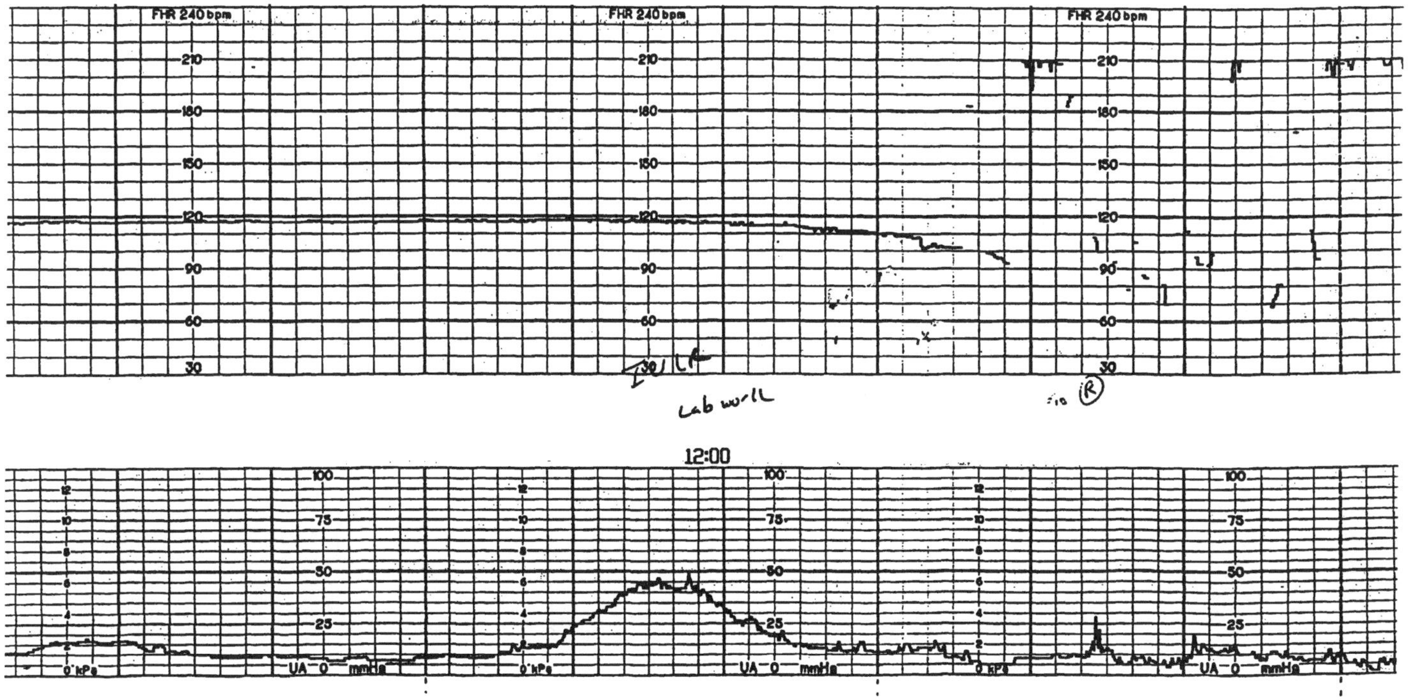

7.3 Short-term variability is absent.

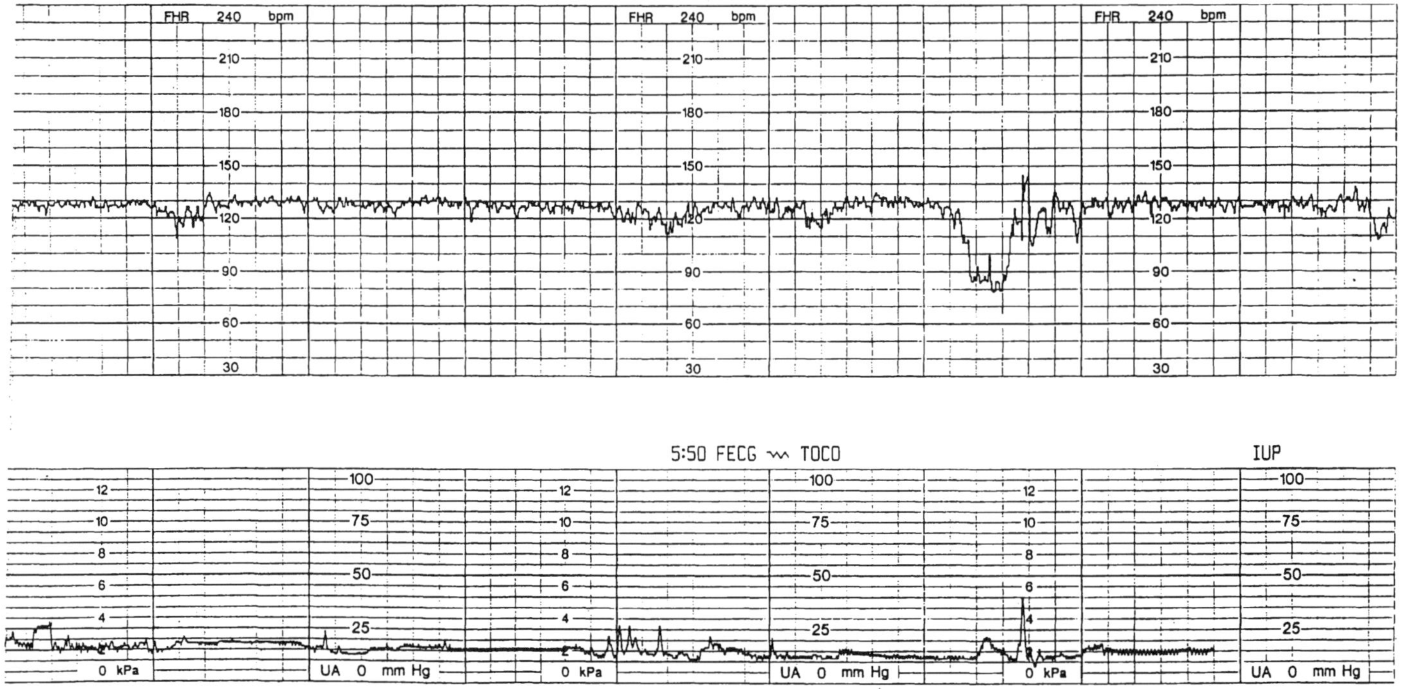

7.4 *Short-term variability is present.*

In the first tracing (7.3), STV is absent. In the second (7.4), STV is present.

Exercises

Record STV for each tracing

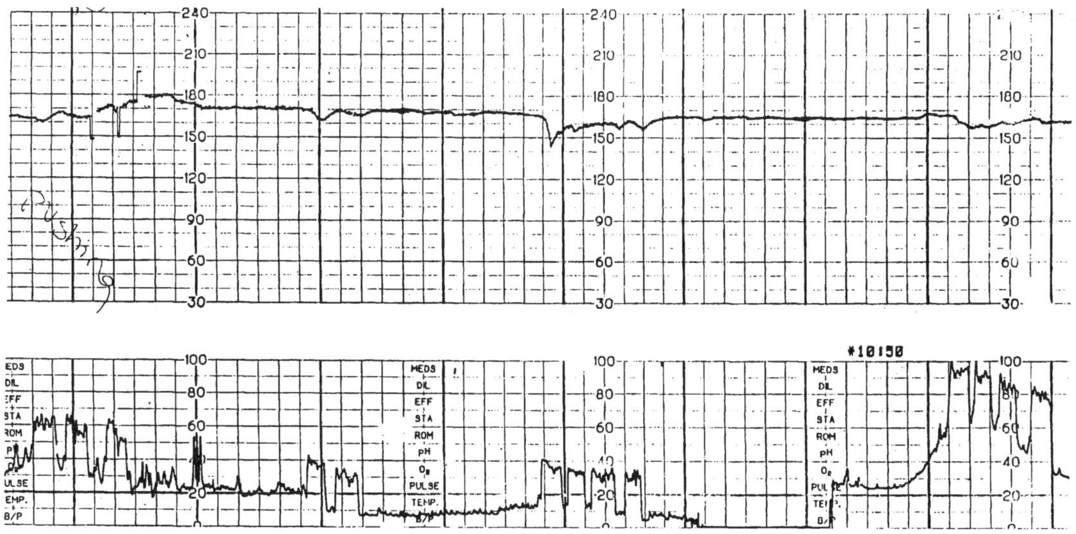

7.5 STV is ______

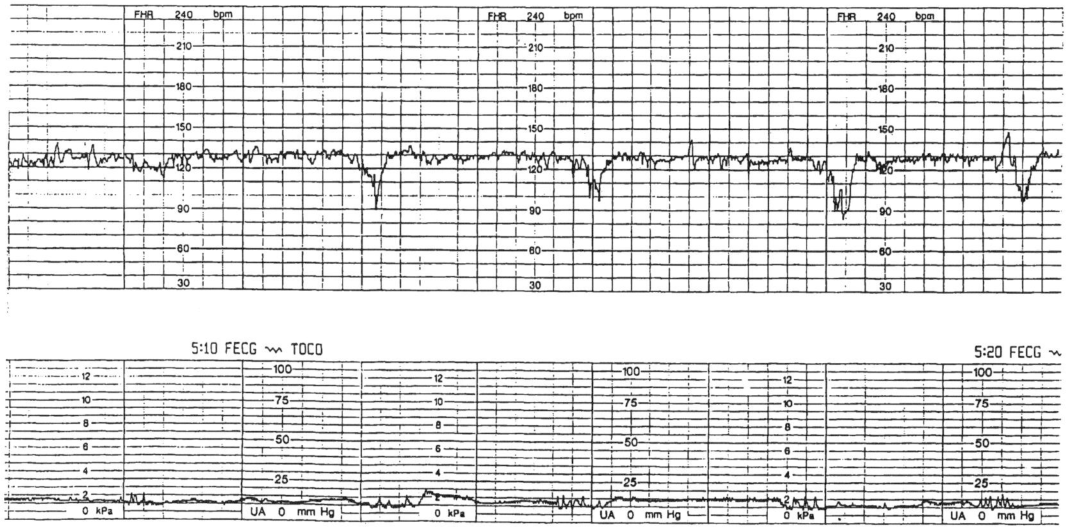

7.6 STV is ______

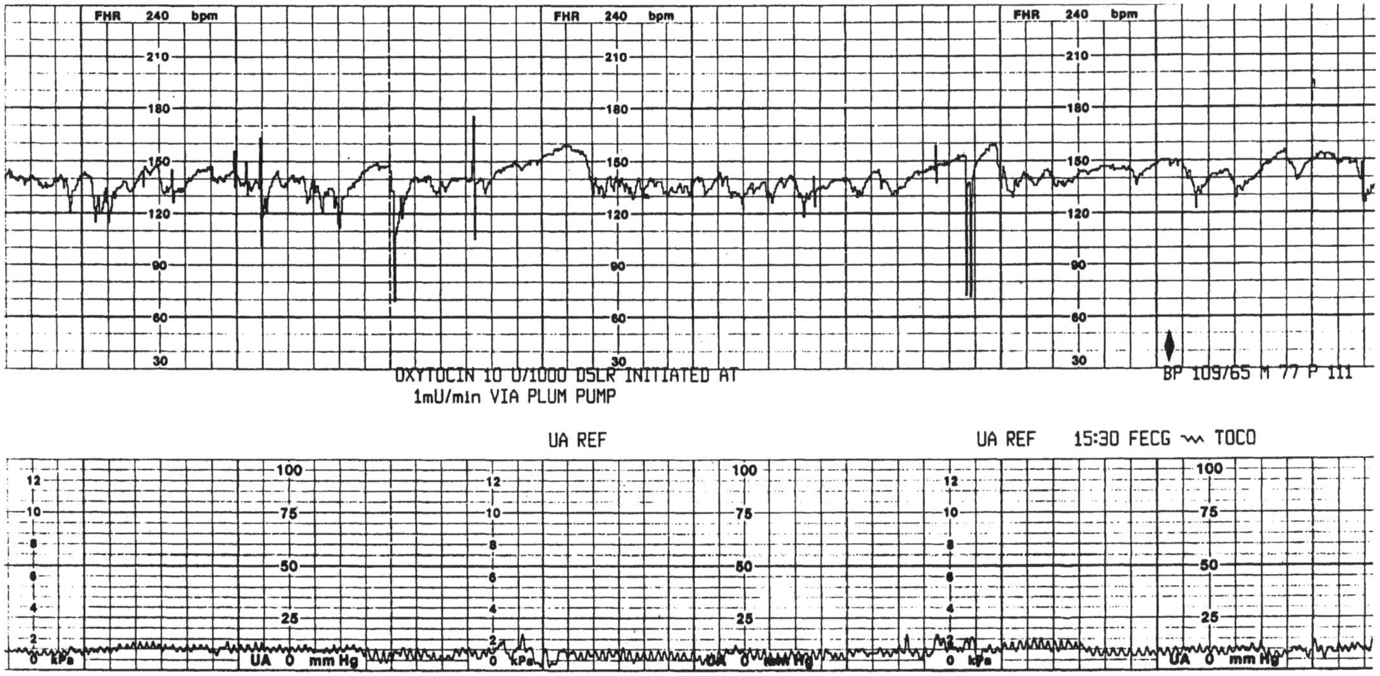

7.7 STV is ______

Did you say 7.5 STV is absent, 7.6 STV is present and 7.7 STV is present? If you did, you're correct! When charting any aspect of the tracing, including STV, the assumption is you viewed the tracing between the last time you charted and the current time you are charting.

SIGNIFICANCE OF STV

Significance of STV

STV exists when there is an intact, oxygenated brainstem, parasympathetic nervous system, and heart conduction system. The vagus exerts a tonic effect and an oscillatory effect on the fetal heart rate (FHR). The tonic effect creates a drop in the baseline, decelerations, and bradycardia. Low voltage, fast electrocortical activity is associated with an increase in vagal tone, which would decrease the bpm change in STV. This happens when fetuses are in an "awake" state. So, while you may see accelerations in the FHR, STV will look small. Fetal vagal tone increases as gestation advances, but even preterm fetuses have STV.

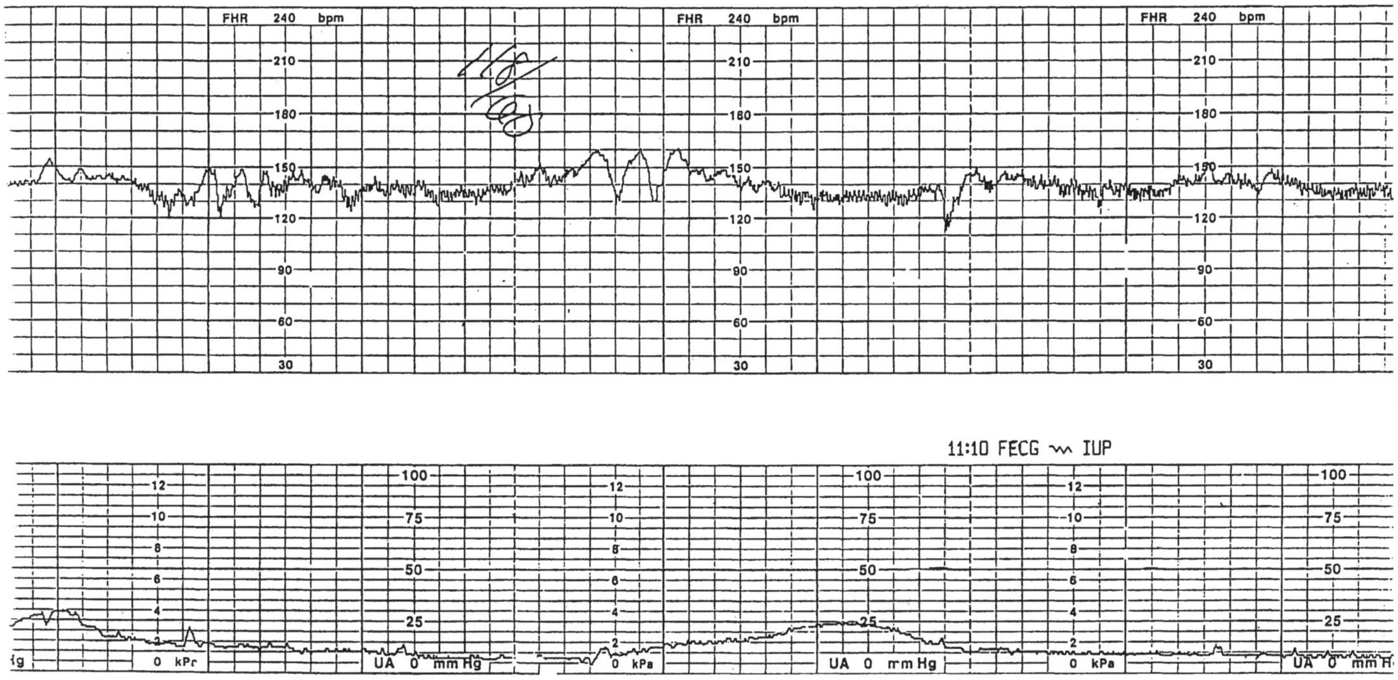

7.8 Accelerations with baseline short-term variability.

When STV is present:

- the vagus is intact and oxygenated
- the brainstem, vagus, and heart are functioning
- STV should fluctuate with fetal breathing movements
- STV is influenced by baroreceptors, chemoreceptors, and catecholamines
- STV will increase or decrease due to fetal brain activity evidenced by changes in fetal “sleep/wake” states
- STV may be exaggerated (> 9 bpm differences) in term and postterm **hypoxic** fetuses who release catecholamines
- drugs, such as atropine, decrease STV
- hypoxia, with the production of fetal adenosine, decreases SA nodal activity, decreasing STV
- drugs, such as narcotics, may decrease neurologic function causing the absence of STV
- fetal infection, trauma, anoxia, asphyxia, brain death, congenital vascular defects, and thrombocytopenia have been associated with absent STV.

The Normal BPM Range of STV

Expect the digital display on the fetal monitor to have bpm differences of 1 to 7 bpm between contractions and 4 to 8 bpm during contractions. STV bpm differences are rarely 9 to 10 bpm and **never** 15 or more bpm.

STV IS GREATER DURING CONTRACTIONS

Why would bpm differences be greater during contractions than between contractions?

Since contractions can squeeze maternal spiral arteries which diminishes blood flow to the placenta, there may be a slight drop in oxygen delivery to the fetus resulting in a chemoreceptor response and possibly a catecholamine response that increases STV. The actual cause of this increased STV is unknown.

STV VS. AN ARRHYTHMIA SUCH AS PACS OR PVCS

When the fluctuation in consecutive FHRs is greater than 15 bpm, suspect premature atrial contractions (PACs) or premature ventricular contractions (PVCs). This is an example of PACs. PACs are the most common fetal arrhythmia.

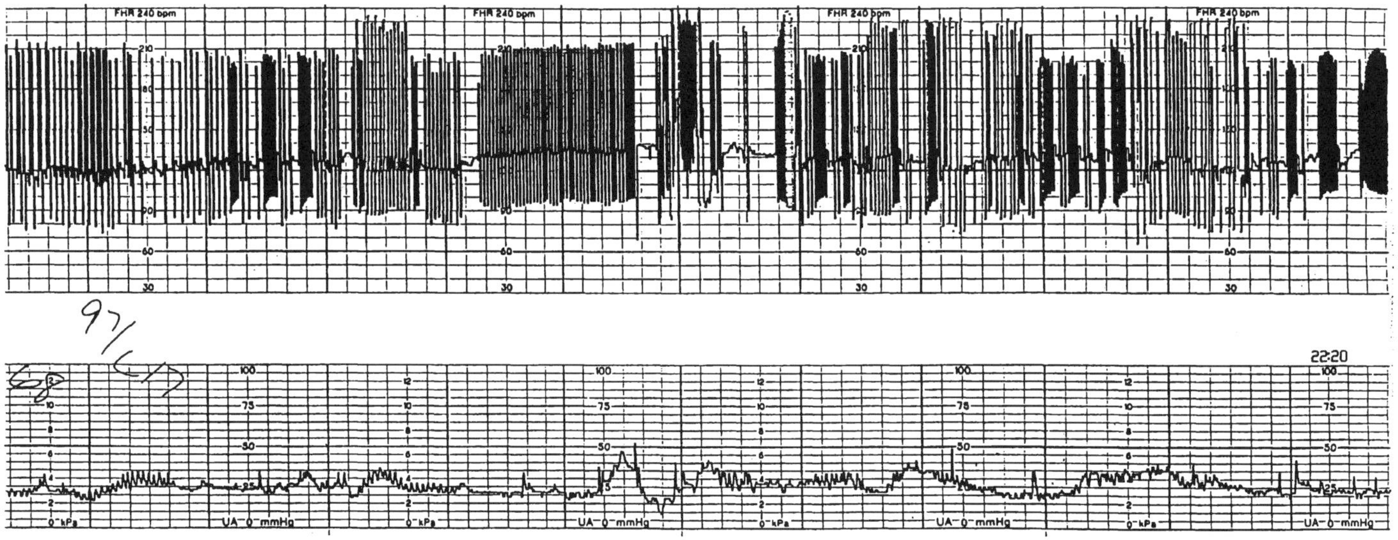

7.9 ***Premature atrial contractions create a line up and the compensatory pause creates an immediate line down. PACs are the most common fetal arrhythmia.***

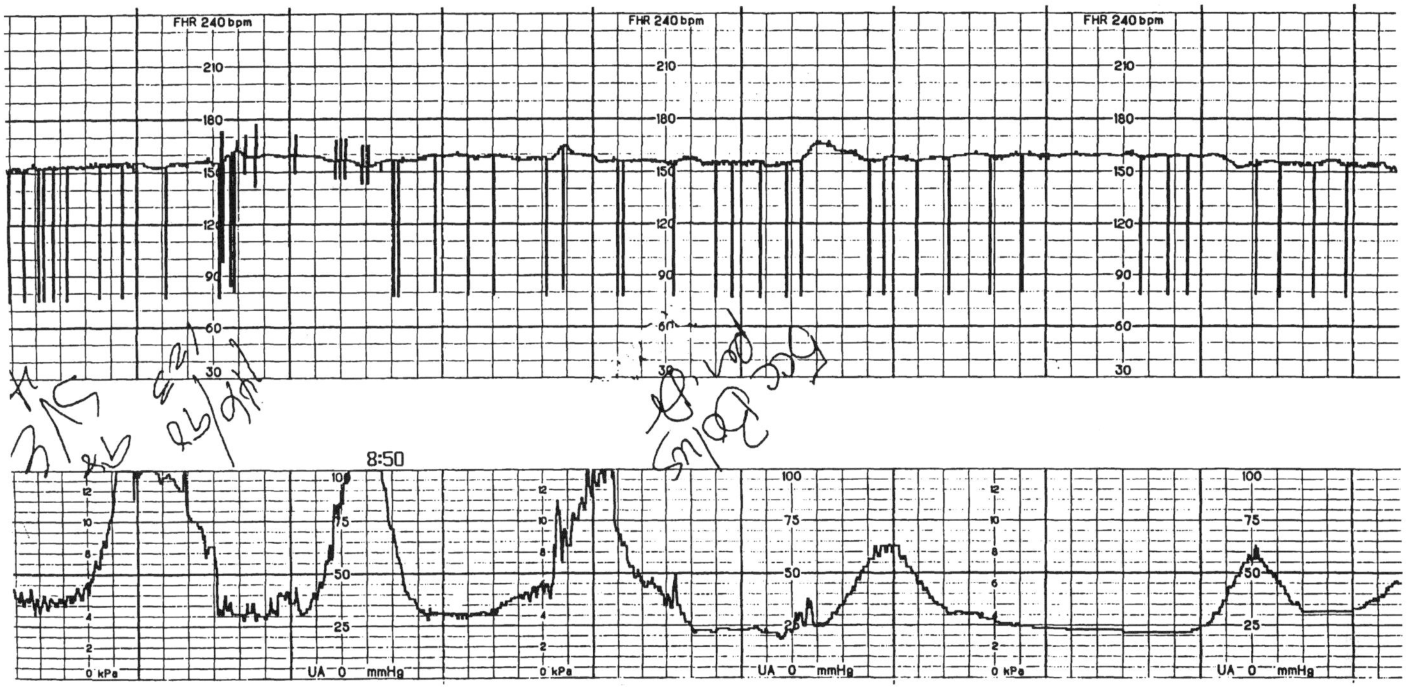

7.10 Dropped beats due to a non-conducted sinoatrial impulse. Note the baseline is near 160 bpm and the bottom of the dropped beats is near 80 bpm (half the rate). Dropped beats reflect a 2 to 1 Mobitz II or second-degree heart block.

An arrhythmia is not the same as STV since STV is the result of normal cardiac electrical conduction and PACs, PVCs, and heart block represent abnormal impulse conduction. If you suspect PACs or PVCs auscultate fetal heart tones with a fetoscope. An irregular rhythm suggests PACs or PVCs. Inform the midwife and/or physician. The pediatrician should also be informed as there is a small risk of a cardiac anomaly.

SAWTOOTH PATTERN

The Oscillatory Effect of the Vagus

The respiratory nerves and the nerves that regulate the vagus are next to each other in the brainstem. When the fetus makes inhalation breathing movements the FHR increases and with exhalation movements the FHR decreases. The result (a respiratory sinus arrhythmia) is called a sawtooth pattern (7.11). A sawtooth pattern is rare and is a sign of fetal well-being.

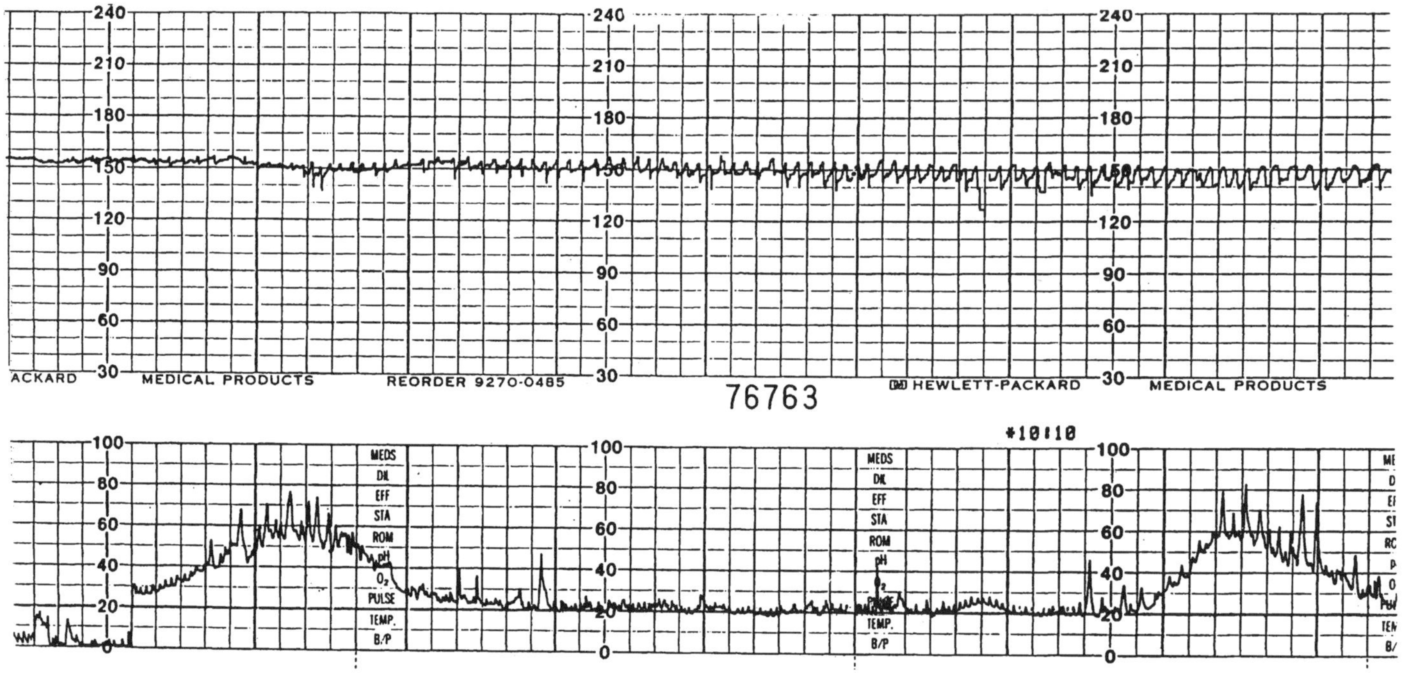

7.11 Sawtooth pattern due to the oscillatory effect of the vagus during fetal breathing movements.

THE ULTRA-SOUND AND STV

The Ultrasound (US) and STV

US signal quality depends on placement of the transducer over the fetal heart, transducer pressure against the maternal abdomen, the quantity of adipose tissue (increasing the distance the US waves must travel), and the amount of coupling gel on the transducer face. If the US signal quality is high, and a fetal monitor with autocorrelation is used, the FHR will be calculated within 2.5 bpm of the true value. The printout will be similar to the printout generated when a spiral electrode is used. It has been said that the US record *very closely* approaches that of STV created when a spiral electrode is used. The tracing is a reasonable representation that is often *virtually identical* to a tracing printed when a spiral electrode is used. Sometimes the US printout has less STV than a printout when the spiral electrode is used. **If it looks good on external, it probably is, but there should be other evidence that the fetus is well, such as a reactive acceleration and fetal movement.**

THE CONCEPT OF STV

STV has been documented by some clinicians as present when the US is used but only when it's presence can be supported conceptually by the presence of a reactive acceleration. A reactive acceleration peaks 15 bpm above the middle of the baseline and lasts 15 seconds at its base (7.12). If the US-generated tracing is smooth and flat, STV has been documented as absent since it is highly probable it is absent.

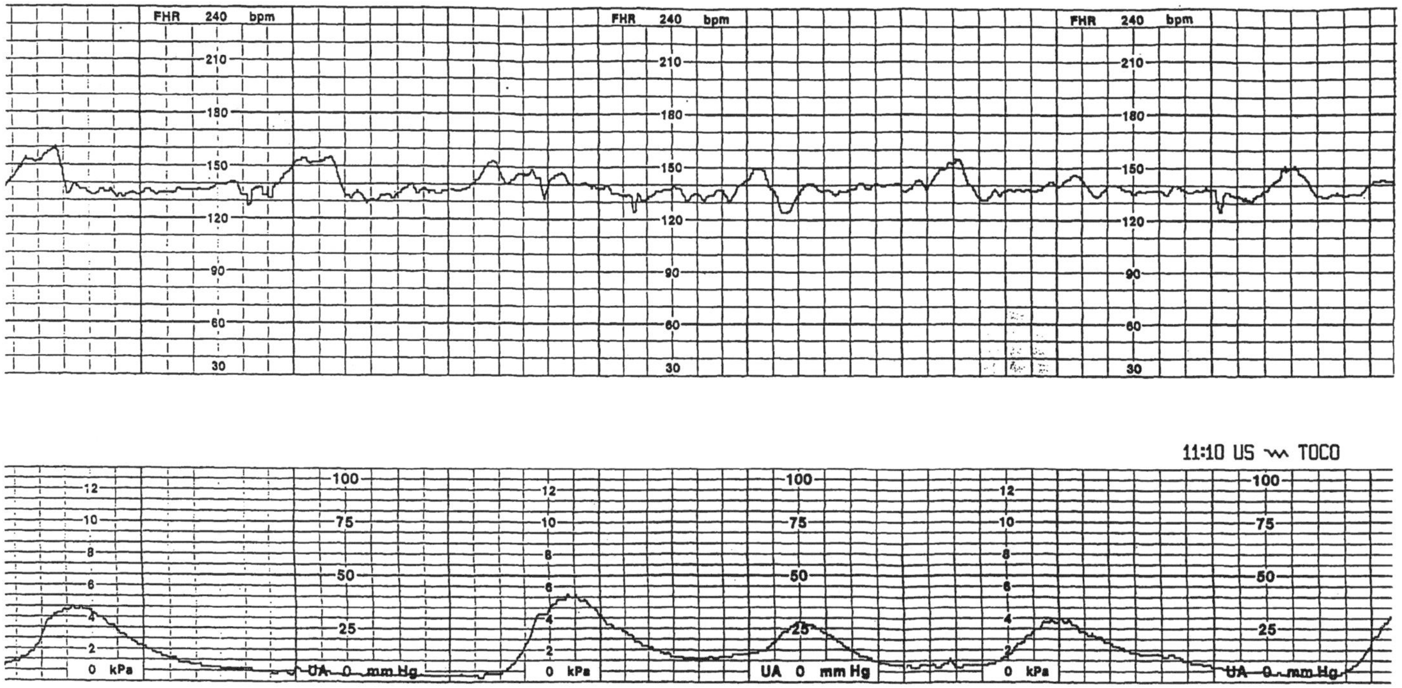

7.12 ***An acceleration that peaks 15 bpm above the baseline and is 15 or more seconds at its base rules out metabolic acidosis. Short-term variability is present when the fetus is not acidotic. Therefore, it may be documented as present. Most nurses hesitate to document STV due to outdated information related to first-genertion monitors.***

A REACTIVE ACCELERATION RULES OUT METABOLIC ACIDOSIS

A reactive acceleration rules out metabolic acidosis. The presence of the reactive acceleration is a reassuring finding. *STV is present when metabolic acidosis is absent* unless there is a congenital defect of the brain, heart, or autonomic nervous system that affects the vagus and prevents STV in spite of normal acid-base balance. Charting STV + is *conceptually correct* if the US-derived tracing has LTV and at least one reactive acceleration.

Another traditional saying is, **"If it looks bad on external, it's probably worse on internal."**

THE ABSENCE OF LTV AND NO ACCELERATION SUGGESTS STV IS ABSENT

When the FHR baseline looks smooth on the US-derived tracing: charting O STV, STV O, or STV – is a good bet. Metabolic acidosis or asphyxia may be one cause of a smooth tracing. Assess fetal movement. If it is present, a tachyarrhythmia with a rate greater than 210 or higher (depending on the paper scale) may be present but the printer is printing at half the actual rate. The fetal monitor is programmed to print up to the top of the paper scale. USA-scaled paper stops at 240 bpm. Therefore, any rate above 240 will print at half that rate.

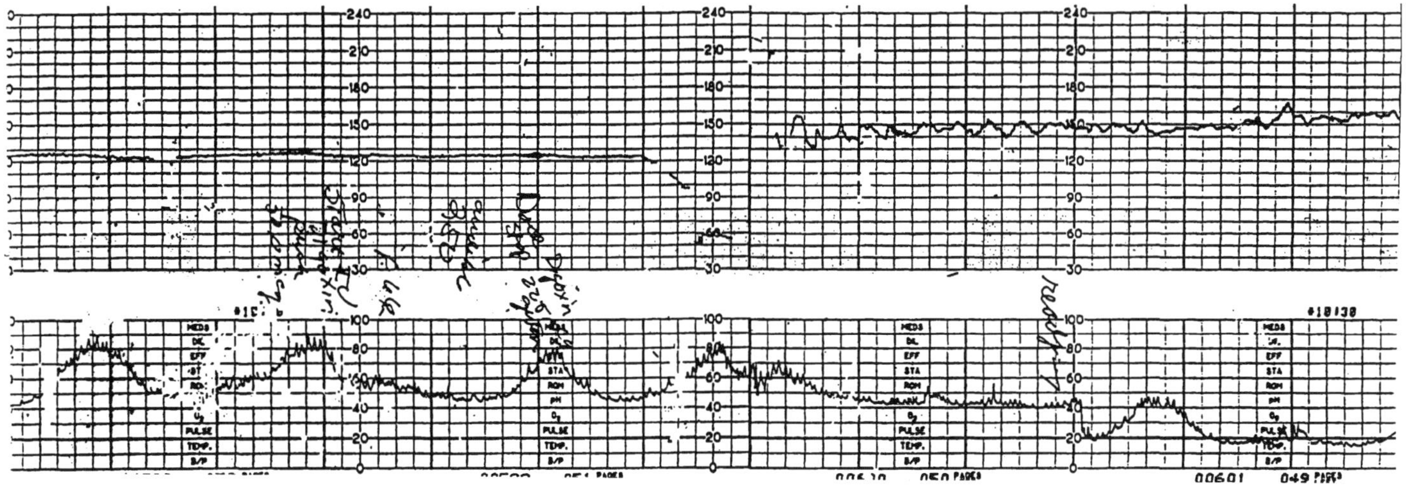

7.13 The FHR due to fetal supraventricular tachycardia printed at half the actual rate before maternal intravenous Digoxin. One and a half minutes later after intravenous Digoxin, there was fetal **cardioversion** *and the FHR returned to a normal rate.*

IF STV IS ABSENT, APPLY A SPIRAL ELECTRODE IF POSSIBLE

If STV is present and the fetus is not moving, and has not moved for more than two hours, fetal decompensation may occur sooner than later. Notify the physician immediately of your assessments. If possible, apply a spiral electrode to 100% accurately *measure* STV.

HEART BLOCK

STV is usually absent when congenital complete heart block (CCHB) or third degree heart block occurs (see 7.14). In this case, the fetus is usually active and well-oxygenated but SA nodal impulses are not transmitted to the AV node. The fetus with CCHB will decompensate as the FHR approaches 50 bpm and hydrops with congestive heart failure develops. Report this FHR to the physician as soon as possible. Try to stay calm. The fetus who is moving is not in any immediate danger. This is an arrhythmia **not** a terminal bradycardia. An ultrasound may be done to rule out hydrops and evaluate cardiac anatomy. The woman will need to be transferred to the care of a perinatologist, and will be delivered where a pediatric surgeon can be present during Cesarean section to instill a temporary pacemaker in the newborn.

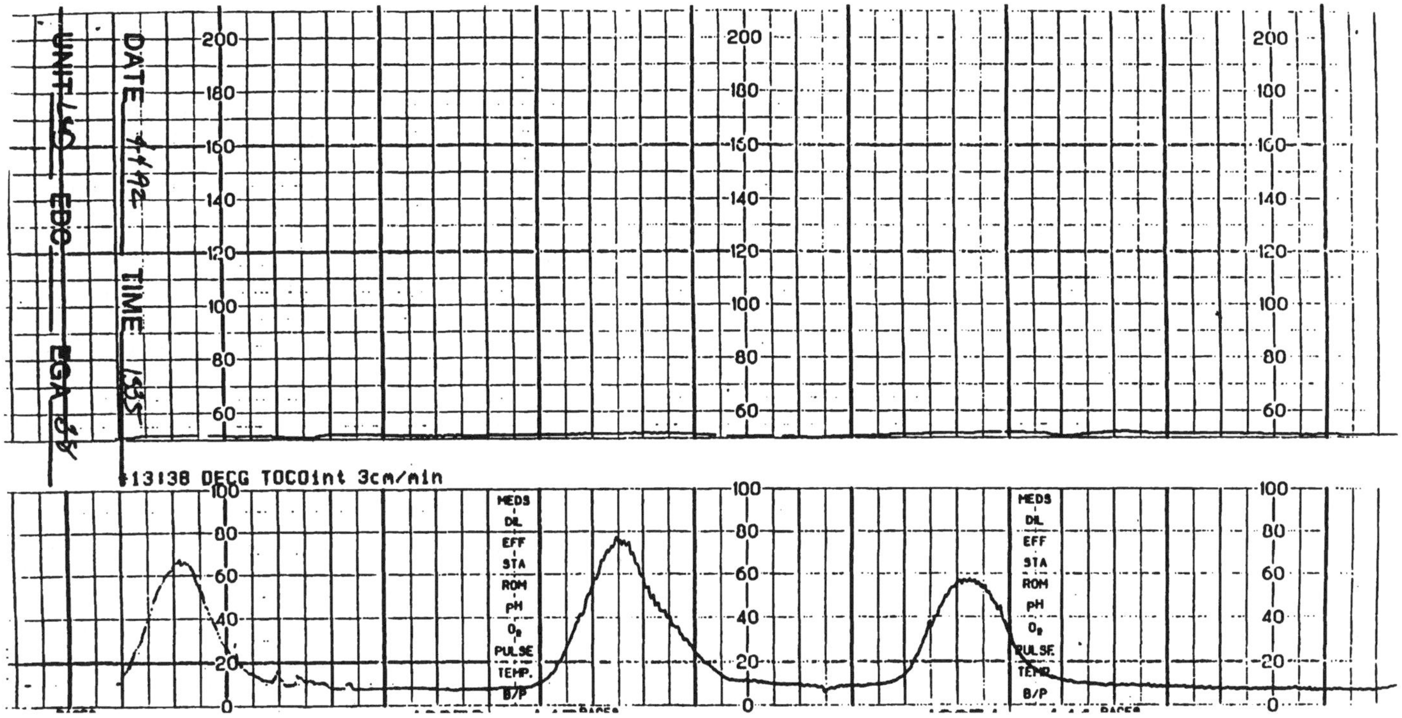

7.14 Complete heart block and European-scaled paper.

The fetal heart rate is 51 to 53 bpm. The Apgars scores were 7 at 1 minute and 7 at 5 minutes and mom was later diagnosed with lupus erythematosus. Half of all newborns with complete heart block have a mother with an antiphospholipid antibody syndrome such as lupus, Sjögren's syndrome, rheumatoid arthritis, Reynard's syndrome or scleroderma. The other half have a congenital heart defect.

What Do You Do When STV is Absent?

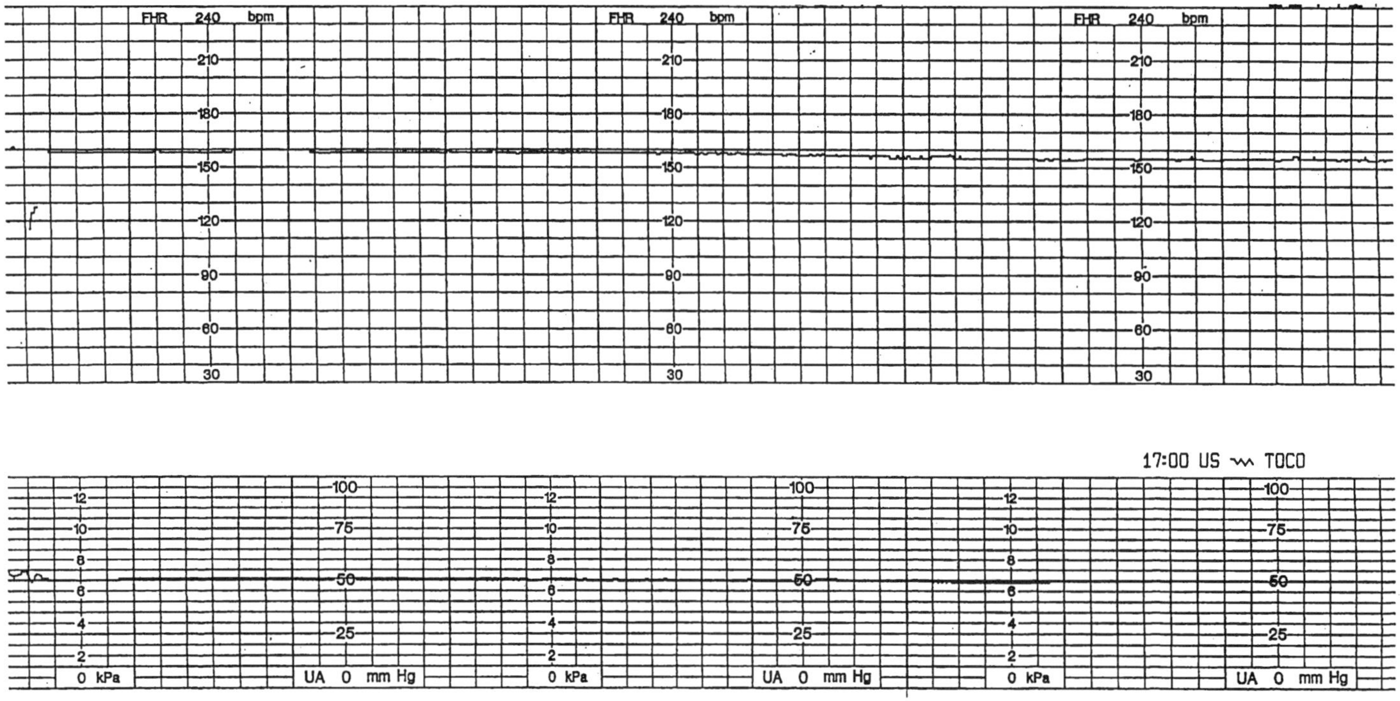

7.15 Absent STV.

Actions in Response to Absent STV

- document O STV, STV O, or STV-
- confirm the fetal monitor test button is not stuck in the in position creating a smooth, flat line
- obtain a maternal drug history and fetal movement history
- palpate fetal movement
- could there be fetal hypoxia, anoxia, metabolic acidosis, and/or asphyxia?
- perform a vaginal examination to determine the possibility of a prompt vaginal delivery
- an ultrasound scan may be done to assess fetal brain and heart development and to confirm the FHR
- no actions are required if STV was present before a central nervous system depressant was given

- is the FHR halving?
- for 100% accurate **measurement** of STV, apply a spiral electrode.

If the baseline looks flat and you suspect the fetus needs oxygen, e.g., due to the lack of fetal movement or accelerations for more than 100 minutes, enhance fetal oxygenation by increasing maternal cardiac output and blood oxygen content. To improve cardiac output and blood flow:

- change the mother's position so she is not supine, avoid Trendelenburg as it decreases cardiac output, avoid knee-chest (elbows and knees) when uterine rupture is suspected
- increase the intravenous fluid flow rate of a nondextrose solution to give a 500 to 1000 ml bolus, avoid this bolus if the woman is at increased risk for pulmonary edema, e.g., she is preeclamptic
- discontinue oxytocic or prostaglandin agents (especially if uterine hyperstimulation occurs)
- if ordered by a physician or midwife, give a tocolytic such as 0.25 mg terbutaline® subcutaneously or intravenously (hold medication if abruption is suspected as this may extend or mask the abruption)

Then, to improve blood oxygen content, apply a tight fitting simple face mask at 8 to 10 liters per minute of 100% oxygen or a partial rebreathing mask (with an oxygen reservoir bag) at 12 liters per minute. Oxygen should reach the fetus in 9 or fewer minutes. Is the FHR better by 10 minutes? Communicate your assessment and actions to the physician. Since the fetus should be out of a quiescent state in 100 minutes, and usually by 60 minutes, look at the tracing to determine when the last acceleration occurred. Evaluate the fetal response. There is a saying when a fetus is metabolically acidotic: **"Once STV is gone, it's too late."**

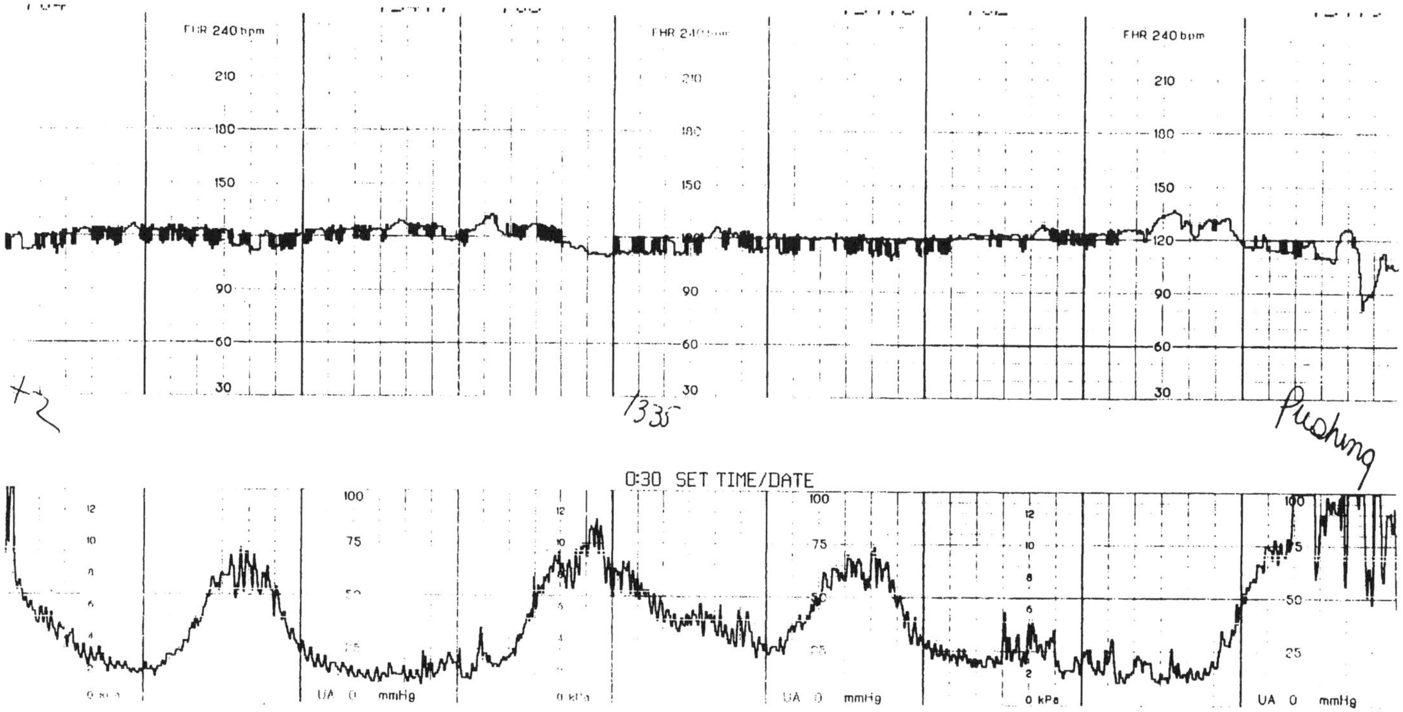

7.16 Exaggerated STV (>9 bpm) may be due to fetal hypoxia. The presence of accelerations rule out metabolic acidosis. Hypoxia in this example may be due to uterine hyperstimulation.

EXAGGERATED STV (>9 BPM)

Actions in Response to Exaggerated STV

Fetal hypoxia may stimulate the release of norepinephrine which will affect sodium ions to increase the excitability of the SA node, increasing its oscillatory effect on the FHR, and exaggerating STV. Assess and record:

- exaggerated STV as STV + or STV present.
- fetal heart tones with a fetoscope to rule out an irregular rhythm (arrhythmia)
- maternal blood pressure to rule out hypo- or hypertension as a cause of hypoxia
- the last acceleration, and fetal movement
- amniotic fluid color, amount, and odor
- if hypoxia is suspected, act to first increase maternal uterine blood flow
- evaluate the fetal response to your actions
- STV should return to a normal range after these actions.

SUMMARY

Summary

- BTBV is the fluctuation in pulse intervals between consecutive heartbeats. It is not visible and it is measured by the fetal monitor in milliseconds. STV is measured in bpm.
- BTBV determines STV.
- STV does not include accelerations or decelerations.
- STV is a baseline characteristic.
- STV is visualized on the FHR printout.
- STV is documented as present or absent.
- STV is chaotic, nonlinear, and may look like small lines 9 to 10 bpm long.
- the baseline appears smooth when pulse intervals are similar.
- the presence of STV is a sign of fetal well-being and brainstem oxygenation.
- the absence of STV suggests possible metabolic acidosis, CNS depression from a drug such as a tranquilizer, narcotic, nicotine, or fetal quiet sleep, anencephaly, injury to the brainstem, a dying fetus, brain death, infection, trauma, vascular defects, or thrombocytopenia.
- when STV is absent, the digital readout will not change most of the time or will be rarely greater than 1 bpm between calculated rates.
- determine the most likely reason for absent STV and intervene accordingly.

Exercises

1. What is the bpm (STV) range expected between contractions? _____ to _____ bpm
2. What is the bpm range expected during contractions? _____ to _____ bpm
3. Document STV as present or absent.

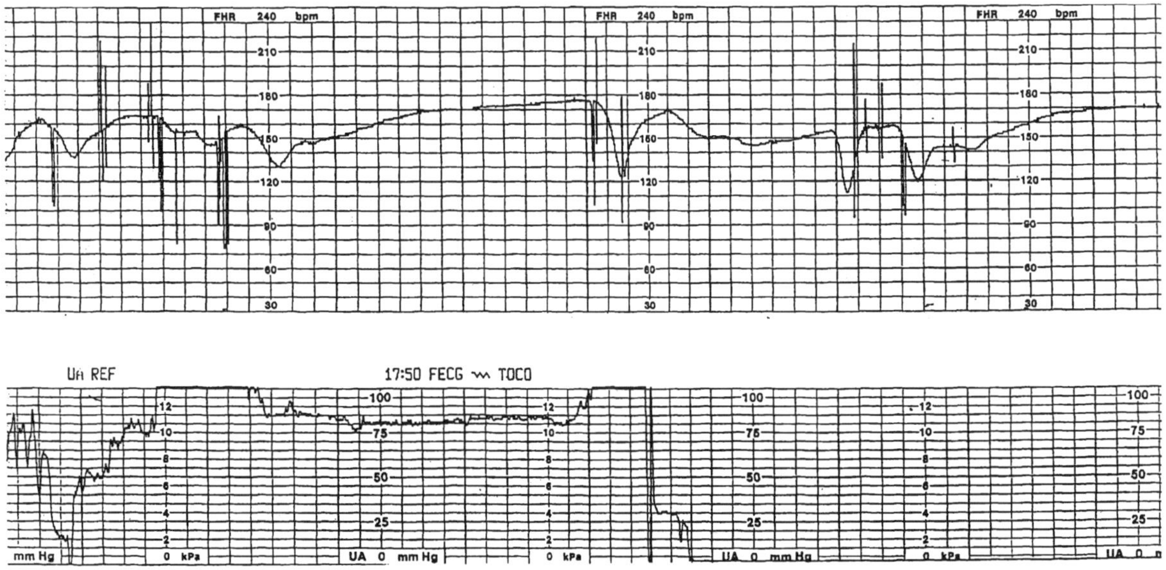

7.17

STV is _______

4. Document STV as present or absent.

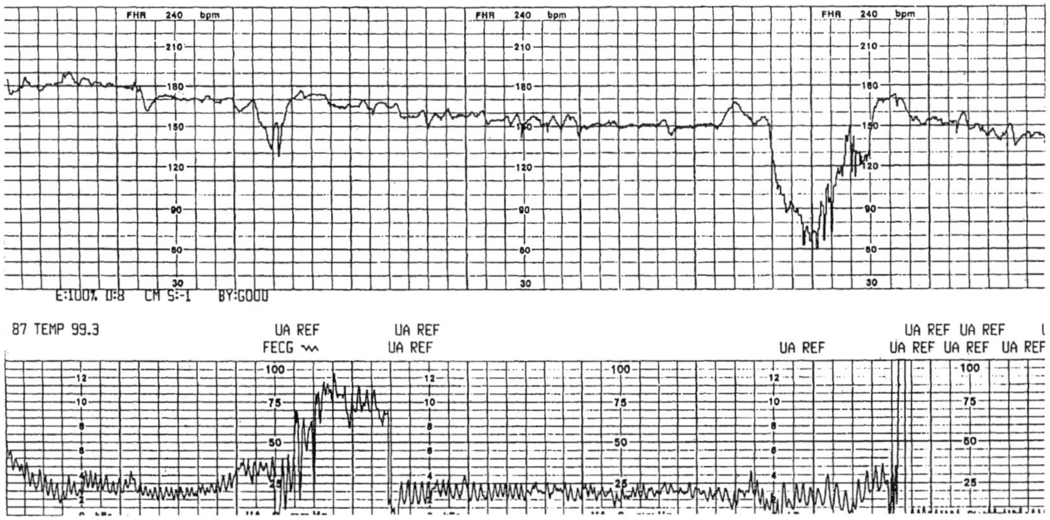

7.18

STV is _______

ANSWERS TO EXERCISES

1. 1-7
2. 4-8
3. absent
4. present

SECTION 7: SHORT-TERM VARIABILITY

QUESTIONS

Directions: Circle T if the statement is true, F if it is false.

QUESTIONS			
T	F	1.	Beat-to-beat variability is measured in beats per minute.
T	F	2.	The presence of a reactive acceleration strongly suggests short-term variability is present.
T	F	3.	A sawtooth pattern is a sign of central nervous system compromise.
T	F	4.	When STV is exaggerated (>9 bpm), the fetus may be hypoxic.
T	F	5.	The absence of STV is always synonymous with metabolic acidosis.
T	F	6.	STV can be 100% accurately *measured* when a spiral electrode is on the fetus.
T	F	7.	STV is a deceleration characteristic.
T	F	8.	Even if the fetus has complete heart block, short-term variability will be present.
T	F	9.	Supplemental oxygen should reach the fetus by 9 or fewer minutes.
T	F	10.	When short-term variability is present, it is never necessary to intervene.

SECTION 8
Acceleration (Accels)

ACCELERATIONS

Variability and accelerations are two separate concepts. Accelerations have been defined as a transient increase in the fetal heart rate (FHR) above the baseline. If the acceleration peaks at least 15 beats per minute (bpm) above the baseline and lasts 15 or more seconds at its base, it is called a **reactive** acceleration.

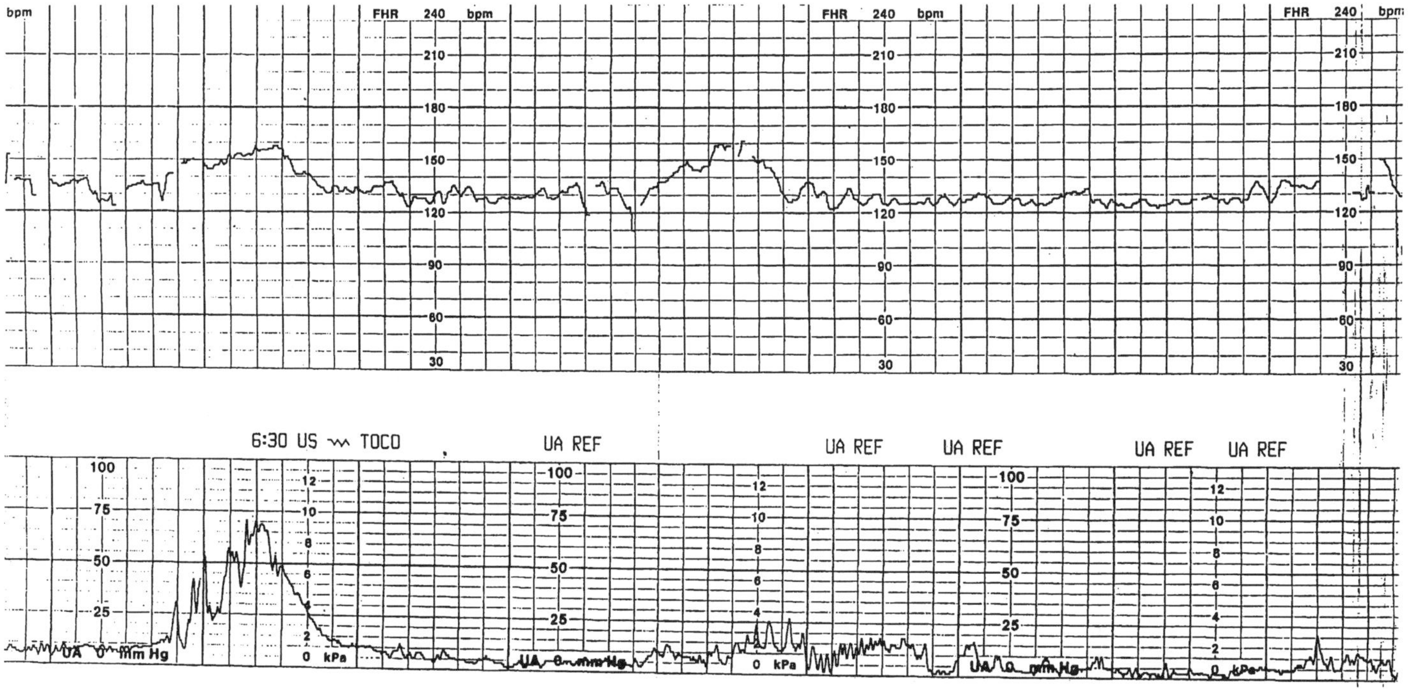

8.1 The baseline is 122 to 134 bpm with spontaneous accelerations to 160 x 60-65 seconds. This is a reassuring pattern.

The rise above the baseline and the duration of accelerations can be measured. A baseline is first identified. Spontaneous accels vary in shape from one to the next. Therefore, the height and duration might be charted using a range, e.g., accels to 160-165 bpm x 55-60 seconds.

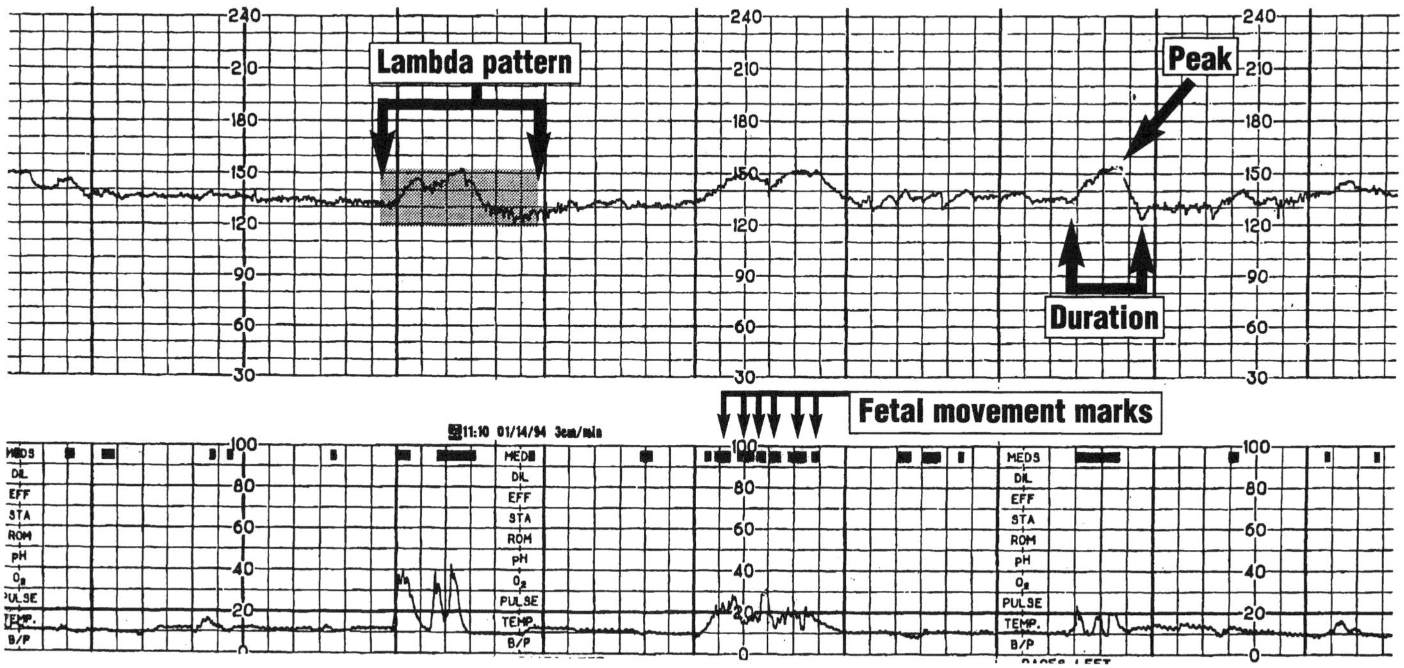

8.2 These spontaneous accelerations peak at 150 to 152 bpm and have a duration of 25-65 seconds. The FHR dips slightly after the first acceleration. This is a normal response and is due to a baroreceptor stimulus and vagal response following the increase in the FHR during the acceleration. It is called a Lambda pattern and is innocuous. Note the fetal movement marks at the top of the uterine activity channel. This was created by a Hewlett-Packard® monitor.

SPONTANEOUS ACCELS

Spontaneous accels usually increase by 10 bpm or more above the BL. They are an obvious "bump" that could stand alone. They vary in shape from one to the next but often look similar as they can have a similar pointed peak.

REACTIVE ACCELS

Reactive accels are defined by their size. They increase at least 15 bpm and last at least 15 seconds. One reactive acceleration rules out metabolic acidosis.

A *reactive* nonstress test (NST) exists when there are at least two reactive accelerations that peak 15 bpm above the baseline and last 15 seconds at their base in a 20 minute tracing. Most people use the middle of the baseline to begin their measurement to the peak of the acceleration. If a NST is not reactive by 40 minutes, the physician should be notified so that additional tests may be ordered. All fetuses should accelerate by the 100th minute of monitoring.

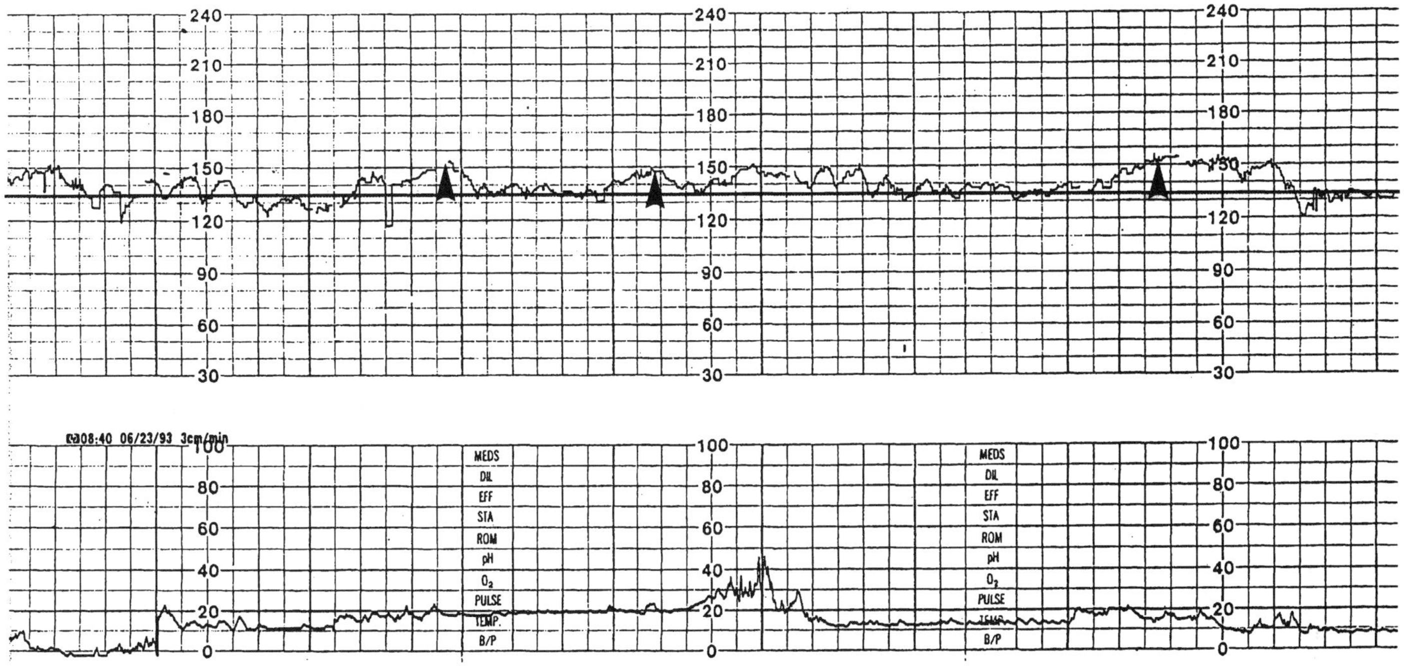

8.3 Select the middle of the baseline prior to measuring acceleration height.

REACTIVITY

Reactivity has been used in some medical articles to mean reactive. However, since there is confusion as to the meaning of reactivity by some who think it means variability is "good," it is best **not** to use this word in communication and documentation.

PREMATURITY AND ACCELS

Prematurity and Accelerations

- accels begin at 15 to 16 weeks of gestation
- the neurologic system is felt to be mature after 30 weeks of gestation and you should expect to see many "15 x 15" accels
- prior to 32 weeks of gestation expect to see many "10 x 10" accels but also some "15 x 15" accels
- "15 x 15" reactive accels are present in 16.7% of 23-27 weeks fetuses
- "15 x 15" reactive accels are present in 65.6% of 28-32 weeks fetuses
- "15 x 15" reactive accels are present in 90.6% of 33-37 weeks fetuses

APPROPRIATE FOR GESTATION AGE

Accelerations (10 bpm x 10 seconds) in a preterm fetus less than 32 weeks of gestation are not usually documented as reactive for gestational age. More research is needed to confirm the relationship between "10 x 10" accels and the lack of metabolic acidosis. Usually prior to 32 weeks of gestation, the tracing is interpreted as "FHR appropriate for gestational age" or "not appropriate for gestational age." A fetus who accelerates is most likely **not** metabolically acidotic. However, a reactive acceleration always rules out metabolic acidosis.

EXERCISE

Exercise

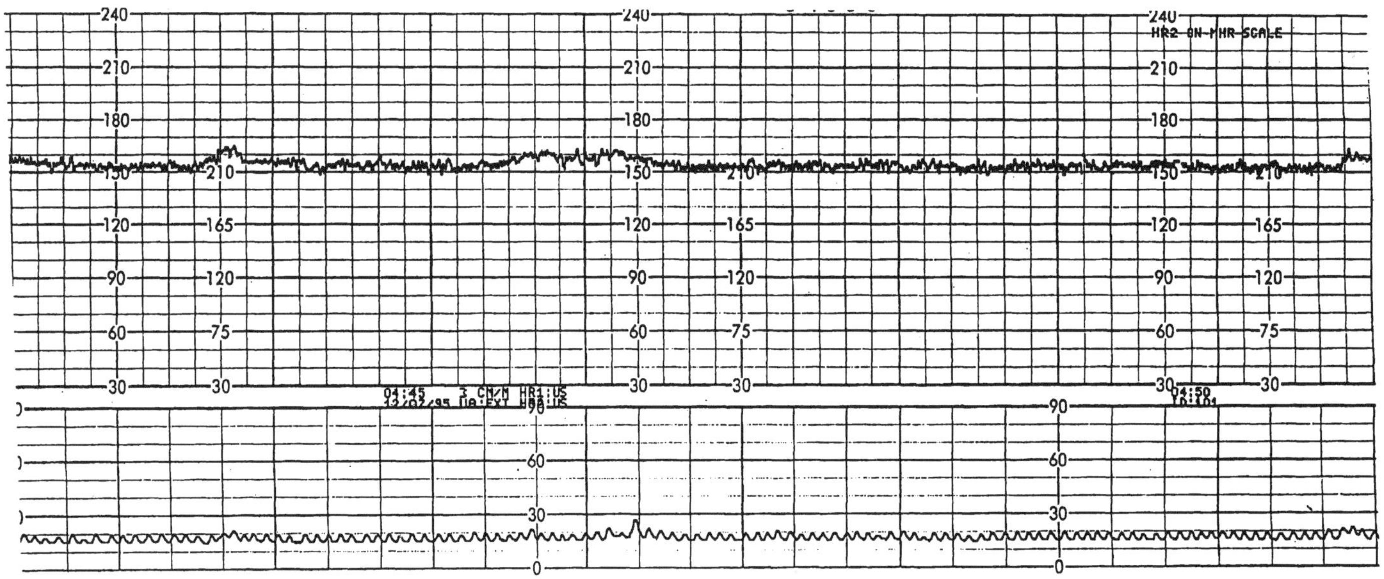

8.4 Baseline 150-154 bpm with accelerations to 162 bpm x 15-50 seconds. The maternal hemoglobin was 6.5 g/dl. The fetus was most likely not metabolically acidotic but may have been hypoxic.

Look at this tracing (8.4). Is it reactive? If you said no, you are correct. You see the accelerations did not meet strict "15 x 15" criteria. This does not mean the fetus is acidotic, it just means the accelerations weren't big enough to call the tracing reactive. Preterm fetuses begin to accelerate their FHR at 15 to 16 weeks of gestation. As the fetus matures, bigger and longer accelerations occur. Research has shown that a "15 x 15" accel rules out metabolic acidosis. More research is needed to determine if smaller accelerations also rule out metabolic acidosis.

ANTENATAL ACCELS

Accels present in a NST have a greater than 99% negative predictive value. That means a reactive NST predicts fetal well-being in 99 of 100 babies at the time of the NST. The frequency and number of NSTs is based on physician preference and maternal/fetal risk factors.

LABOR ACCELS

Accelerations During Labor

A spontaneous reactive accel indicates the absence of a metabolically acidotic fetus at the time of the acceleration.

Expect spontaneous accels during labor. Well fetuses during labor move 30 to 40 times an hour and should accelerate each and every hour. If concern exists regarding fetal well-being, a spiral electrode (SE) could be applied to accurately measure short-term variability. If the cervix is not dilated enough to insert the SE or if there is a contraindication to rupture of membranes, a real-time ultrasound may be needed to assess fetal movement, fetal breathing movements, fetal anatomy, and amniotic fluid volume to demonstrate fetal well-being. No woman should leave your facility until fetal well-being is firmly established, even if the woman is not in labor or is in false or early labor. Remember to react to the fetal physiology. If the vertex is accessible, scalp rubbing, known as scalp stimulation, could be used to create a sensory nerve/sympathetic nerve stimulus to elicit an acceleration to rule out metabolic acidosis.

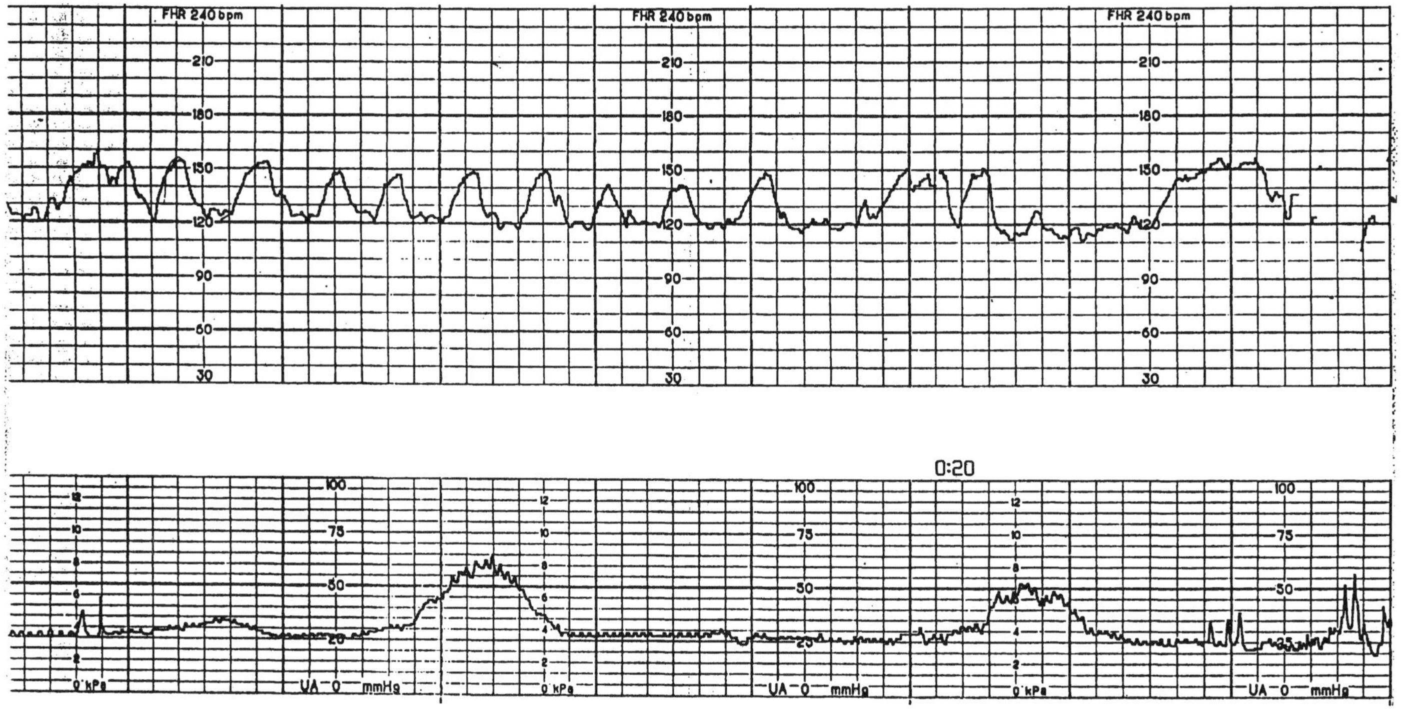

8.5 Fetus in an active awake (4F) state with multiple spontaneous accelerations and a baseline near 120 bpm.

PROLONGED ACCELS

Prolonged accels may be confused with tachycardia when the FHR stays above 160 bpm. Fetuses with a prolonged accel, one that lasts 2 or more minutes, should be actively moving. Abdominal palpation confirms fetal movement. Some fetuses can stay in the active awake state up to two hours which delays baseline identification. As long as there are no decelerations, prolonged accelerations strongly suggest an uncompromised, well-oxygenated fetus.

SUMMARY

Summary

Accelerations are a transient, obvious increase in the FHR above the baseline. A reactive nonstress test (NST) has at least two accelerations that peak 15 bpm above the baseline and last 15 seconds at their base in a 20 minute period. Most people use the middle of the baseline then measure 15 bpm above it. A reactive NST predicts a well-oxygenated fetus at the time of the test. NSTs are usually called reactive or nonreactive at 32 or more weeks of gestation. Prior to 32 weeks, the test is usually interpreted as FHR "appropriate for gestational age" or "not appropriate for gestational age." An NST ends at 40 minutes and the physician should be notified if it is nonreactive. All fetuses should accelerate by the end of 100 minutes of monitoring. If a spiral electrode cannot be applied or scalp stimulation cannot be done to rule in fetal well-being, a real-time ultrasound should be done to assess fetal status.

"Reactivity" is poorly defined in the literature and should not be used in communication or documentation. The presence of accelerations that do not meet "reactive" criteria still suggests a nonhypoxic fetus. More research is needed to determine if smaller accelerations also rule out metabolic acidosis. Fetuses can accelerate for two or more minutes when they are in an active awake state. The presence of fetal movement and the lack of decelerations suggests fetal well-being.

SECTION 8: ACCELERATIONS

QUESTIONS

QUESTIONS

Directions: Circle T if the statement is true, F if it is false.

T F 1. Nonstress tests are reactive if they have two "10 x 15" accelerations in a 20 minute period.

T F 2. It is not an acceleration unless it is 15 beats above baseline and lasts 15 seconds at it's base.

T F 3. Acceleration height for a nonstress test is usually measured from the bottom of the baseline.

T F 4. Accelerations are related to fetal acid-base status.

T F 5. Reactive accelerations must be sustained at the top for 15 or more seconds.

T F 6. By 33 weeks of gestation, 90% of fetuses have reactive accelerations.

T F 7. If one acceleration lasts 2 minutes, you can classify the tracing as reactive.

T F 8. If two "10 x 15" accelerations are present in 20 minutes and the fetus is 26 weeks of gestation, the NST is not appropriate for gestation age.

T F 9. More than half of fetuses less than 27 weeks of gestation have "15 x 15" accelerations.

T F 10. "Reactive for gestational age" is acceptable language to document the NST result of a preterm fetus.

SECTION 9
Early Decelerations (Early decels)

PERIODIC DECELERATIONS

Early Decelerations are Periodic in Timing

Decelerations that occur in response to pressure exerted during contractions are called periodic decelerations. The three types of periodic decelerations are early, late, and variable decelerations. Variable decelerations can also occur between contractions.

PERIODIC DECELERATIONS/WITH CONTRACTIONS	
Pressure is on the	Type of Deceleration
• **fetal head**	• **early**
• uterine vessels	• late
• umbilical cord	• variable

PHYSIOLOGY OF EARLY DECELERATIONS

Early decelerations are rare. They occur in approximately 3% of all labors and never occur prior to labor. They reflect a vagal response as a result of *increased* intracranial pressure and *decreased* blood flow through blood vessels in the brain. There may also be a squeeze on carotid arteries preceding the vagal slowing of the fetal heart rate (FHR). When early decels occur, the baby's body is well-oxygenated but the brain is compressed more than normal. Expect to see accelerations and short-term variability as a sign of fetal well-being. Abnormally strong head compression could result in a brain bleed if it becomes persistent. For example, the baby may suffer from a subdural hemorrhage and/or a cephalohematoma. In rare cases, the brain hemorrhage may cause brain damage and cerebral palsy. Therefore, although early decelerations suggest the fetus is not hypoxic nor metabolically acidotic, we must be concerned about the risk of brain trauma.

4 TO 7 CM

Early decelerations are usually apparent when the cervix presses on the anterior fontanel between 4 to 7 centimeters of dilatation. Therefore early decelerations will not exist between 0 and 4 cm. You will never see early decelerations during an antepartal test such as a nonstress test. Early decelerations may occur between 7 and 10 cm if enough force is exerted on the fetal head to cause a vagal response. However, usually at and after 10 cm of dilatation, the vagal response from head and cord compression produces sharp drops in the FHR or variable decelerations.

CPD RISK BUT NOT HYPOXIA

Fetuses who have increased caput and molding and who are adapting the shape of their head to the maternal pelvis are at an increased risk of cephalopelvic disproportion (CPD). Document and communicate caput and/or molding. Early decelerations are associated with CPD. Observe the descent of the vertex during labor. The lack of descent may be associated with CPD, especially if the vertex never engages in the pelvis.

REASSURING PATTERN, EMOTIONALLY CONCERNED

Increased caput and overriding sutures can occur in the fetal head. Even though early decelerations are part of a reassuring (nonhypoxic) FHR pattern (accelerations should exist too), nurses, midwives, and physicians should still be concerned about the risk of CPD. Will the baby fit? Is a vaginal route of delivery probable or improbable? What signs of fetal well-being are still in evidence?

CAPUT

Caput or caput succedaneum is scalp edema due to subcutaneous serum collection and scalp edema. The pressure on the scalp from the cervix obstructs venous return and creates caput. Caput only occurs *after* rupture of the membranes. Increasing caput is an indicator for reassessing the labor situation to rule out CPD. Caput crosses the sutures. It is indentable. Caput usually resolves by 24 to 36 hours after birth.

MOLDING

Molding is the ability of the fetal head to change shape to fit the maternal pelvis. Molding ideally takes place slowly so no brain damage occurs. Excessive molding can cause extreme compression and potentially damage the brain as a result of hemorrhage. Therefore, molding is a greater concern than caput. Molding is determined by palpating overriding skull bones (overlapping bony plates of the skull) and noting the fontanels may be compressed.

CAPUT, MOLDING, CERVICAL EDEMA, AND LABOR PROGRESS

Actions in Response to Early Decelerations

Early decelerations should be reported to the midwife and/or physician. In addition, the clinician may:

- plot a labor curve (see Section 4)
  - is progress delayed?
- assess the cervix
  - 4 to 7 cm?
  - swollen?
- assess station and the fetal head
  - caput?
  - molding?

RECOGNITION CRITERIA

Recognition Criteria

Early decels begin 10 to 20 seconds after the contraction begins, their lowest point or nadir is less than 18 seconds after the peak of the contraction. Therefore, the nadir lag time for early decels is < 18 seconds. Early decels have a slanted onset and offset, they have a saucer or bowl shape. Early decels are back to the baseline close to the end of the contraction (see 9.1). To reiterate, the contraction peak to decel nadir duration is known as lag time. The lag time for early decels is < 18 seconds.

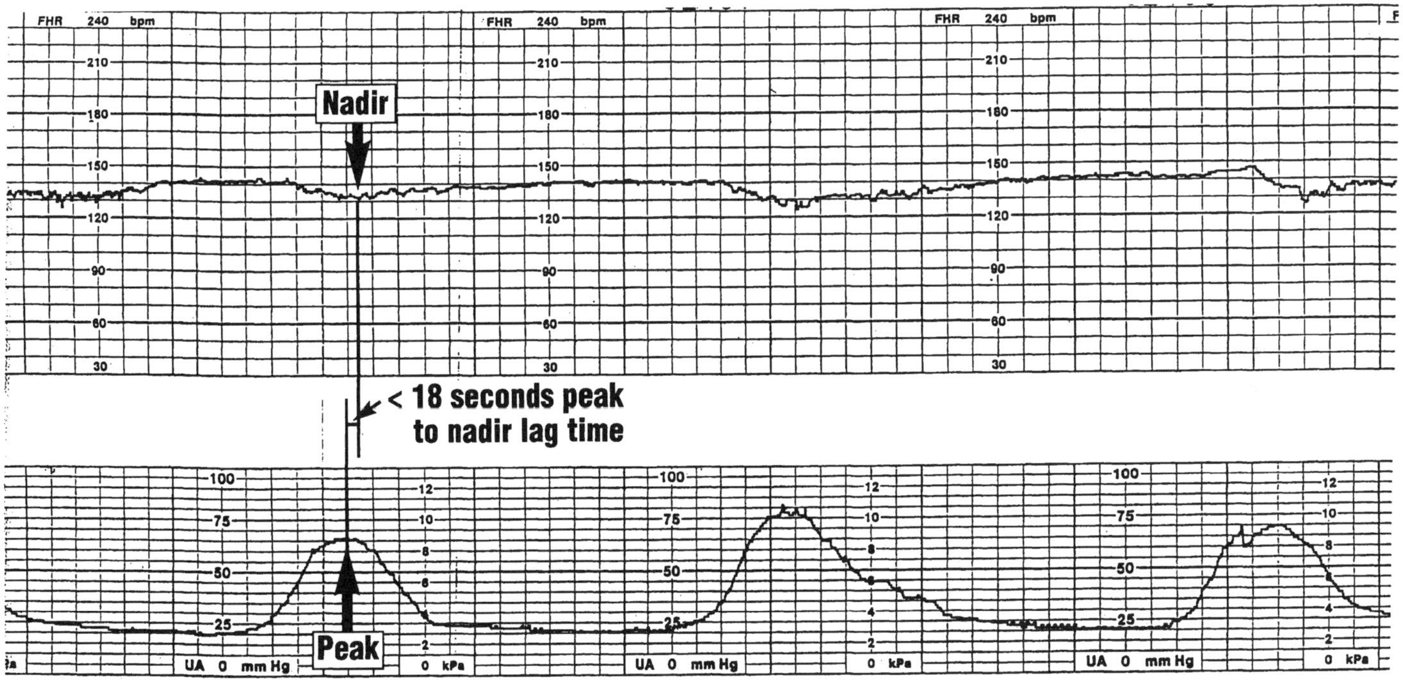

9.1 ***The baseline is 140-143 bpm. Short-term variability and early decelerations are present. Note the nadir (lowest point) of the decelerations occurs within 18 seconds from the contraction peak.***

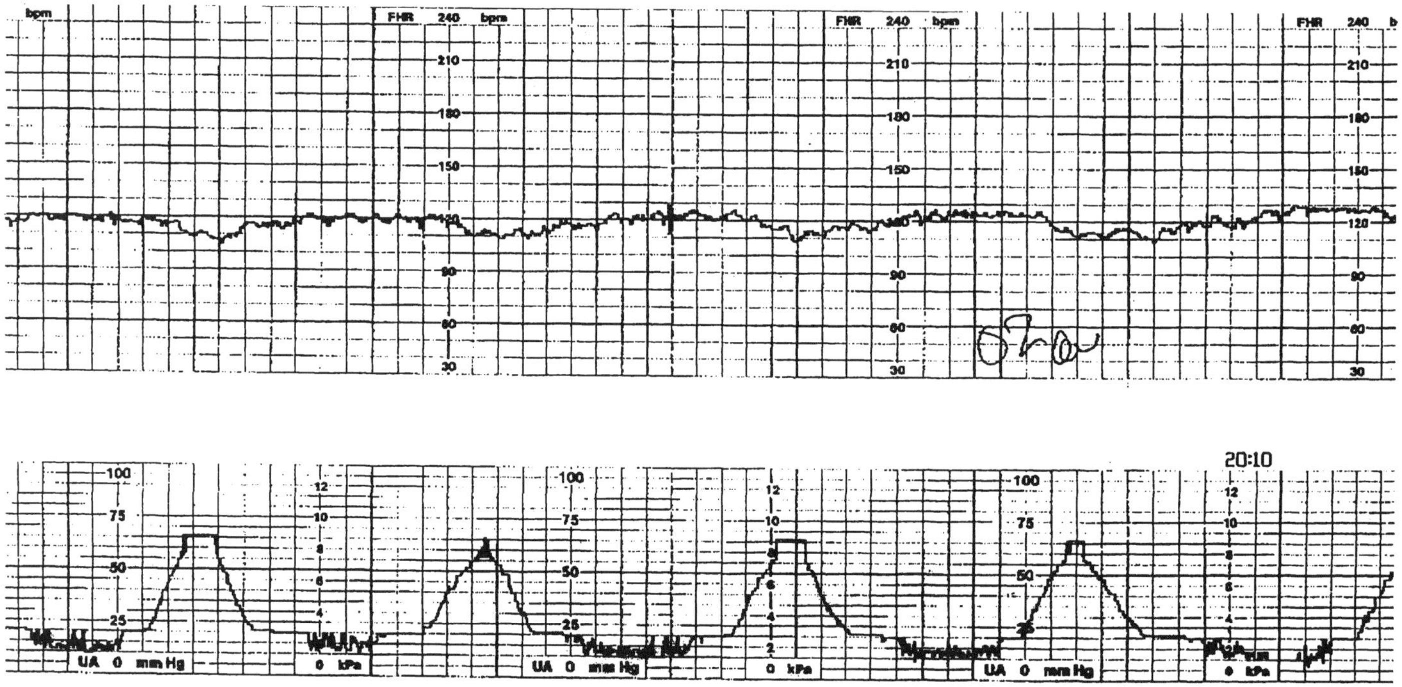

9.2 The baseline is 118-120 bpm and 120-125 bpm. Short-term variability and early decelerations are present. Was oxygen needed? Note the contraction peak to deceleration nadir lag time is less than 18 seconds.

DOCUMENTATION

Document "early decels." Since all early decelerations represent head compression, their duration and depth are not clinically significant. Therefore, there is no need to document duration and depth. Oxygen is not needed since the fetus is not hypoxic. Be sure to document signs of fetal well-being such as fetal movement, accelerations, and short-term varibility.

Review the prenatal record. Has there been a greater than 40 pound weight gain or diabetes during this pregnancy? Is she small in stature? Could there be CPD? Estimate fetal weight. Does it suggest the possibility of macrosomia? Measure fundal height. Does it seem high for gestational age?

Plot a labor curve. (See Section 4). Is descent delayed? If so, there may be CPD.

Document your findings regarding dilatation, effacement, station, caput, and molding. Notify the midwife or physician of caput and/or molding and any concerns you may have regarding fetal fit. For example, "Early decels. 5' 3", 185 lbs., EFW (estimated fetal weight) 8 lbs., 5/90%/0 with caput, no molding. Midwife notified of early decels and SVE (sterile vaginal examination) findings. No further orders at this time. Plan is to continue observation of dilatation and descent."

WHEN EARLY DECELS ARE DOCUMENTED BUT THE HEAD IS NOT COMPRESSED

What if after your SVE you decide the fetal head is high and not compressed? Or, what if she is only dilated 2 to 3 cm? Then the most likely cause of the vagal response or deceleration was cord compression. If "early decels" was charted, don't change your entry. We document the picture we see then confirm with our actions. A logical assumption is the cord is compressed. Try a position change to see which position results in smaller decelerations. Then look for short-term variability. Palpate fetal movement, and note any accelerations (all signs of fetal well-being). Document these signs of fetal well-being, i.e., fetal movement, accelerations, and short-term variability.

SUMMARY

Summary

Early decelerations are a vagal response. They usually occur during contractions and between 4 to 7 cm of dilatation. They are associated with CPD and as long as there are accelerations, fetal movement, and STV, the overall pattern is a reassuring pattern reflective of a nonhypoxic fetus. Be concerned about CPD, arrested labor progress, caput, and molding. If the head is not compressed, the vagal response is most likely caused by umbilical cord compression.

SECTION 9: EARLY DECELERATIONS

QUESTIONS

Directions: Circle T if the statement is true, F if it is false.

QUESTIONS			
T	F	1.	Early decelerations occur during the antepartal period.
T	F	2.	Early decelerations often occur when the cervix is dilated 1-3 cm.
T	F	3.	Early decelerations are associated with cephalopelvic disproportion.
T	F	4.	Caput can occur before rupture of the membranes.
T	F	5.	It is important to document the depth and duration of early decelerations.
T	F	6.	If the fetal head is not compressed but the decelerations meet all the criteria of early decelerations, the next most likely cause of the decelerations is cord compression.
T	F	7.	Early decelerations result from decreased intracranial pressure and increased blood flow through the cerebral blood vessels.
T	F	8.	Early decelerations may be the result of pressure on the posterior fontanel.
T	F	9.	Early decelerations are a precursor of possible brain trauma.
T	F	10.	Early decelerations only occur when there is caput and molding.

SECTION 10
Late Decelerations (Late decels)

PERIODIC DECELERATIONS/WITH CONTRACTIONS	
Pressure is on the	Type of Deceleration
• fetal head	• early
• **uterine vessels**	• **late**
• umbilical cord	• variable

A late deceleration is caused by fetal hypoxia due to diminished blood flow through uterine or placental vessels. This diminished blood flow is called uteroplacental insufficiency. Late decelerations are periodic in their timing, i.e., they only occur in response to contractions which squeeze maternal spiral arteries (arteries in the uterus) decreasing oxygen to the placenta. Late decelerations may also be a response to placental abruption. There can be just one late deceleration, an intermittent appearance of a late deceleration, or repetitive late decelerations. Five or more late decelerations in a row is called a pattern of late decelerations.

RECOGNITION CRITERIA

Recognition Criteria

Late decelerations are usually similar in shape from one to the next. Some are curved, some are shaped like a U or V, and some may appear "boxy." Late decelerations last up to 2 minutes. A deceleration that lasts longer than 2 minutes is called a prolonged deceleration. Prolonged decelerations are discussed in Section 12. You do **not** need internal monitors to determine if a late deceleration exists. You just need to recognize them and document them as late decelerations.

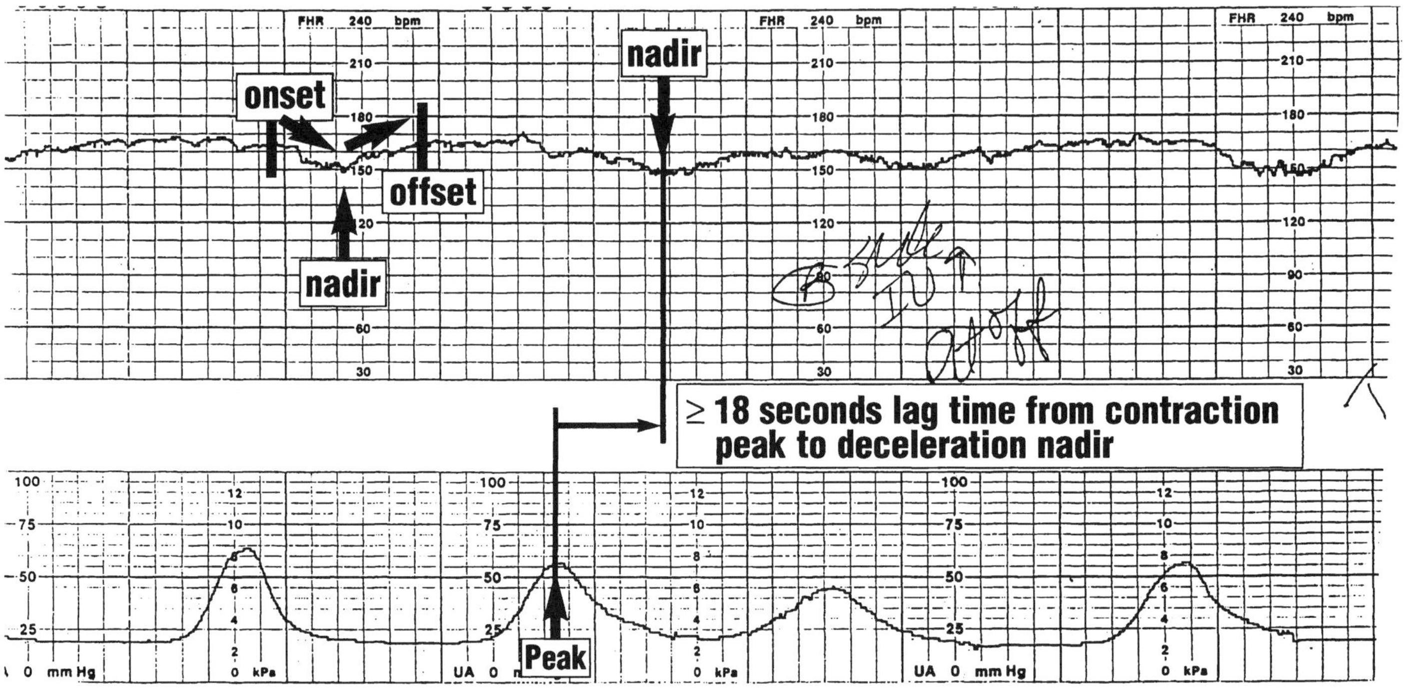

10.1 Late decelerations. The nurse responded appropriately by turning the woman to her right side, increasing the intravenous fluid flow rate, and discontinuing pitocin®.

A late deceleration has a slanted, gradual onset but may have an abrupt recovery or offset. **Late decelerations begin after the contraction begins. The lowest point of the deceleration or nadir is always ≥ 18 seconds after the contraction peak.** When a tocotransducer is used to assess contractions, the uterine activity waveform may last longer than the actual contraction. As a result, the late deceleration appears to return to the baseline (BL) before the contraction ends, even though all late decelerations return to the baseline after the contraction ends. The appearance of a contraction that lasts longer than its actual duration may be due to the woman arching her back or tightening her abdominal muscles which increases abdominal pressure on the tocotransducer. Palpate the uterus. Adjust the TOCO. Document on the tracing the actual end of the contraction if you can.

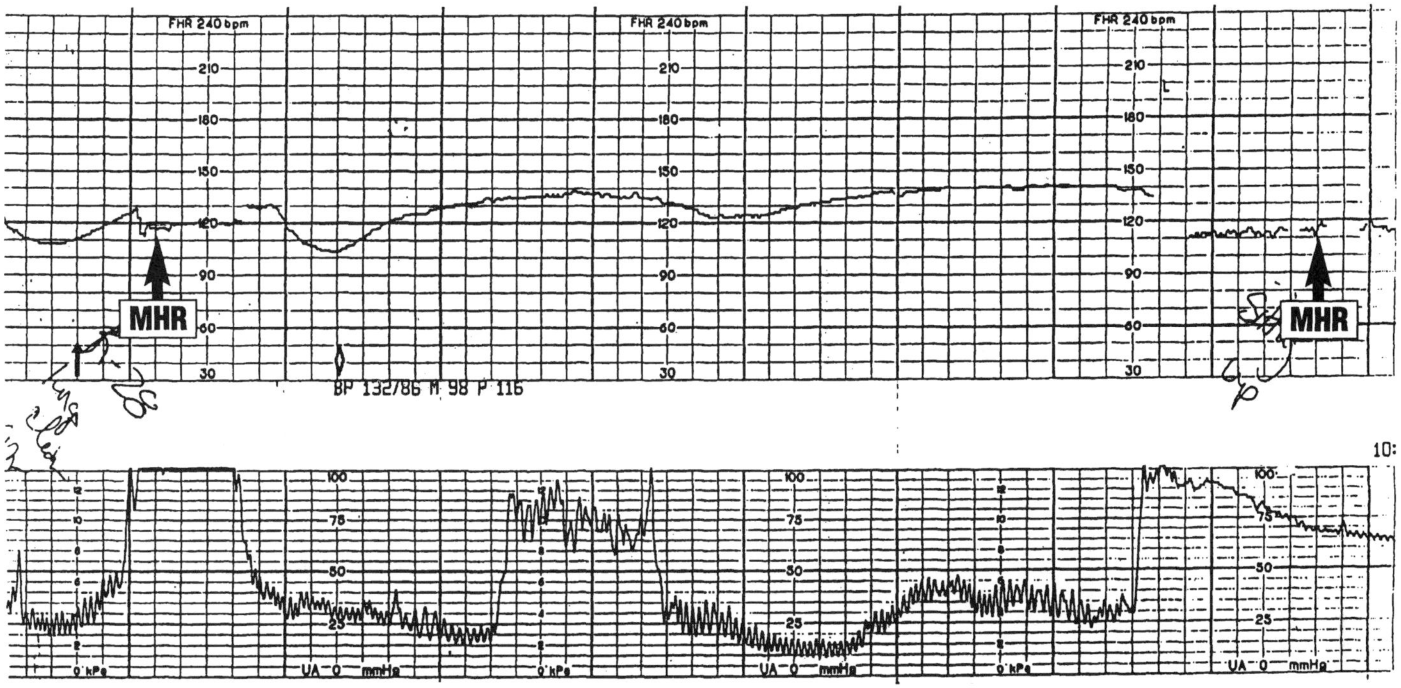

10.2 During pushing with the first contraction, the maternal heart rate (MHR) of approximately 120 bpm is recorded. It is also recorded in the last minute of the strip. These late decelerations reach their nadir in 20-25 seconds. The nadir is ≥ 18 seconds after the contraction peak. The deceleration is back to baseline after the contraction ends. The decelerations are similar in shape.

PHYSIOLOGY

During a contraction, especially those stronger than 35 mm Hg, oxygen delivery to the fetus is significantly curtailed. Well-oxygenated fetuses have oxygen reserves and maintain a normal FHR during and after contractions. When a fetus has borderline oxygen reserves, a late deceleration may appear. Inadequate oxygen delivery to the fetus is called *uteroplacental insufficiency*. **The fetus is hypoxic**. The presence of a reactive acceleration does not rule out a late deceleration but merely demonstrates the fetus is not metabolically acidotic yet.

The lack of oxygen may originate from a maternal cause such as uterine hyperstimulation and/or hypertonus, or a placental cause such as villous edema, avascular villi, or placental calcifications or infarcts which can occur in women who smoke or who have diseases such as anticardiolipin antibody syndrome or lupus erythematosus. If hypoxia persists, eventually there will be a loss of accelerations and short-term variability. At that point, the fetus is probably acidotic. Contractions cut off the oxygen supply and the metabolically acidotic fetal heart rate slows in response.

This flow diagram illustrates an example of a maternal cause of late decelerations.

Insufficient cardiac output

▼

Decreased uterine perfusion

▼

Deficient placental perfusion

▼

Decreased oxygen delivery

▼

Late deceleration(s)

ONE OR MORE LATE DECELERATIONS

There can be just one late deceleration, especially if only one contraction occurs. Usually, a series of late decelerations are seen. Five or more late decelerations are called a *pattern of lates*. Late decelerations may occur in response to maternal hypotension. If so, accelerations and short-term variability (STV) may be seen with late decelerations. Assess the maternal blood pressure (BP). If a drug such as ephedrine is needed to increase BP, call the anesthesia provider.

RULES ABOUT LATE DECELERATIONS

Rules

- there can be just one late deceleration
- accelerations and short-term variability (STV) may exist, even with late decelerations (nonacidotic but hypoxic fetus)
- if there is a "shoulder" before or after the decel, it is NOT a late deceleration (it is a variable deceleration)
- late decelerations only occur with contractions
- late decels are *usually* similar in shape from one to the next
- an intrauterine pressure catheter is NOT needed to call a deceleration a late deceleration
- a deceleration $\geq$ 2 minutes is a prolonged deceleration not a late deceleration.

When late decelerations first appear, the fetus may be well-oxygenated, i.e., accelerations, movement, and STV are present.

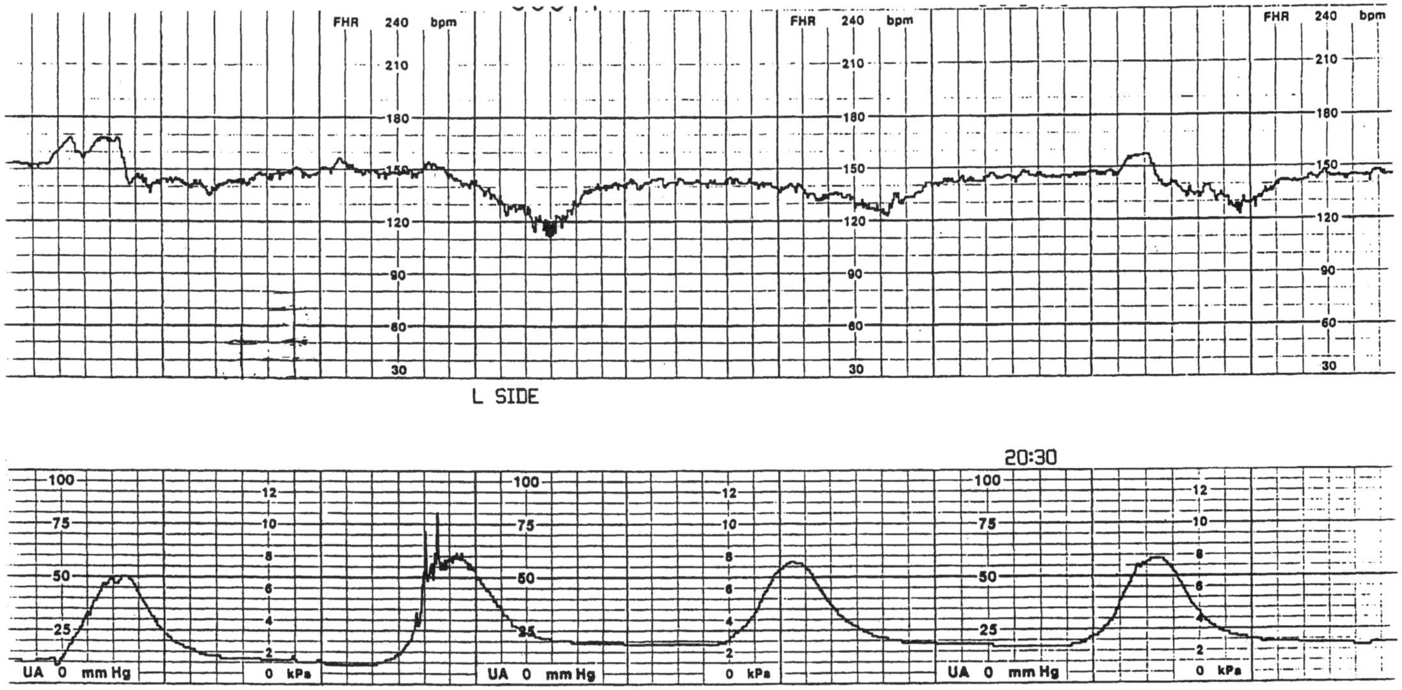

10.3 Accelerations, short-term variability, and three late decelerations.

There may be hypotension due to a supine position or after epidural medication. After repositioning the woman off her back, e.g., to her side, assess blood pressure. If not contraindicated, a bolus of lactated Ringer's solution should increase blood pressure, improve uterine perfusion, and alleviate late decelerations. Supplemental oxygen may be needed if the late decelerations do not quickly disappear, and the physician or midwife should be promptly notified.

As the hypoxic stressor continues (and late decels continue), accelerations cease. As the risk of metabolic acidosis increases, long-term variability and short-term variability decrease. Then the baseline may rise or fall. If there is a reactive acceleration, the fetus is hypoxic but not metabolically acidotic (see 10.3). Since the risk of metabolic acidosis is high, the FHR pattern demands prompt action to improve fetal oxygenation. So, as the fetus becomes more hypoxic you will see:

- 1st late decels
- 2nd loss of accels
- 3rd loss of variability
- 4th baseline rises or falls.

ACTIONS

Actions in Response to Late Decelerations

To improve fetal oxygenation, actions are directed at finding the source of hypoxia and increasing *maternal blood flow* to the uterus while increasing *blood oxygen content.* If the placenta is abrupting, an expeditious delivery is required.

The first action is to position the woman off her back. She may lie on either her right or left side as either side produces a similar cardiac output. Once repositioned, pitocin® and amnioinfusion should be discontinued. Blood pressure should be assessed. If hypertension exists prior to late decelerations, position her on her side where her BP is lowest. Do not place her in Trendelenburg as this position decreases cardiac output. Avoid the elbows and knees (knee-chest) position if you think the uterus is rupturing as gravity may cause the fetal weight to extend the rupture.

Actions Related to Improving Maternal Blood Flow and Fetal Oxygen Delivery
• **change position**
• **discontinue oxytocics** or prostaglandins if possible
• **discontinue amnioinfusion**
• **take blood pressure**
• provide **a fluid bolus** (≥ 400 ml of lactated Ringer's solution is common) unless a fluid bolus is contraindicated due to an increased risk of pulmonary edema, e.g., preeclampsia or heart disease
• **administer supplemental oxygen** by a tight-fitting mask
• **ephedrine®** 5-10 mg IVP slowly as ordered for hypotension
• **terbutaline®** as ordered (0.25 mg IV push slowly or subcutaneous) if there is no abruption

If late decelerations began just after the amnioinfusion was initiated, discontinue the infusion. Sometimes fluid pressure on the inside uterine wall impedes oxygen delivery as vessels in the uterus are compressed.

Once the woman is on her side and pitocin® and/or prostaglandins are discontinued, apply a tight-fitting face mask. Ask her to breathe deeply and slowly. If a simple mask is used, oxygen (0_2) should flow through the mask at 8 to 10 liters per minute. If, on the other hand, an oxygen mask with a reservoir (partial rebreathing mask) is used, 0_2 should flow at 12 liters per minute (to prevent carbon dioxide from entering the reservoir bag). A simple 0_2 mask is most common.

It takes 1 to 9 minutes for oxygen to reach the fetus. Observe the FHR pattern 10 minutes after you initiated oxygen. An improvement in the FHR pattern, e.g., late decels disappear or decrease in number or accelerations reappear, tells you the 0_2 reached the fetus. Of course, a worsening of the pattern tells you otherwise and delivery may need to be expedited. Nurses should promptly inform the midwife or physician of the FHR pattern and actions taken.

ASSESS FETAL WELL-BEING: SCALP STIMULATION

Assess Fetal Well-being

Scalp stimulation may be done instead of scalp pH sampling. Scalp stimulation should be done **between** contractions and **between** decelerations to assess fetal acid-base status. If a 15 seconds x 15 bpm (reactive) acceleration occurs, the fetus is not yet metabolically acidotic at that time.

pH sampling has inherent errors. pH results depend on the presence of caput, timing of the blood collection, and the physician's skill and technique. Most hospitals do not have the equipment to perform a scalp pH. A normal pH may exist even when the fetus is hypoxic. **A reactive acceleration following scalp puncture is a more accurate reflection of acid-base status than a normal pH**, since maternal hyperventilation or slow collection of the sample may result in an erroneously high pH when the fetus is not well.

SPIRAL ELECTRODE TEST

Another noninvasive technique to assess fetal status is to pull on the spiral electrode five times. If the fetus has a reactive acceleration, metabolic acidosis is not present.

DOCUMENTATION

When you observe late decelerations, it is common to document "late decels." All late decels, regardless of their depth, represent fetal hypoxia due to uteroplacental insufficiency. Some research suggests *"The deeper the late, the lower the pH."* After documenting "late decels," record all the actions you initiated, the maternal and fetal response, and your communications.

You might chart something like:

Following epidural placement, late decels noted @ 1428. Mom to L side. BP 90/58. CRNA notified. 5 mg ephedrine IVP per CRNA. LR IV ⇑d via IV pump. pitocin® DCd. 0_2 @ 10 LPM. 1440 no lates noted, BP 120/80. 0_2 mask removed. FM (fetal movement) +, STV +. N. Nurse RNC

Another note might read:

Late decels noted @ 1700 following 5 minutes of uterine hyperstimulation. Complains of sharp, unrelenting abd pain, 5 cm blood clot noted. To R side, 0_2 at 10 LPM. Dr. Caring paged to come to L & D stat. IV started in L cephalic vein with #18 cath. LR bolus initiated. Charge nurse notified of FHR pattern and suspected abruption. N. Nurse RNC

Ideally, uterine contractions should appear as a waveform in the uterine activity channel. If decelerations appear but contractions are not recorded, palpate for uterine activity. Reposition the tocotransducer. It may also be necessary to insert an intrauterine pressure catheter (IUPC). However, an IUPC is not needed to see or document late decelerations.

Examples of Late Decelerations

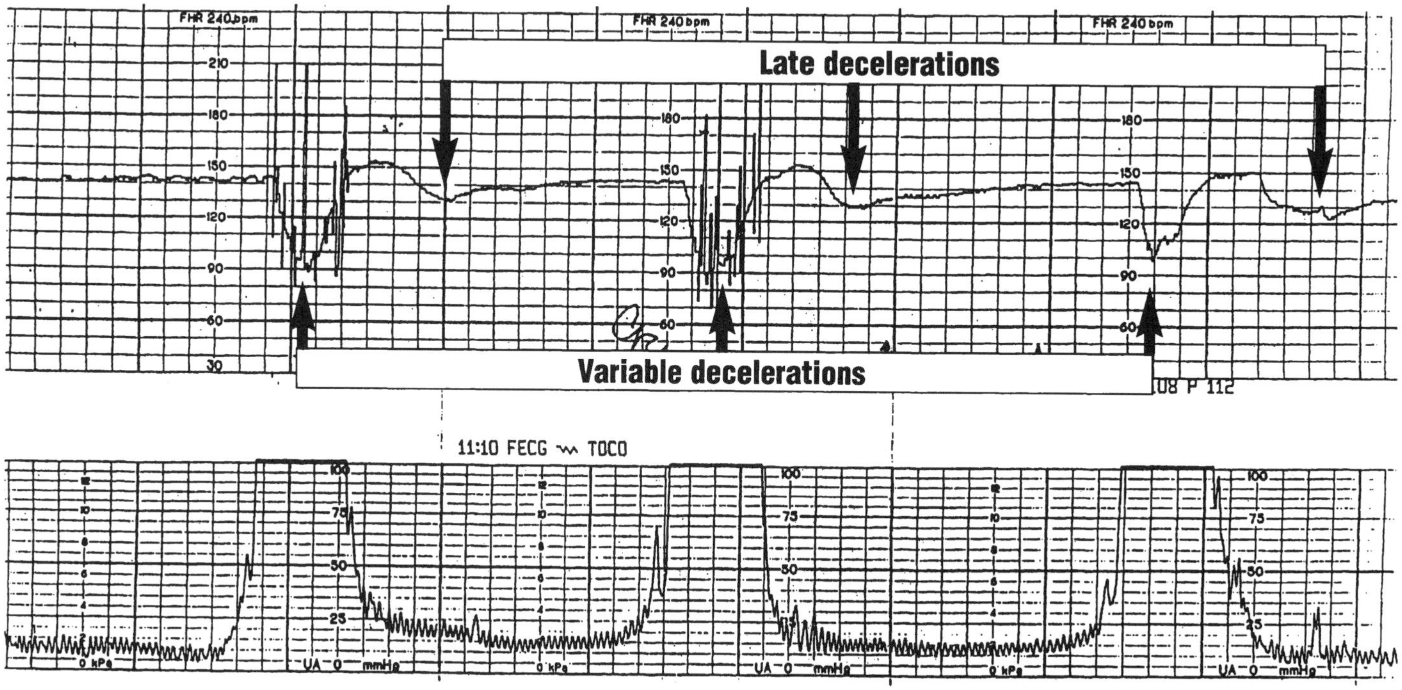

10.4 ***Note that the onset to nadir duration of these late decelerations lasts 15 to 30 seconds and the contraction peak to nadir lag time is ≥ 18 seconds. When two types of decelerations occur in a repeating sequence, this is a mixed deceleration pattern or a combination or combined deceleration pattern.***

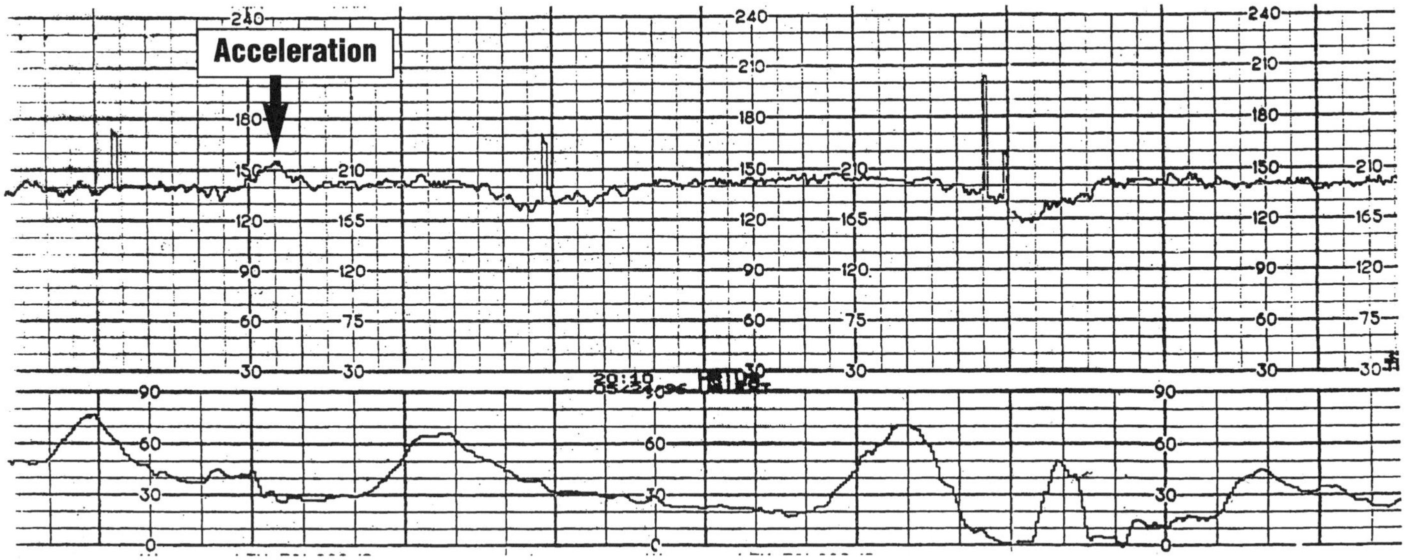

10.5 A nearly reactive acceleration with late decelerations suggests the fetus is hypoxic but not metabolically acidotic.

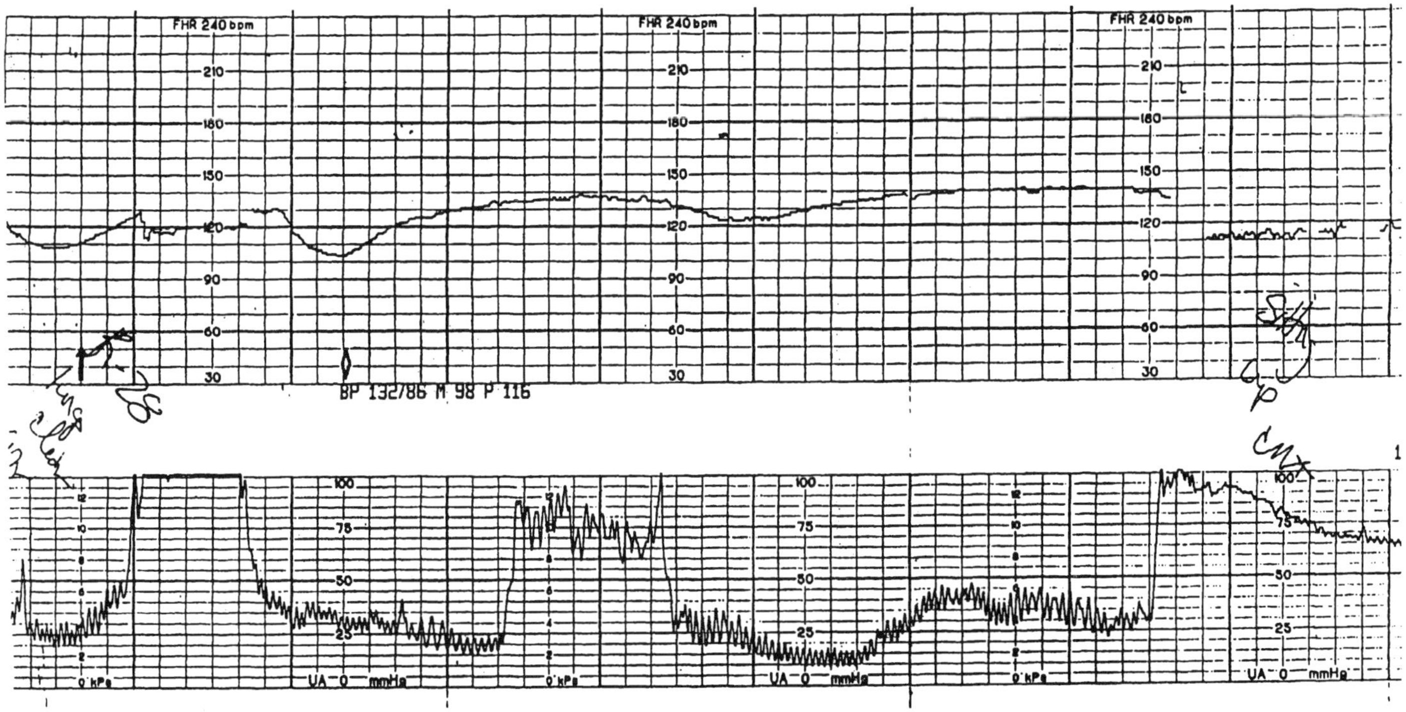

10.6 ***During the first contraction, the maternal heart rate is recorded near 120 bpm followed by a late deceleration to 105 bpm at its nadir. The next late deceleration drops to 122 bpm. After the last contraction, the woman sits up and the ultrasound transducer moves to her aorta. The maternal heart rate is recorded at 100-118 bpm.***

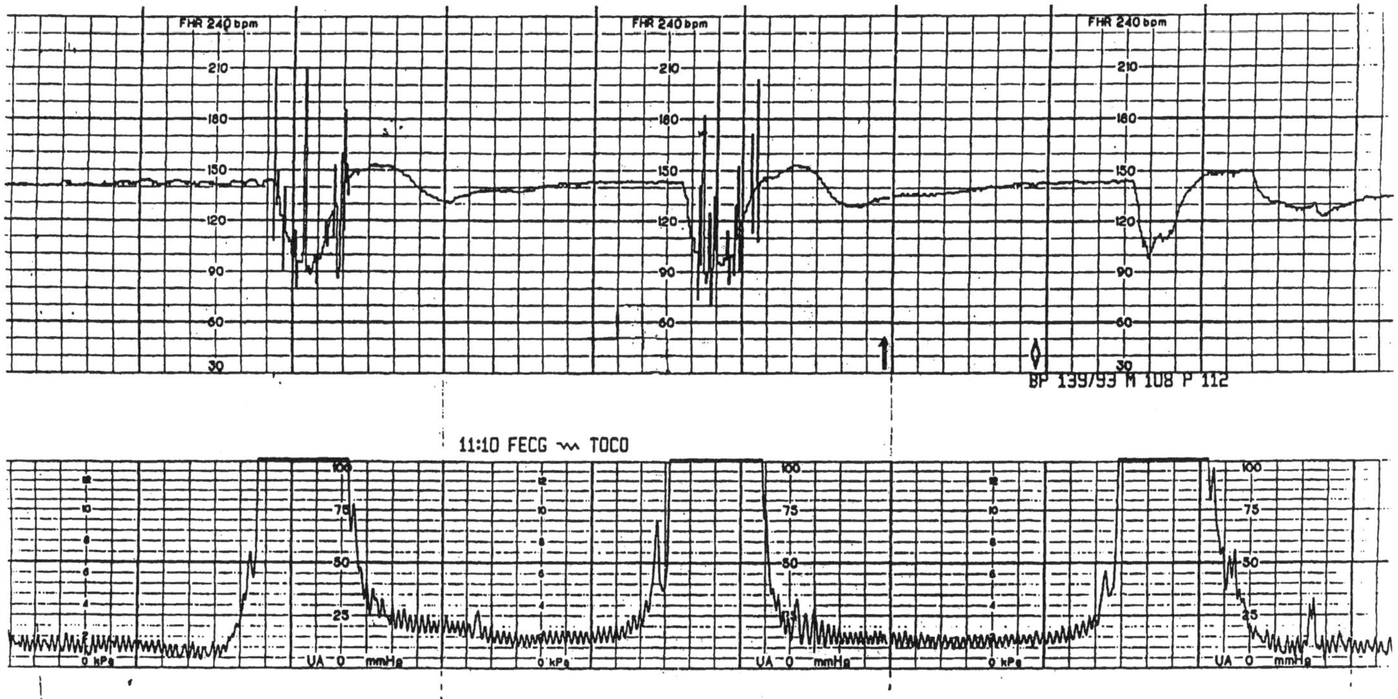

10.7 After the spiral electrode was applied, variable decelerations are evident during contractions, followed by late decelerations. There is absent short-term variability and absent to minimal long-term variability. When two types of decelerations consecutively occur, this is called a mixed, combination or combined deceleration pattern.

CORD/ PLACENTAL GASES

To confirm the fetal and placental status just prior to birth, blood gases are obtained. Umbilical cord artery or placental artery blood reflects fetal blood gases or fetal status and venous blood reflects placental blood gases or placental status prior to birth. A syringe heparinized with 1000 U/ml heparin is used. Using 10,000U/ml heparin produces erroneous results. Usually only 1 ml of blood is needed but it is best to ask laboratory personnel what they need. The blood gases are stable in the syringe at room temperature up to one hour after their collection. However, laboratory standards require the blood be analyzed within 60 minutes after their collection. Laboratory personnel also like the syringe to be placed in a slush of ice. To not do so does not change results.

PLACENTAL PATHOLOGY

Since an abnormal placenta may be the primary cause of uteroplacental insufficiency, it may be helpful to send the placenta to pathology. On the request, include pertinent risk or history information and indications for the pathology study. The physician may request **center cuts** of the placenta as the placenta ages from the external edges, and/or the physician may request **cross cut sections** of the umbilical cord. These requests ensure quality slides for accurate placental diagnosis by skilled pathologists. Never place the placenta in formalin because it discolors the tissue when meconium staining is present. Record the location of newborn staining, e.g., the fingernails, vernix, or cord, and amniotic fluid as the staining reflects the length of time the fetus was exposed to meconium.

Reflex Late Decelerations

Dr. Julian Parer has suggested there are two kinds of late decelerations: reflex late decelerations and hypoxic myocardial failure late decelerations.

REFLEX LATE DECELERATIONS

A reflex late decel accompanies a stable baseline with short-term variability. The offset of reflex late decelerations may be gradual or abrupt. Accels may precede or follow this type of late deceleration pattern. The fetus is hypoxic but not metabolically acidotic.

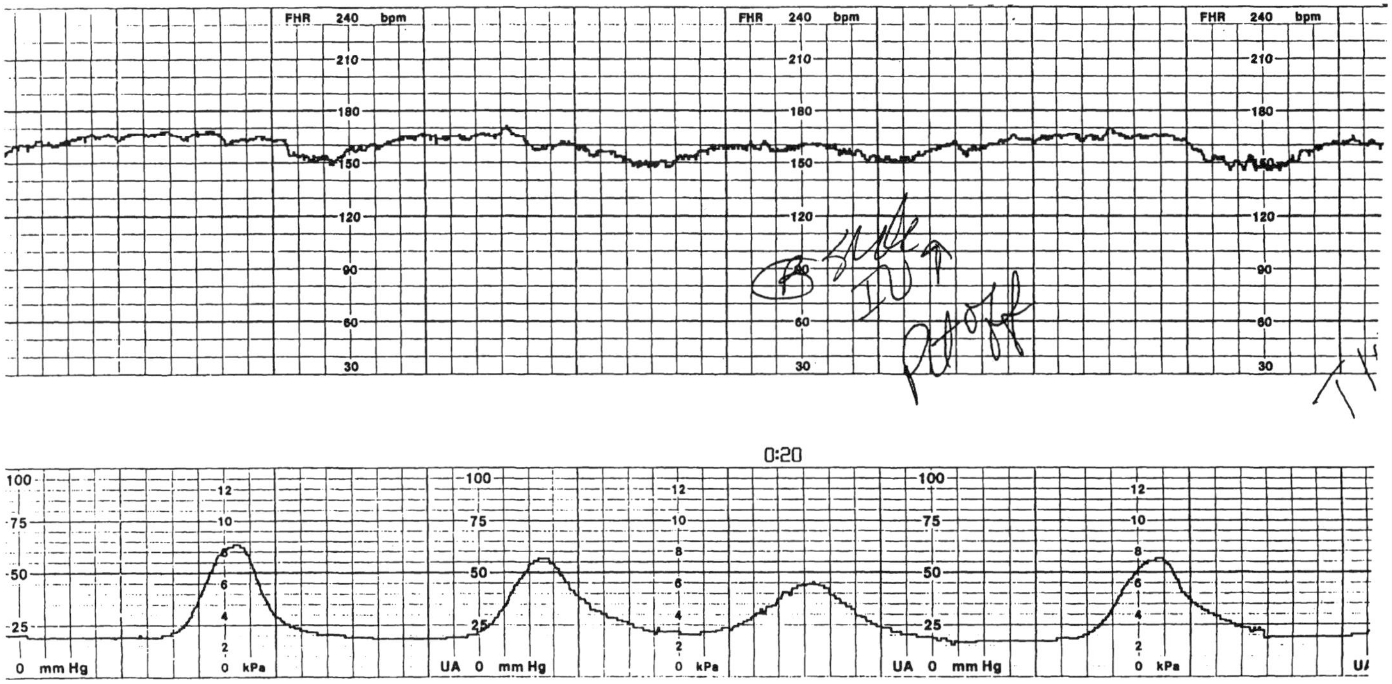

10.8 ***Short-term variability in the baseline suggests the fetus is hypoxic but not metabolically acidotic. These are reflex late decelerations. Note the contraction peak to deceleration nadir lag time is ≥ 18 seconds. The baseline is tachycardic. Appropriate actions were to position the woman on her right side, increase the intravenous fluid flow rate, discontinue pitocin®, and call the midwife and/or physician.***

HYPOXIC MYOCARDIAL FAILURE LATE DECELERATIONS

Hypoxic Myocardial Late Decelerations

When lates appear and short-term variability is absent, the fetus is metabolically acidotic and should be promptly delivered. This pattern is called hypoxic myocardial failure late decelerations.

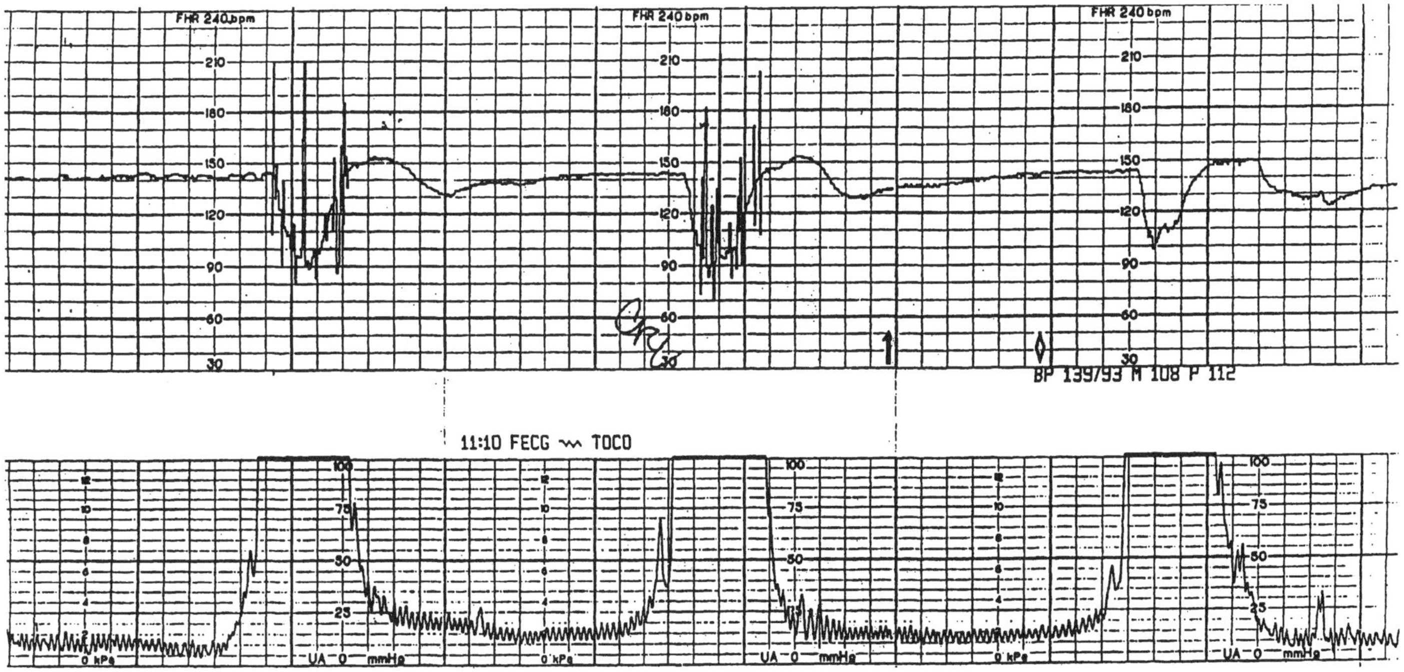

10.9 ***Hypoxic myocardial failure late decelerations. This child suffered permanent, irreversible brain damage and has cerebral palsy.***

SUMMARY

Summary

Late decelerations are periodic decelerations associated with hypoxia. They have a slanted onset, reaching their nadir in as little as 15 seconds but often in 30 or more seconds. They may have a boxy, U, or V shape. They usually last less than 2 minutes. If short-term variability is present or accelerations are present the fetus is hypoxic but not metabolically acidotic. These are classified as reflex late decelerations but are documented as "late decelerations, STV present." If short-term variability is absent, the pattern of late decelerations reflects metabolic acidosis and has been called hypoxic myocardial failure late decelerations. They are documented as "late decelerations, STV absent." Whenever late decelerations occur, actions to improve oxygen delivery to the fetus should be initiated. These include a position change; discontinuance of oxytocics, prostaglandins, and amnioinfusion; assessment of blood pressure, providing ephedrine as ordered, an intravenous bolus of a non-glucose solution, oxygen by a tight-fitting face mask, and terbutaline® as ordered provided there is no abruption. Terbutaline® can mask an abruption or extend the abruption. Oxygen should be in the fetus by 10 minutes after it is initiated. Document late decelerations and other FHR pattern characteristics, all actions, communications, and the fetal and maternal response.

SECTION 10: LATE DECELERATIONS

QUESTIONS

Directions: Circle T if the statement is true, F if it is false.

QUESTIONS			
T	F	1.	Late decelerations all have a gradual onset and offset.
T	F	2.	All late decelerations begin at or after the peak of the contraction.
T	F	3.	Late decelerations are often similar in shape.
T	F	4.	If short-term variability is present, they are not late decelerations.
T	F	5.	If accelerations are present, they are not late decelerations.
T	F	6.	It takes 15 minutes for supplemental oxygen to reach the fetus.
T	F	7.	Hypotension may precede late decelerations.
T	F	8.	Late decelerations may last more than 2 minutes.
T	F	9.	Late decelerations are indicative of fetal hypoxia.

SECTION 11
Variable Decelerations (Variable decels)

Pressure on	Type of Deceleration
• fetal head	• early
• uterine vessels	• late
• **umbilical cord**	• **variable**

Variable decelerations vary in shape, depth, and duration and can occur with or between contractions.

DEFINITION AND RECOGNITION CRITERIA OF A VARIABLE DECELERATION

A variable deceleration is a U, V, or W shaped drop in the fetal heart rate that lasts 15 or more seconds and drops 15 or more bpm. The deceleration duration is the time between the descent and the recovery at the baseline level. A prompt recovery is a nadir to baseline time of 8 to 27 seconds. Since it is hard to see 27 seconds, a slow recovery is 30 or more seconds.

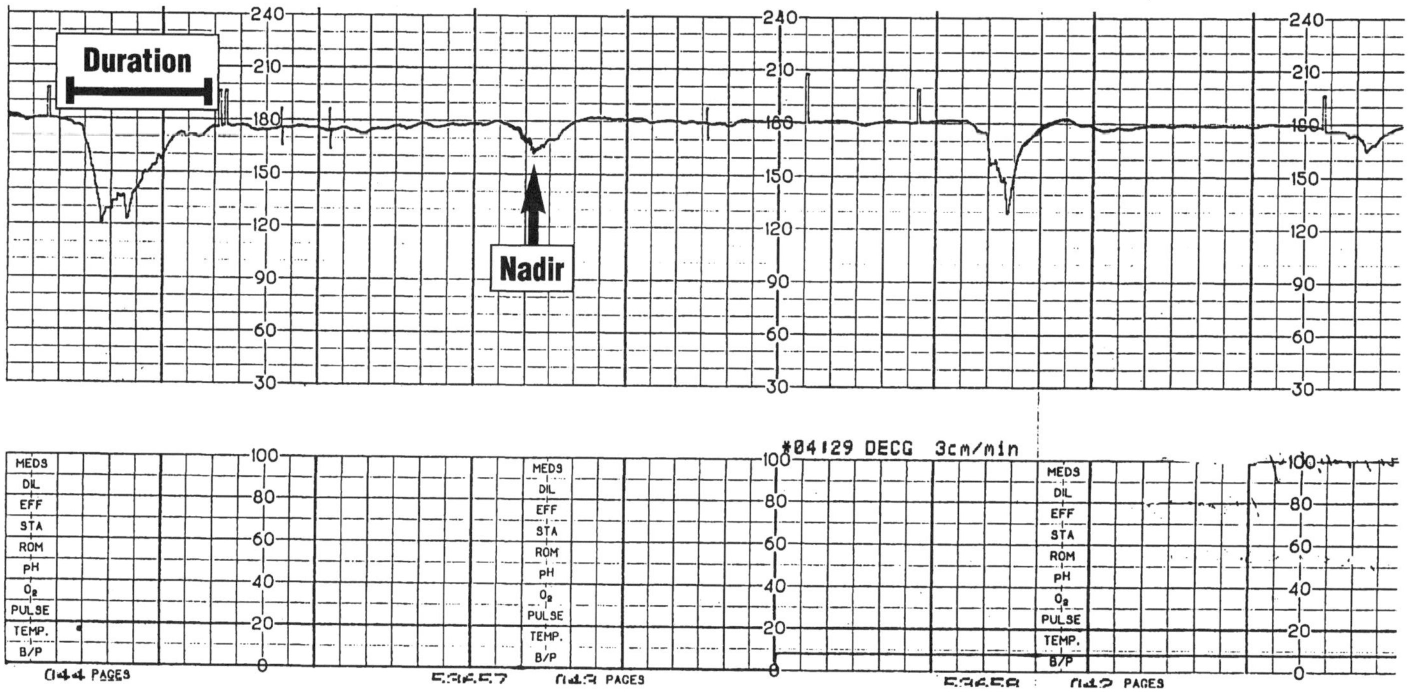

11.1 The nadir is the lowest point of a deceleration.

Anything smaller than 15 bpm x 15 seconds is called a "dip." Dips are more common in preterm fetuses. Dips have no clinical significance.

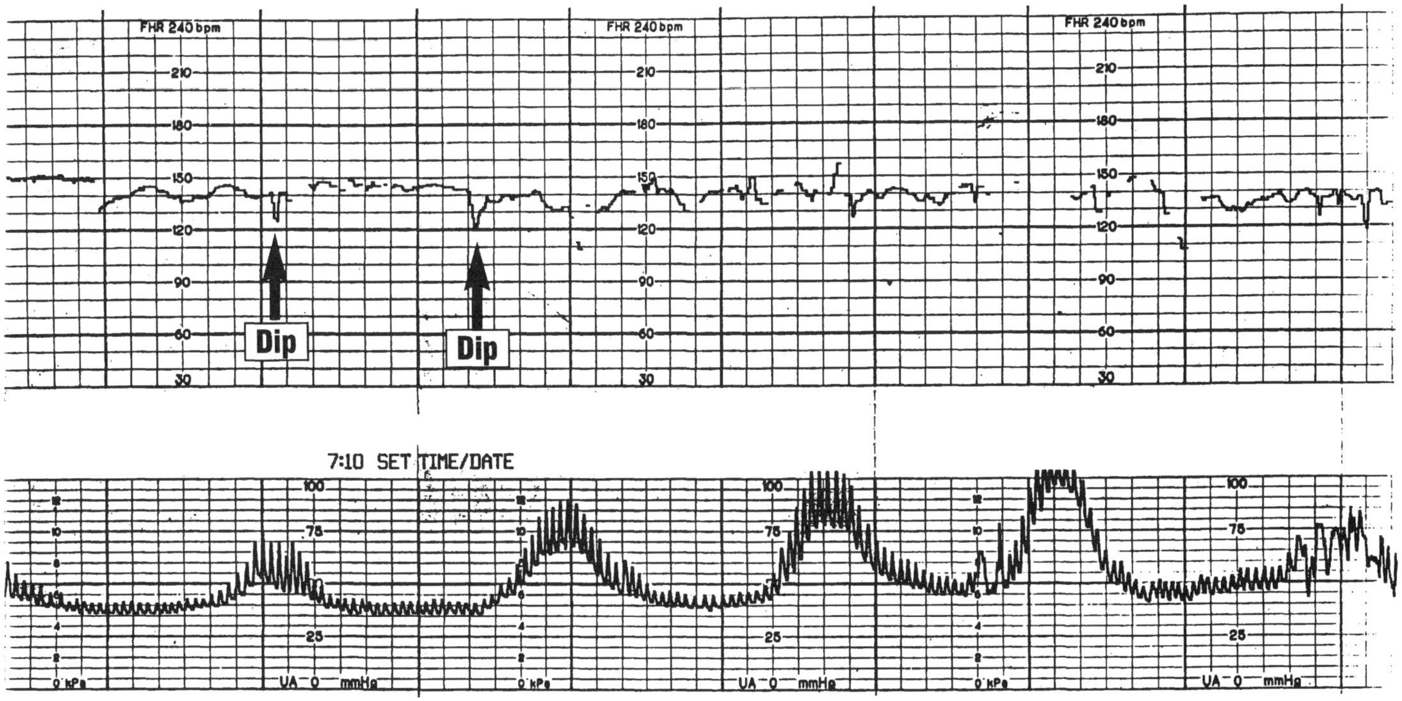

11.2 There are multiple dips present, but not decelerations. This fetus was 26 weeks of gestation and was delivered preterm.

CLINICAL SIGNIFICANCE OF VARIABLE DECELERATIONS

The clinical significance of a variable deceleration depends on the stability of the baseline, the presence or absence of baseline long-term variability (LTV) and short-term variability (STV), the presence of accelerations, and the timing of the deceleration, i.e., with or between uterine contraction.

Variable decelerations are usually a response to umbilical cord compression. Variable decels usually abruptly fall and recover.

During cord compression there is a change in fetal blood pressure and a decrease in fetal PaO_2, an increase in $PaCO_2$, a decrease in pH, which activates specialized nerves called baroreceptors and chemoreceptors. When recovery is slow, lasting 30 or more seconds, there is hypoxia. The fetal heart is slower to respond and the fetus needs more oxygen.

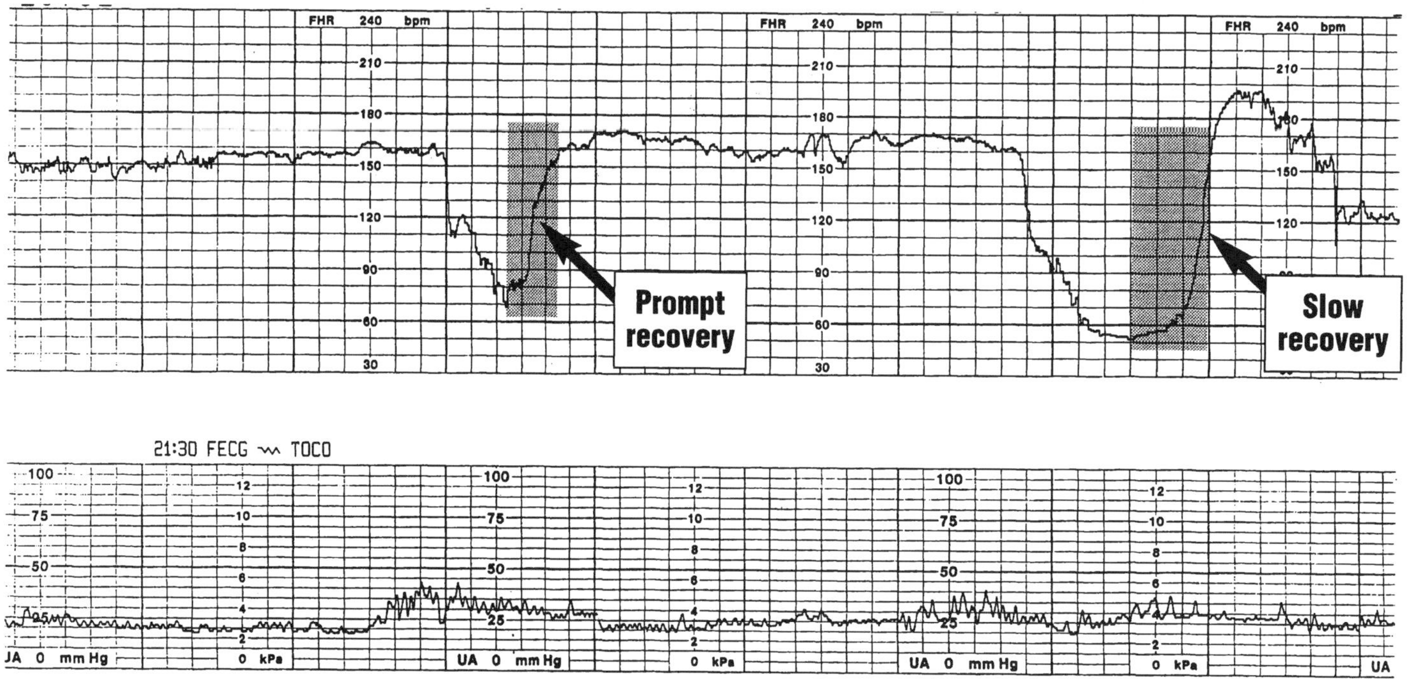

11.3 Recovery (from the nadir to the baseline) is prompt when the recovery is < 30 seconds and is slow if it is > 30 seconds. This illustration shows each type of recovery.

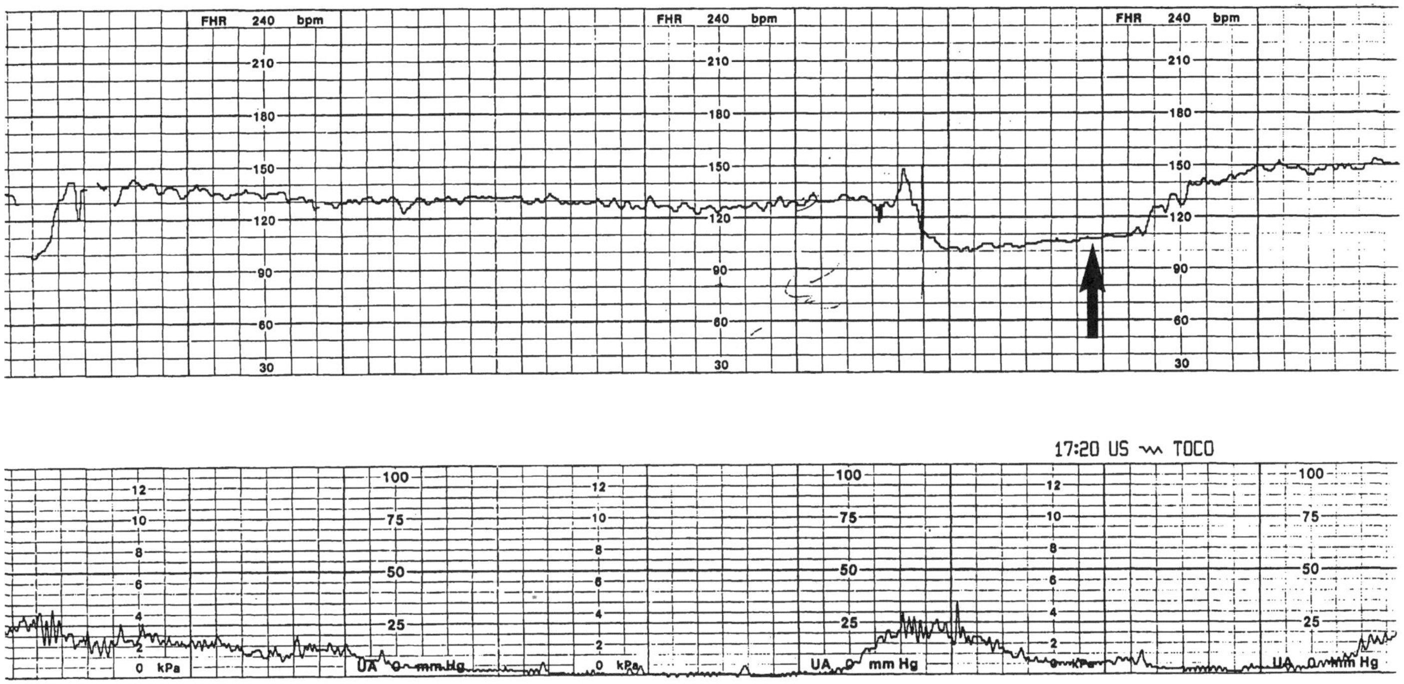

11.4 Slow recovery of a variable deceleration reflects fetal hypoxia.

SHAPES OF VARIABLE DECELERATIONS

A variable deceleration is a transient decrease in the FHR with a U, V, or W shape. A W shape has been associated with a cord that is 50 cm or longer.

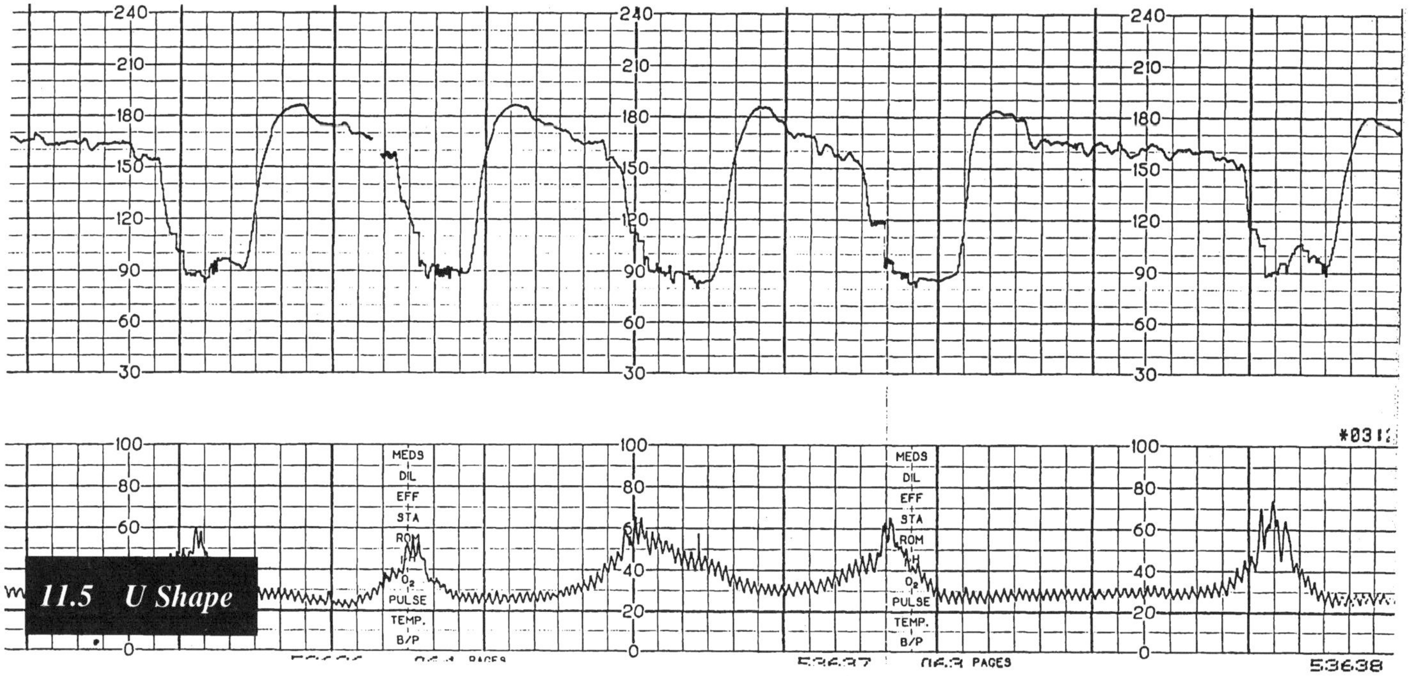

11.5 U Shape

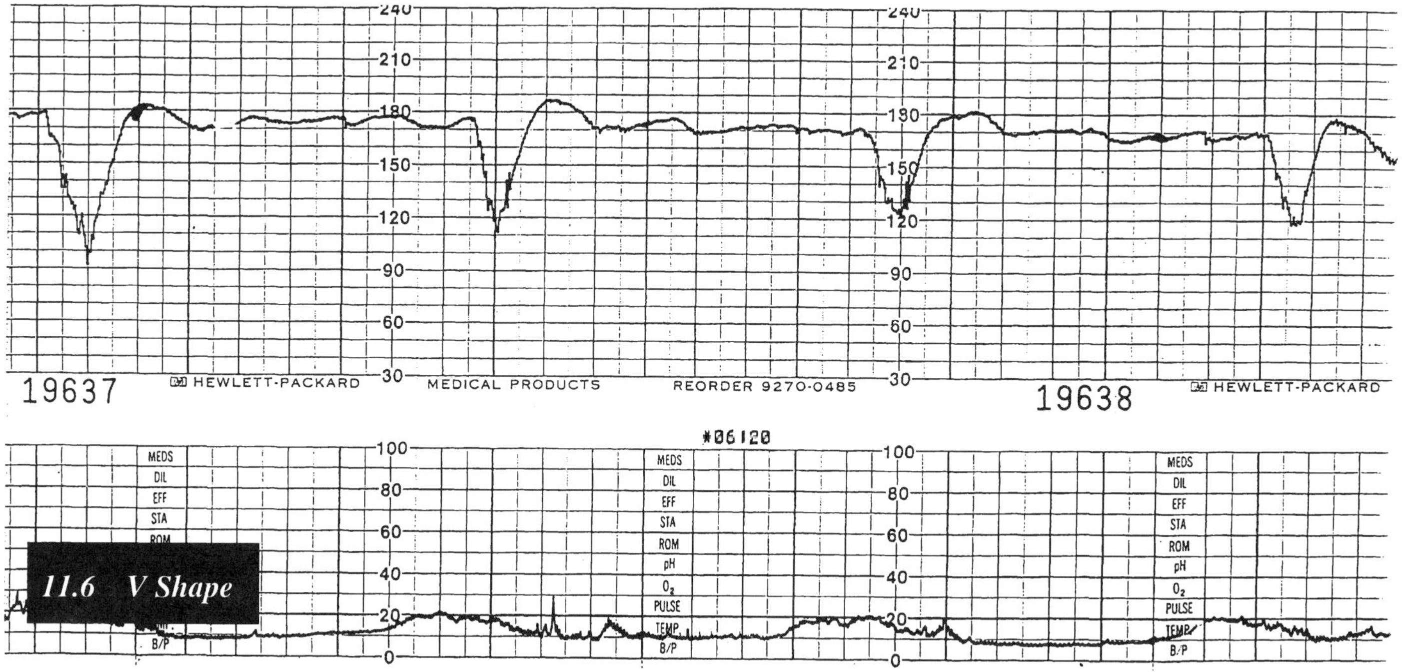

11.6 V Shape

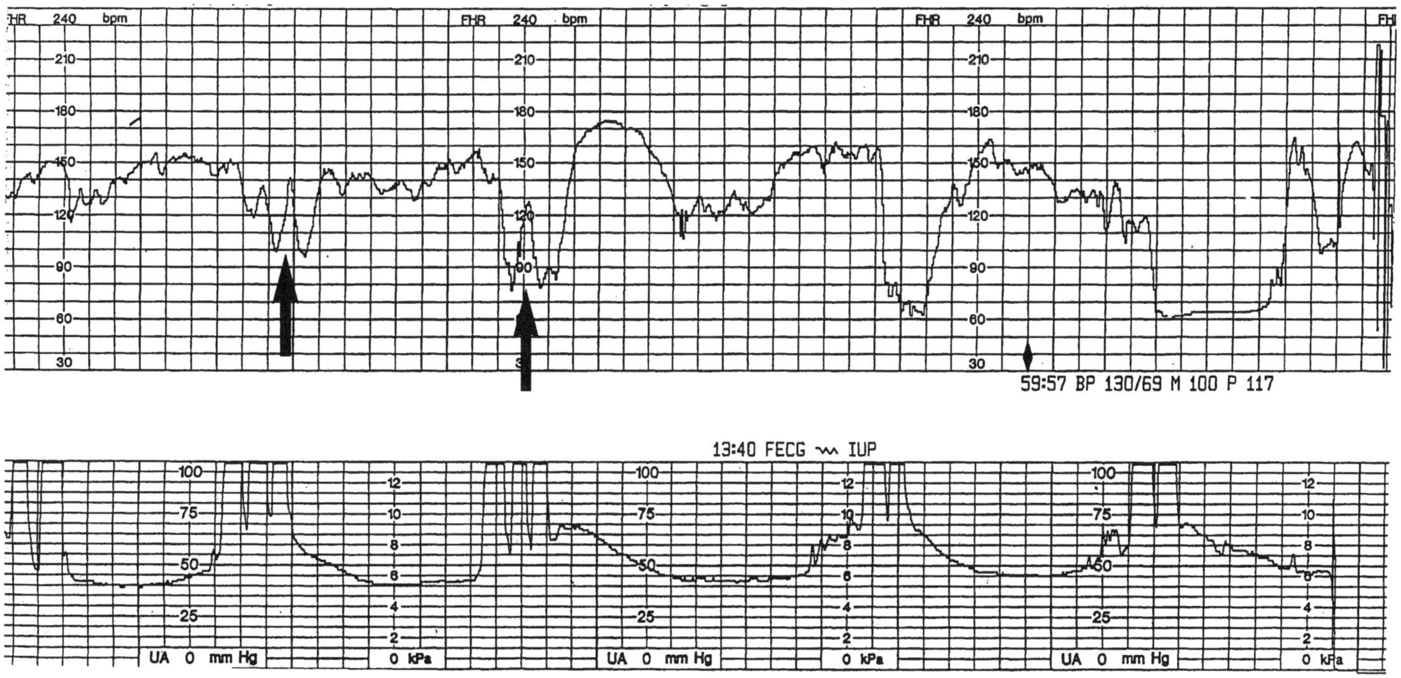

11.7 W Shape

The depth and duration of a variable decelerations is less significant in predicting Apgar scores or fetal scalp pH than the presence or absence of baseline short-term variability. The incidence of low Apgars and a compromised neonate increases when there is also

- tachycardia
- bradycardia
- decreased long-term and short-term variability
- presence of atypical variable deceleration features and/or the
- absence of accelerations.

The fetus who has any deceleration to a rate less than 80 bpm has an increased risk of hypoxia. As the rate falls, so does the fetal blood pressure and the fetus' ability to perfuse its brain. In illustration 11.3 the decelerations fell to 52 to 70 beats per minute and were less than 80 bpm for up to almost 50 seconds during the second deceleration. Hypoxia is reflected by the slow recovery and an overshoot. The fetus in this illustration is attempting to survive. Epinephrine and norepinephrine are released by the adrenal glands which produces the overshoot.

TYPICAL VARIABLE DECELERATIONS HAVE "SHOULDERS"

Typical variable decelerations are also known as classic or pure variable decelerations. They have "shoulders" on either side of the variable deceleration.

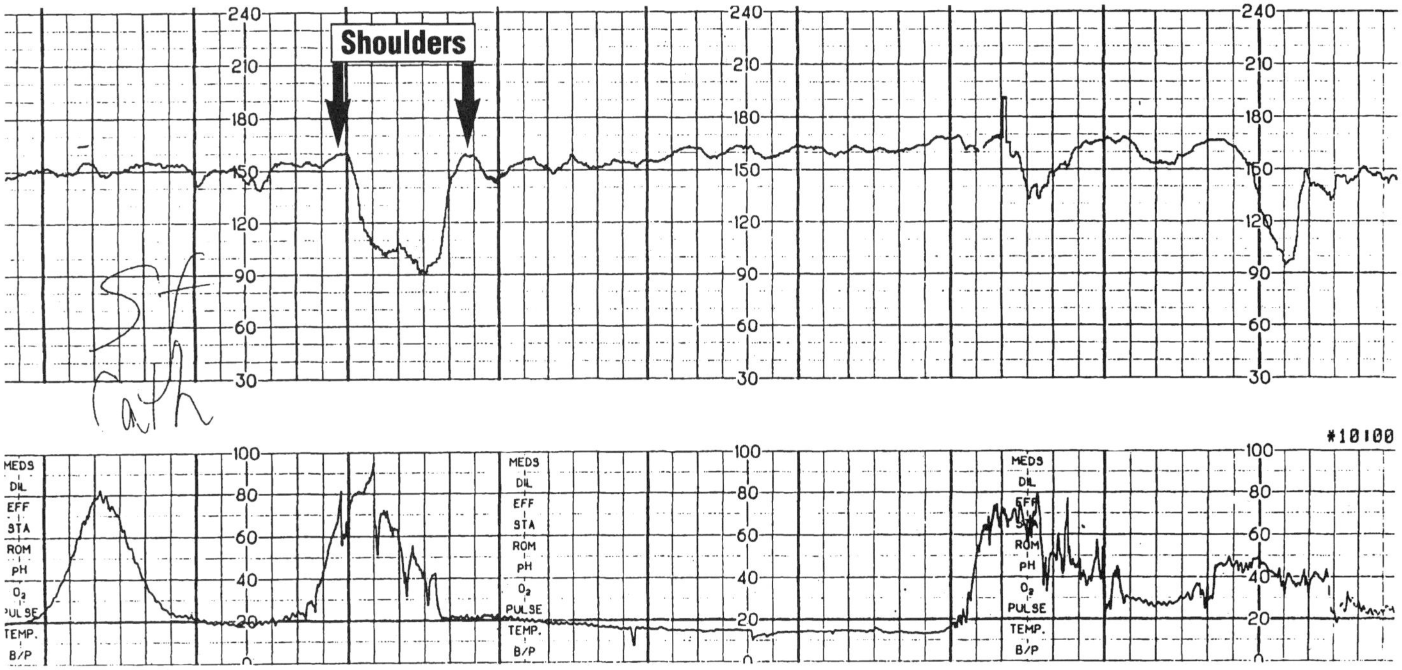

11.8 Pure variable decelerations with "shoulders."

A shoulder or increase in the FHR preceding and/or following a variable deceleration is a compensatory sign and a fetal response to umbilical **overshoots** compression.

A nonreassuring sign is an increase in the size or duration of the secondary "shoulder" following a variable deceleration. Shoulders are usually no higher than 20 bpm above the baseline and are less than or equal to 20 seconds in duration. An overshoot may be more than 20 bpm above the baseline or last longer than 20 seconds.

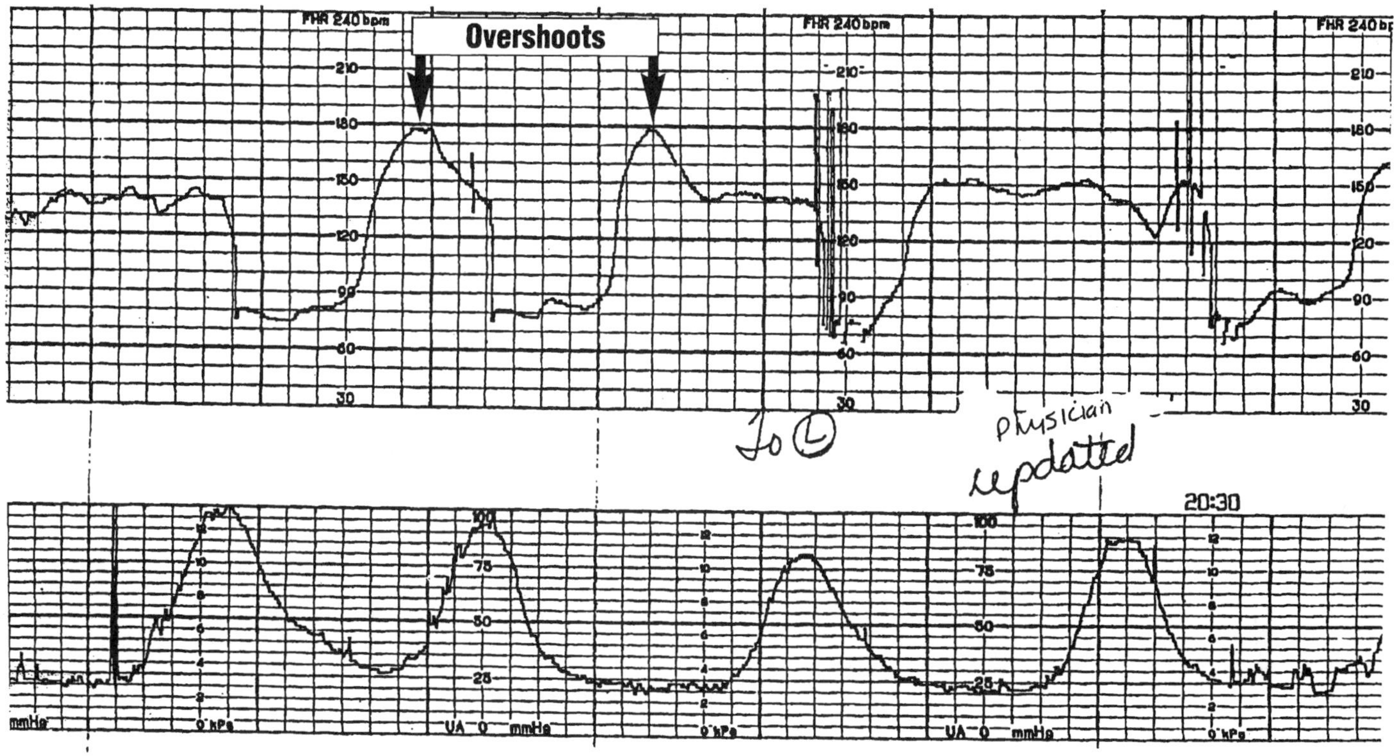

11.9 Two overshoots following variable decelerations. Note uterine hyperstimulation. Actions to decrease uterine activity and relieve cord compression, such as a position change to the left side, are needed.

Overshoots suggest fetal hypoxia. Actions to improve fetal oxygenation are needed. Overshoots are **not** spontaneous accelerations. Recurring variable decelerations with overshoots are **not** a reassuring sign. They are associated with a low fetal pH. Look at the baseline. If short-term variability is present, it rules out metabolic acidosis but not hypoxia. Since overshoots are nonreassuring, the midwife and/or physician should be promptly informed.

ATYPICAL VARIABLE DECELERATIONS

Atypical Variable Decelerations

Atypical variable decelerations are identified by their shapes. Some variable decelerations are missing one or both shoulders. Others look smooth. The significance of the pattern depends on the presence of baseline short-term variability, accelerations, and a baseline at a normal level. Atypical variable decelerations during the 30 minutes preceding birth often precede significant fetal hypoxia with a PO_2 less than 15 mm Hg.

Atypical features within a variable deceleration create an increased risk of fetal hypoxia, especially in combination with a smooth appearance, tachycardia, bradycardia, and/or a duration of 45 or more seconds.

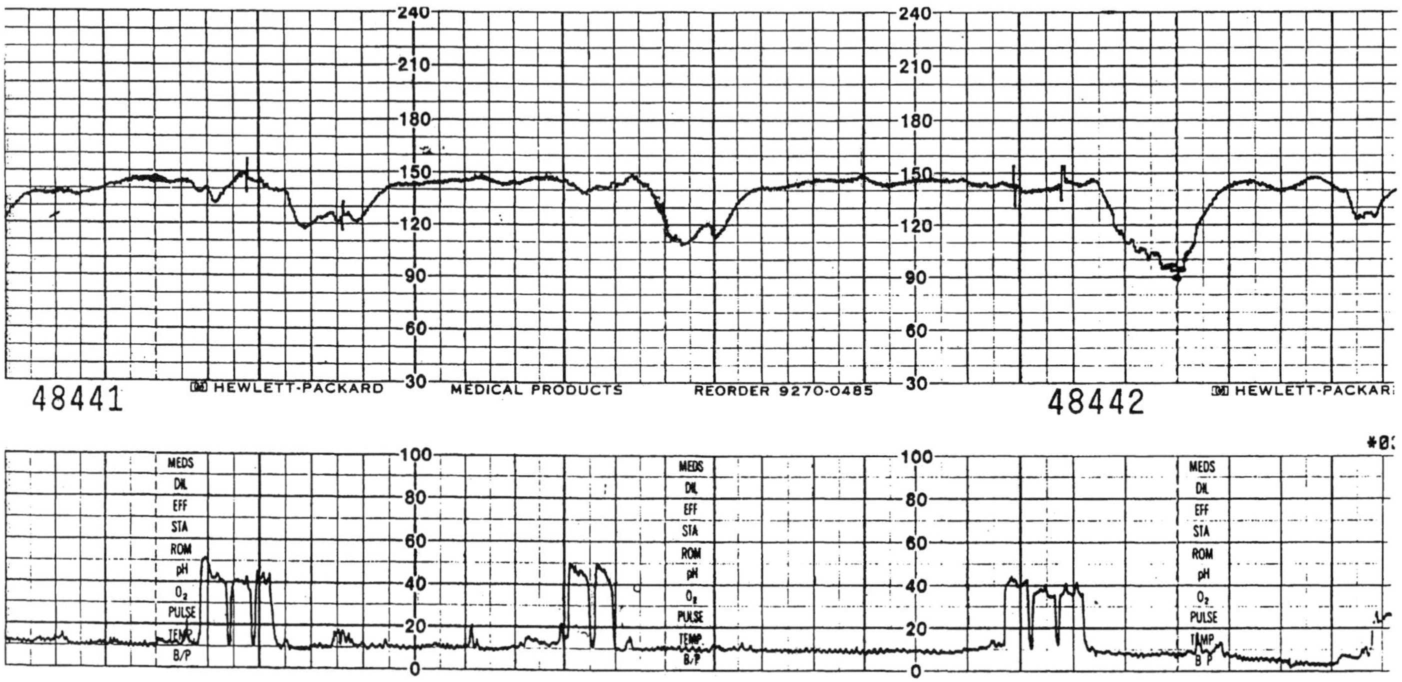

11.10 Atypical feature: loss of initial and secondary shoulders. Note the absence of normal long-term and short-term variability, and there are no accelerations.

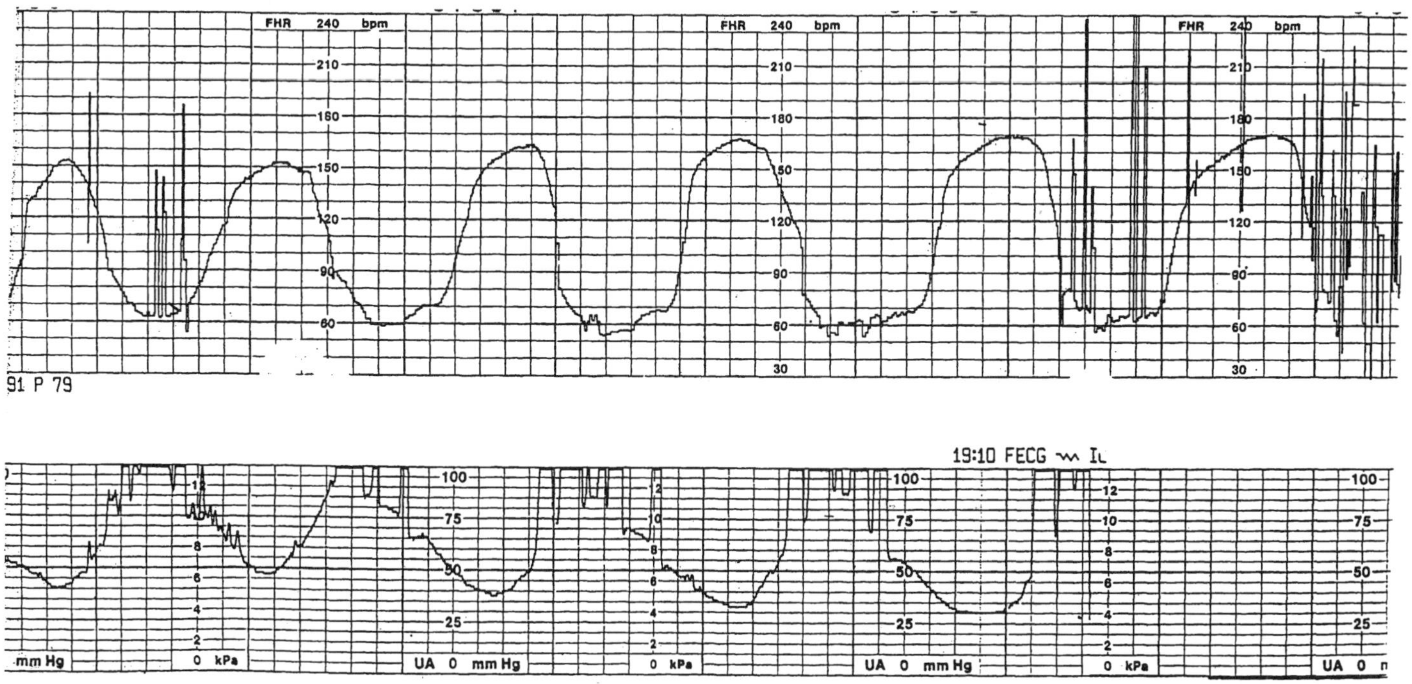

11.11 Atypical feature: smooth decelerations. Note uterine hyperstimulation, hypertonus, and pushing during contractions.

Smooth decels predict the highest incidence of low apgar scores. The smooth decelerations in this example are significant because of the additional slow recovery and overshoots. There is less than one minute between contractions. This is an inadequate amount of time to reoxygenate the fetus. Fetal decompensation can be expected.

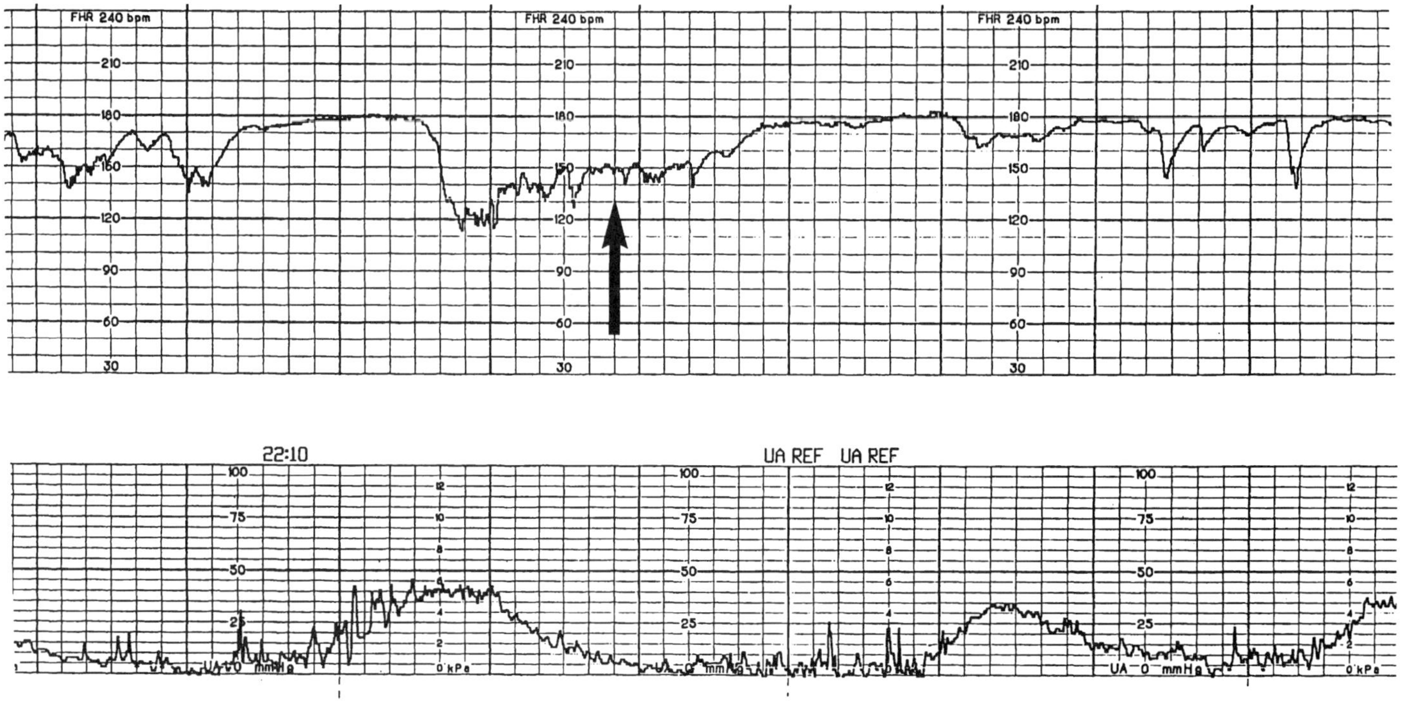

11.12 Atypical feature: continuation of the baseline at lower level. Note at about 2211 a variable deceleration to 115 bpm, followed by a baseline at 140-150 bpm that increases to the 170s.

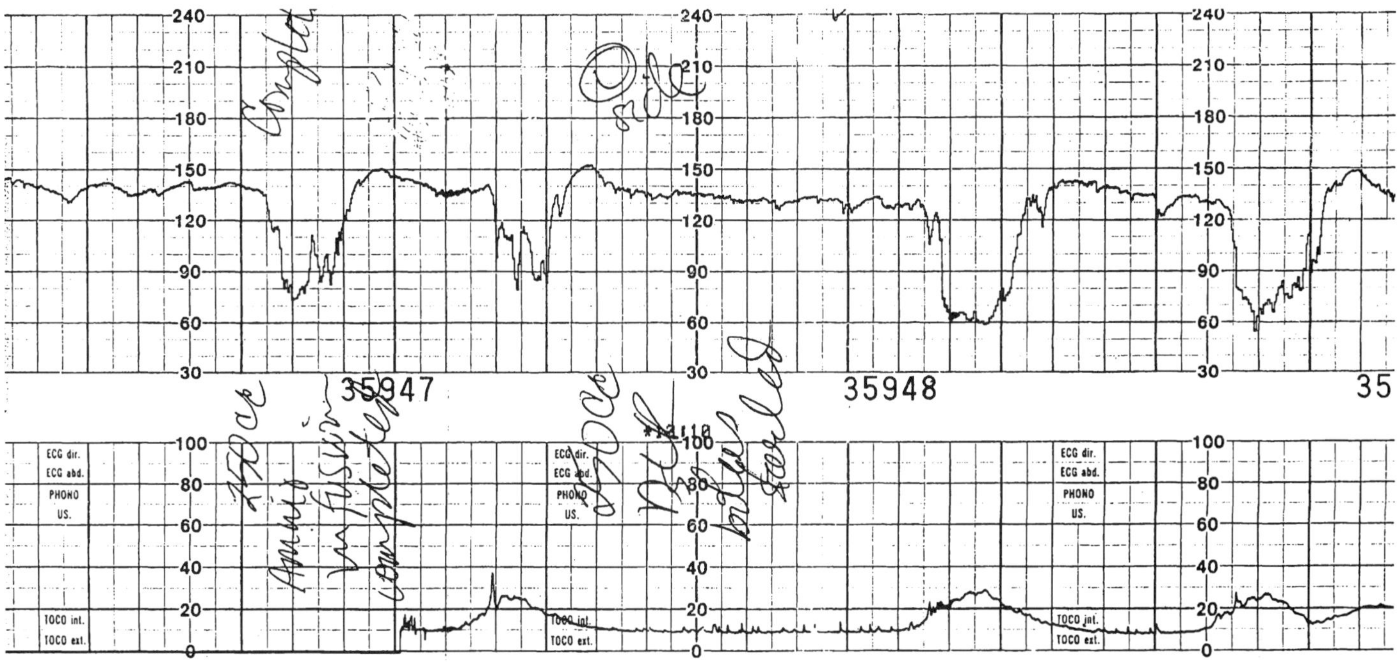

11.13 Atypical feature: biphasic variable deceleration or W shape.

A W shaped variable deceleration is also called a biphasic variable and has been considered atypical (see 11.13). However, the W shape is never as significant as the baseline level, short-term variability, and accelerations in predicting fetal status. A W shape decel with accelerations and a normal baseline and variability is reassuring. A W shape decel wtih tachycardia and no accelerations and decreased to absent variability is nonreassuring.

CLASSIC CLASSIFICATION OF VARIABLE DECELERATIONS

Classification of Variable Decelerations

How you document variable decelerations will depend on your hospital's chart forms. Some chart forms provide the following classifications:

It is essential to record the duration and depth of the variable decelerations if there is no chart form legend.

	Duration	Depth
Mild variable deceleration:	< 30 seconds	any depth but not < 70 to 80 bpm
Moderate variable deceleration:	if 30-60 seconds	and < 70 bpm **or**
	if > 60 seconds	and 70 to 80 bpm
Severe variable deceleration:	> 60 seconds	< 70 bpm

PHYSIOLOGY

Physiology of Variable Decelerations

The depth of variable decelerations indirectly reflects the degree of fetal hypotension and the response to cord compression. The decelerations occur due to slowing of sinoatrial nodal impulses. As the fetal heart rate drops, the fetal blood pressure also drops. This may affect the ability of the fetus to perfuse its brain. Fetal oxygen reserves can become depleted. Severe variable decels (> 60 seconds, < 70 bpm) were associated with fetal acidemia and a scalp pH less than 7.20.

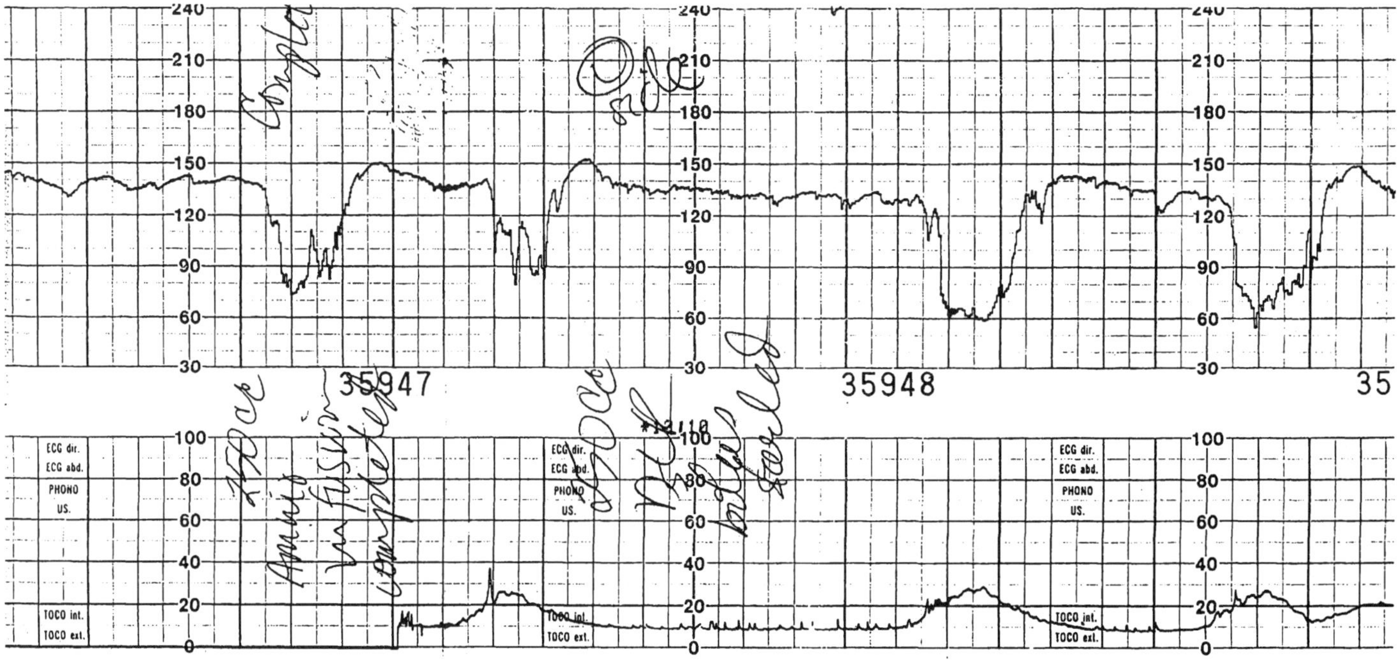

11.13 Baseline 130-142, LTV minimal to average. STV present. No accelerations. Variable decelerations x 30-40 seconds ⇓ 60-88 bpm. Amnioinfusion was completed and IV bolus of D_5LR was started. The woman was placed on her left side. Which intervention was inappropriate?

ACTIONS

Actions in Response to Variable Decelerations

The response to variable decelerations depends on where the fetus is on the continuum between nonhypoxic and asphyxiated.

Variable decelerations are usually due to umbilical cord compression. However, head compression, especially during the second stage, may contribute to variable decelerations by making them deeper.

Nursing Actions for Cord Compression

- change maternal position and observe the fetal response
- IV bolus with dextrose-free solution such as lactated Ringer's solution
- hyperoxygenate with a simple face mask at 8-10 L/minute or a partial rebreathing mask at 12 L/minute
- observe for an improvement within 1 to 9 minutes
- vaginal exam to rule out cord prolapse
- communicate and document assessments and interventions to the midwife and/or physician.

DOCUMENTATION

Documentation

Variable decelerations vary in configuration, duration, and depth. Document the range of variable decel duration in seconds and depth as the level in bpm. If more than one variable deceleration is present, the range of durations and depths is recorded, e.g., "variable decels 35-45 seconds, ⇓ 80-110 bpm." If the recovery is slow (≥ 30 seconds) it would be important to document it, e.g., "return to baseline 45 seconds." This slow return to baseline is indicative of hypoxia and nursing interventions should include hyperoxygenation with a tight-fitting face mask. Usually, "atypical" is not used in documentation to describe variable decelerations. Document compensatory signs such as "variable decelerations with primary shoulder" or signs of fetal well-being such as "STV present, accels ⇑ 170 x 30 sec."

SUMMARY

Summary

Variable decelerations are transient decreases in the FHR with a U, V or W shape. Variable decelerations last at least 15 seconds, decreasing 15 or more beats per minute. The heart rate abruptly falls (usually in less than 30 seconds), depth varies, and the offset usually is abrupt (8-27 seconds). However, if the offset is slow (≥ 30 seconds), it suggests a hypoxic fetus with myocardial depression.

The primary and secondary acceleratory phases of the variable deceleration pattern (shoulders) are a compensatory response to cord compression. When a variable deceleration is preceded and followed by a shoulder it is considered a classic, pure or "typical" variable deceleration. When shoulders are missing, or the deceleration is smooth or the baseline after the deceleration is lower, or there is an overshoot or a W shape variable deceleration, the deceleration is called atypical. If the deceleration falls below 80 bpm, fetal brain perfusion is compromised. Act to improve blood flow through the cord and oxygen delivery to the fetus.

SECTION 11: VARIABLE DECELERATIONS

QUESTIONS

Directions: Circle T if the statement is true, F if it is false.

QUESTIONS			
T	F	1.	Variable decelerations are uniform in shape and size.
T	F	2.	Variable decelerations are only a periodic pattern.
T	F	3.	Low Apgar scores are likely when variable decelerations are associated with decreased long-term variability.
T	F	4.	An atypical feature of a variable deceleration is a shoulder.
T	F	5.	An overshoot is an increase in the fetal heart rate following a variable deceleration. The increase is 15 bpm above the baseline which lasts 15 seconds.
T	F	6.	A low fetal pH is associated with repetitive variable decelerations with overshoots.
T	F	7.	A biphasic variable deceleration is related to an umbilical cord less than 50 cm in length.
T	F	8.	Utilizing descriptors or mild, moderate, and severe adequately documents variable decelerations.
T	F	9.	A nadir less than 80 bpm has no clinical significance.
T	F	10.	Variable decelerations lasting 60 or more seconds and falling to 70 bpm or lower are associated with fetal acidemia.

SECTION 12
Prolonged Decelerations

PROLONGED DECELERATION DEFINITION

A prolonged deceleration is a deceleration lasting 2 to 10 minutes with an abrupt onset and usually a gradual recovery. If the fetal heart rate stays down, bradycardia begins and a prolonged deceleration ends after 10 minutes.

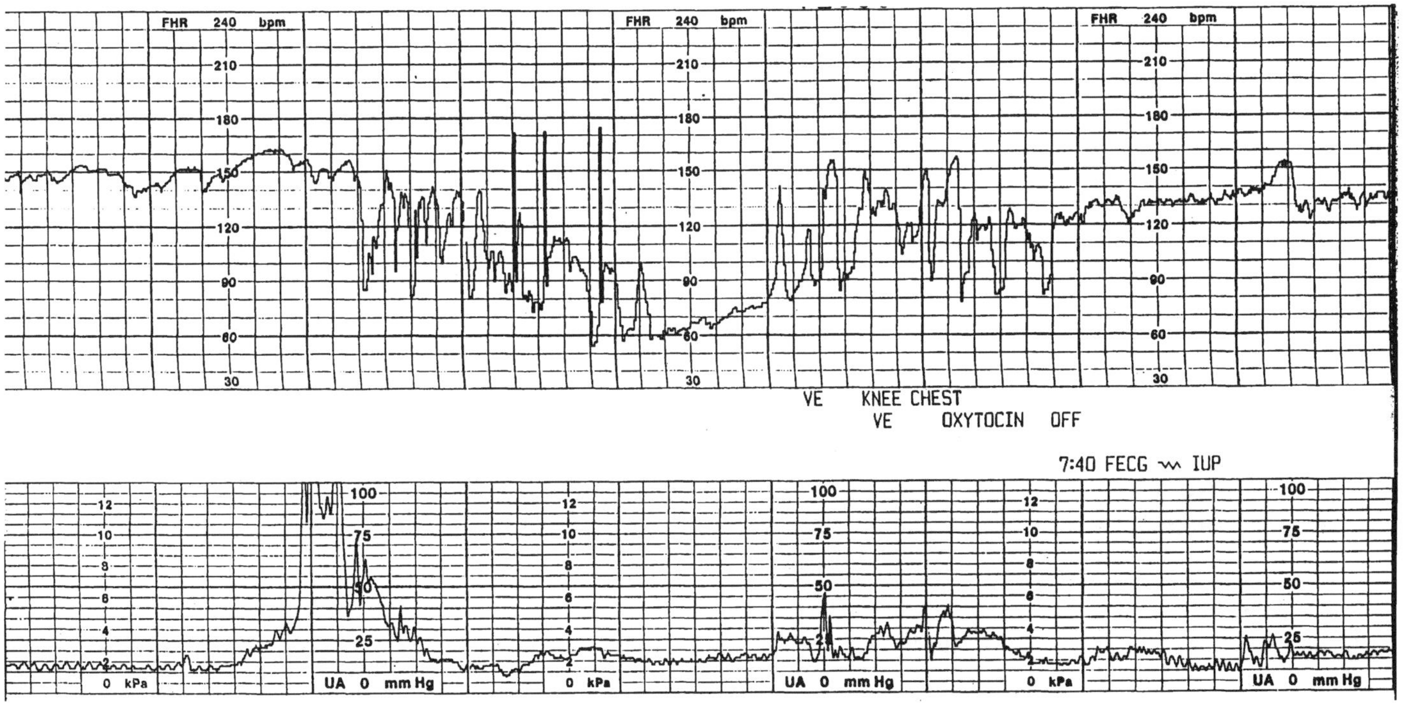

12.1 Document this as "decel x 6 minutes ⇓ 60 bpm." Note short-term variability and a 15 second spontaneous acceleration is present after the prolonged deceleration. The presence of marked long-term variability suggests this prolonged deceleration was due to umbilical cord compression.

Determine the etiology of the prolonged decel. Usually it's maternal hypotension or umbilical cord compression.

CAUSES OF PROLONGED DECELERATIONS

Causes of Prolonged Decelerations

Maternal Causes	Fetal Causes
• hypotension • excessive uterine activity • seizure	• umbilical cord compression • hypoxia, e.g., due to maternal hypotension or uterine hyperstimulation • direct anesthetic response

As long as tissue oxygen (O_2) reserves exist, fetal hypoxemia will not progress to tissue hypoxia, acidemia or acidosis. Fetal O_2 reserves become depleted when the FHR is less than 80 bpm. The FHR less than 80 bpm is a reflection of fetal hypotension and the lack of fetal brain perfusion. When fetal O_2 reserves become depleted, metabolic acidosis can occur. The evidence of metabolic acidosis is absence of short-term variability, long-term variability, and accelerations. Following a prolonged deceleration with the development of metabolic acidosis, the FHR will be less than 80 beats per minute (bpm) and may become an agonal pattern or terminal bradycardia from which the fetus will not recover.

REBOUND TACHYCARDIA

Fetal tachycardia following a prolonged deceleration is reflective of a response to hypoxia and is called rebound tachycardia. This is not considered a reassuring sign. This is a compensatory sign. While one prolonged deceleration may be a fetal compensatory response to a temporary asphyxial insult, two or more prolonged decelerations are nonreassuring and raise one's suspicion of occult cord prolapse, hypotension, and/or a potential need to expedite delivery by cesarean section.

ACTIONS

Actions in Response to a Prolonged Deceleration

- maximize maternal cardiac output and umbilical cord blood flow, turn the woman to her side, observe for improvement in the FHR
- discontinue pitocin® or prostaglandins
- discontinue amnioinfusion if the pattern worsened after initiating amnioinfusion
- increase maternal circulatory volume and cardiac output by giving an intravenous (IV) bolus of a non-glucose solution such as lactated Ringers (LR) solution
- ephedrine® 5 to 10 mg slow IV push for maternal hypotension
- hyperoxygenate maternal plasma, provide oxygen by a tight-fitting face mask at 8-10 or 12 liters per minute depending on mask type
- perform a vaginal examination to rule out cord prolapse
- administer a tocolytic if it is ordered by the physician or midwife and the placenta is not abrupting
- communicate with the charge nurse, midwife and/or physician

To gently flush the vagina of intravaginal prostaglandin gel, attach a 20 cc syringe filled with normal saline to a red robinson (straight) catheter and irrigate the vagina or attach IV tubing to a bag of normal saline and insert the tubing into the vagina. Interventions need to be done in a rapid fashion as time is of the essence. Notify the midwife or physician of the deceleration as soon as actions are initiated.

EVALUATE FETAL STATUS AND DOCUMENT

Evaluate Fetal Status and Document

Following actions in response to a prolonged deceleration, the fetus needs to be resuscitated within the uterus if possible.

- Did a position change help? Document the response of the fetus.
- Has the FHR recovered to the previous baseline? Document actions related to chain of command activation, physician or midwife communication, neonatal and resuscitation team notification.
- Evaluate the strip for evidence of fetal well-being. Is the amniotic fluid clear?

- Document signs of fetal well-being beyond a stable FHR such as:
    - accelerations
    - short-term variability
    - fetal movement.
- A prolonged deceleration may reoccur.
    - Discontinue pitocin® until the midwife and/or physician have evaluated the woman and the fetus.
    - Is a tocolytic necessary?

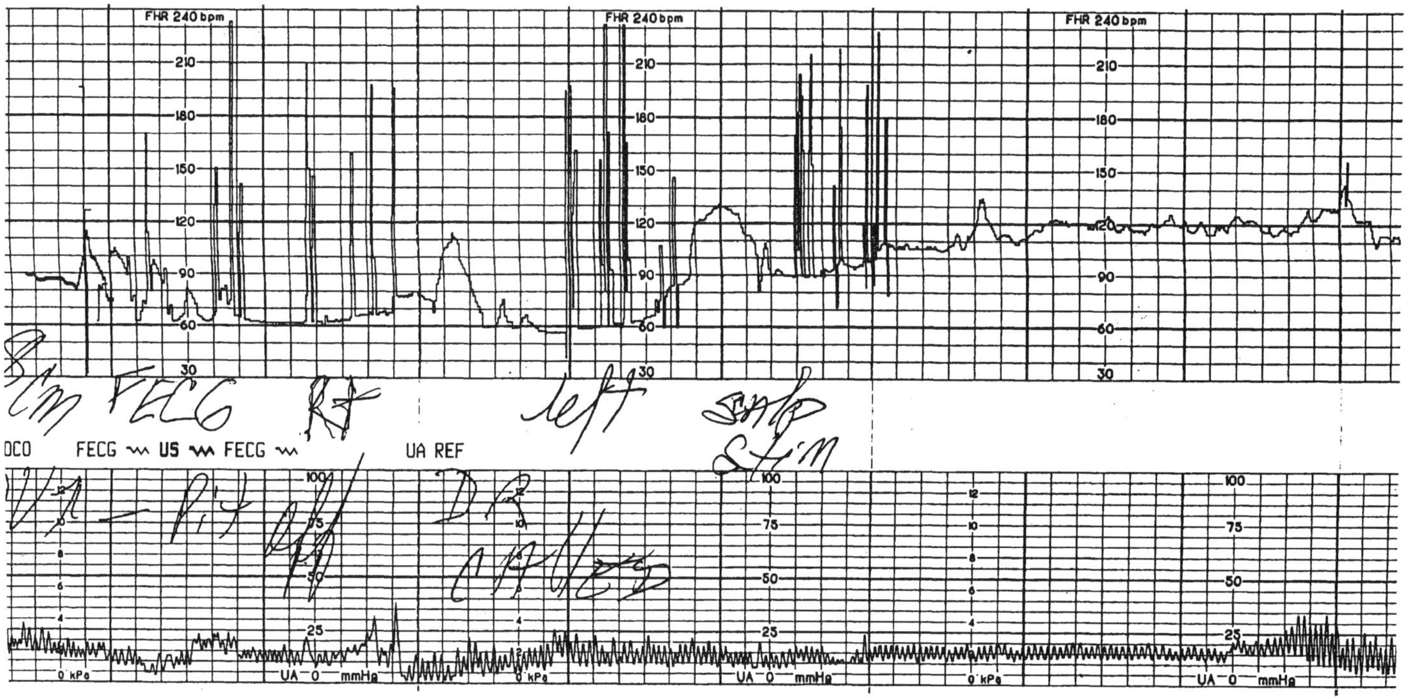

12.2 Scalp stimulation is NOT useful during a fetal deceleration or bradycardia as the vagal response overrides any sympathetic nerve stimulus.

SCALP STIMULATION IS AN ASSESSMENT METHOD NOT AN INTERVENTION

Scalp stimulation during a deceleration is inappropriate. It may create a vagal response. It delays appropriate actions. The fetus needs oxygen not touch. Scalp stimulation should be done between contractions and between decelerations when there is a baseline, to elicit a reactive acceleration and rule out metabolic acidosis.

SUMMARY

Summary

A prolonged deceleration lasts 2 to 10 minutes. Its duration and depth are documented versus the words "prolonged deceleration." The most common cause of prolonged decelerations is umbilical cord compression. Some prolonged decelerations occur as a result of maternal hypotension and the resultant, transient fetal hypoxia. Actions to improve fetal oxygen delivery are done first, e.g., a position change, an intravenous bolus of a non-glucose solution, discontinuation of a pitocin® drip and/or amnioinfusion and supplemental oxygen administration. Actions are also directed at determining the cause of the prolonged deceleration. These include assessing blood pressure and ruling out an umbilical cord prolapse. If hyperstimulation is evident, oxytocics are discontinued and intravaginal prostaglandins are flushed from the vagina. Communicate assessments and actions to the midwife or physician. Document the signs of fetal well-being following the prolonged deceleration. Signs of fetal well-being include accelerations, short-term variability, and fetal movement. Scalp stimulation during the deceleration is an inappropriate action since this is an assessment technique to rule out metabolic acidosis which is done in lieu of scalp pH sampling **between** decelerations and between contractions.

SECTION 12: PROLONGED DECELERATIONS

QUESTIONS

Directions: Circle T if the statement is true, F if it is false.

QUESTIONS			
T	F	1.	A prolonged deceleration lasts 2 to 15 minutes.
T	F	2.	Fetal tachycardia following fetal bradycardia is a reassuring sign.
T	F	3.	A prolonged deceleration may be due to fetal head compression.
T	F	4.	Maternal hypotension may precede a prolonged deceleration.
T	F	5.	Actions in response to a prolonged deceleration include fetal scalp stimulation.
T	F	6.	Following a prolonged deceleration, the return to a baseline within the normal range in and of itself is reassuring.
T	F	7.	Supplemental oxygen is not useful when a prolonged deceleration occurs.
T	F	8.	The presence of long-term variability following a prolonged deceleration confirms fetal well-being.
T	F	9.	Two or more prolonged decelerations preceded by a normal baseline with accelerations and short-term variability create a nonreassuring fetal heart rate pattern.

SECTION 13
Strip Evaluation and Categorization

In this section, you will evaluate your knowlege and visual assessment skill. Fill in the blanks after each question then look at the correct responses on pages 185 and 186. Remember, visual assessment rarely has 100% agreement, so the numbers we feel are correct may be slightly different from yours.

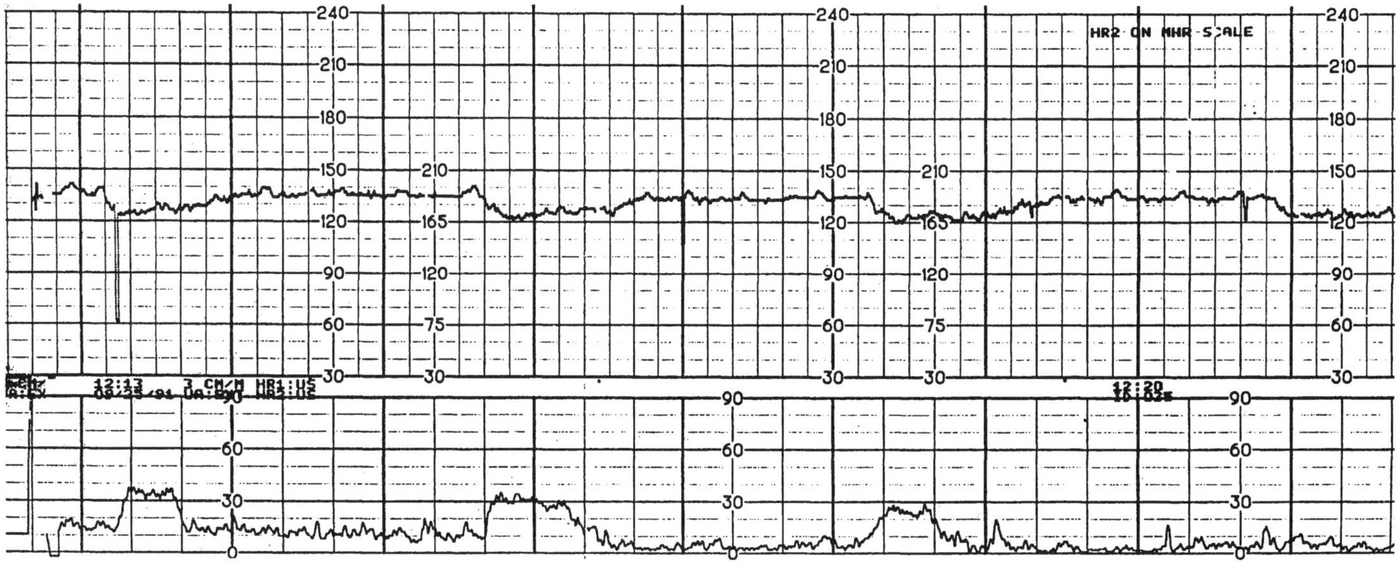

13.1 Strip 1.

1. What is the depth of the nadirs in bpm? _____-_____ bpm

2. Is the contraction peak-to-deceleration nadir lag time greater or less than 18 seconds? ______________

3. What is the recovery time from nadir to baseline? _____-_____ seconds

4. What kind of decelerations are these?

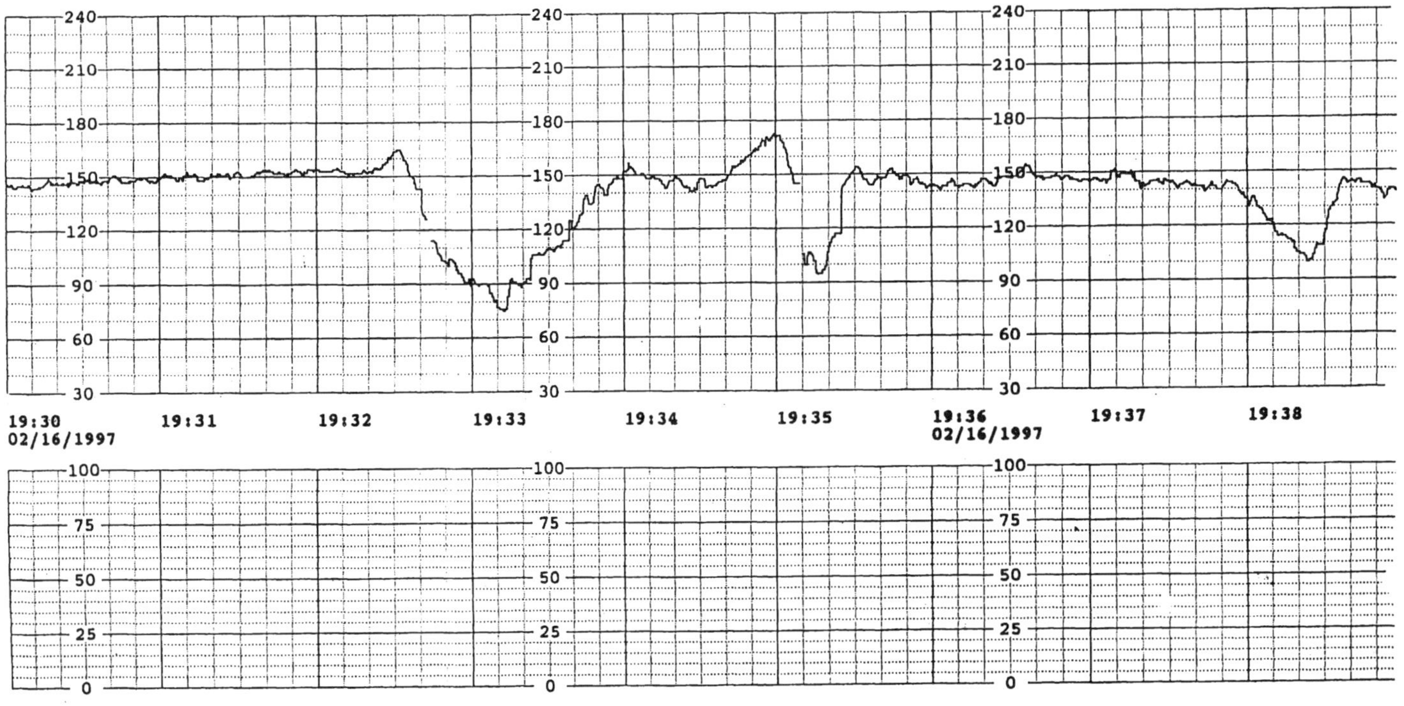

13.2 Strip 2.

5. What is the duration of the decelerations in seconds? _____-_____ seconds

6. What is the depth of the nadirs in bpm? _____-_____ bpm

7. What is the recovery time from nadir to baseline? _____-_____ seconds

8. What kind of decelerations are these?

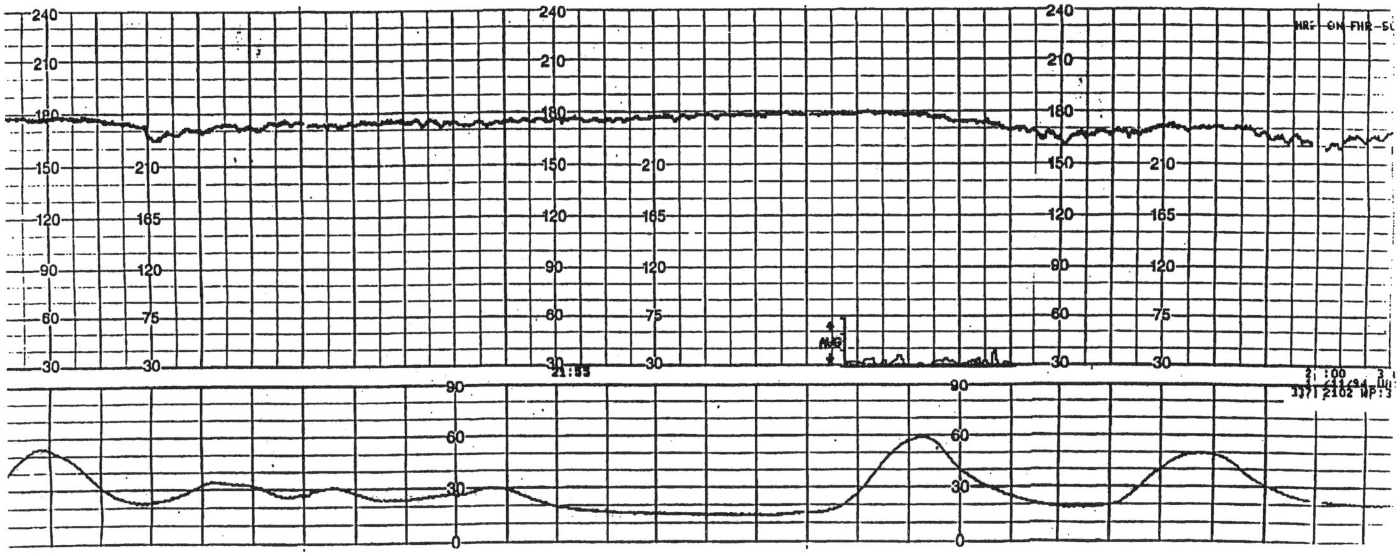

13.3 Strip 3.

9. How long is the onset from baseline to nadir? ________ seconds

10. What is the lag time between the contraction peak and the nadirs in seconds? _____-_____ seconds

11. What is the recovery time from nadir to baseline? ______ seconds

12. What kind of decelerations are these?

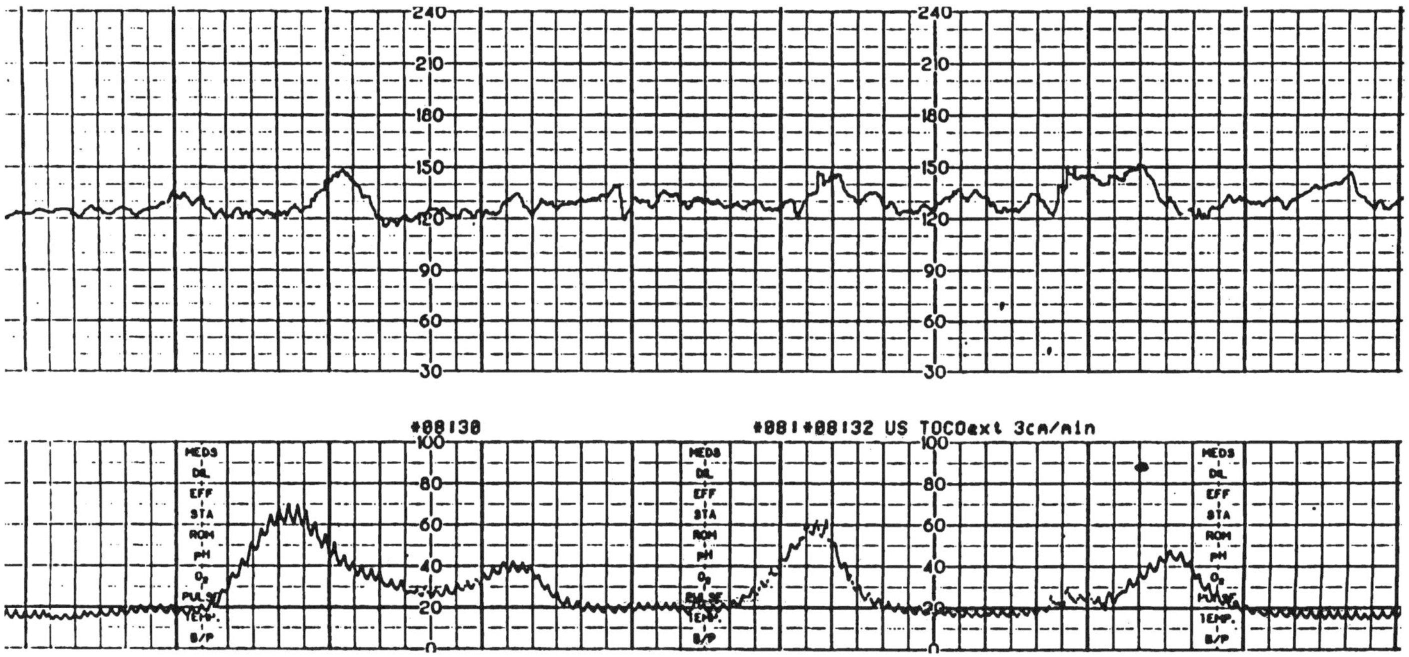

13.4 Strip 4.

13. What is the baseline range? _____-_____ bpm

14. Is short-term variability present or absent? ______________

15. Classify long-term variability. ______________________

16. What is the level of the height of the accelerations? _____-_____ bpm

17. What is the duration of the accelerations? _____-_____ seconds

18. Are any of these reactive accelerations? ❑ Yes or ❑ No

19. Is this fetus metabolically acidotic? ❑ Yes or ❑ No

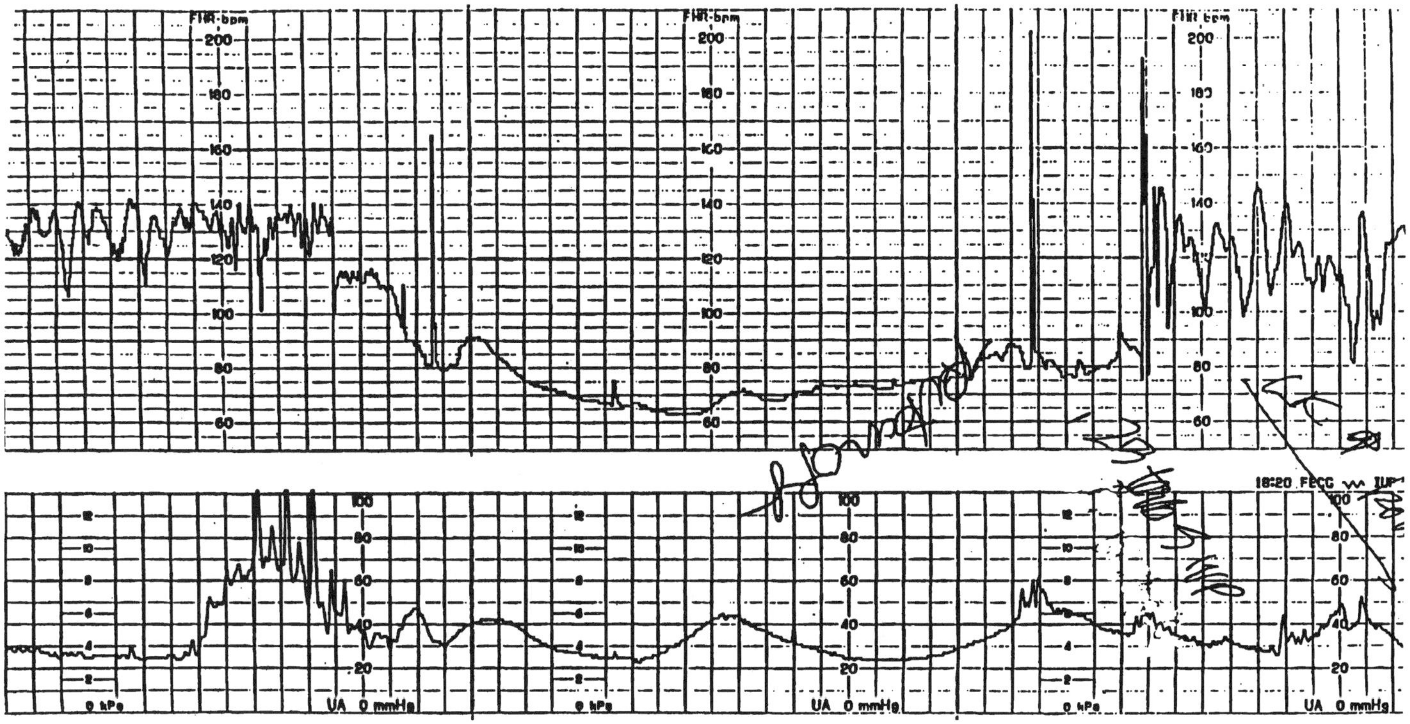

13.5 Strip 5.

20. Is this a periodic or episodic (nonperiodic) deceleration? ______________________________

21. What is the duration of the deceleration? __________ minutes

22. What is the level of the nadir of the deceleration?_______ bpm

23. What are the two most likely causes of this deceleration?

1. ____________________ 2. ____________________

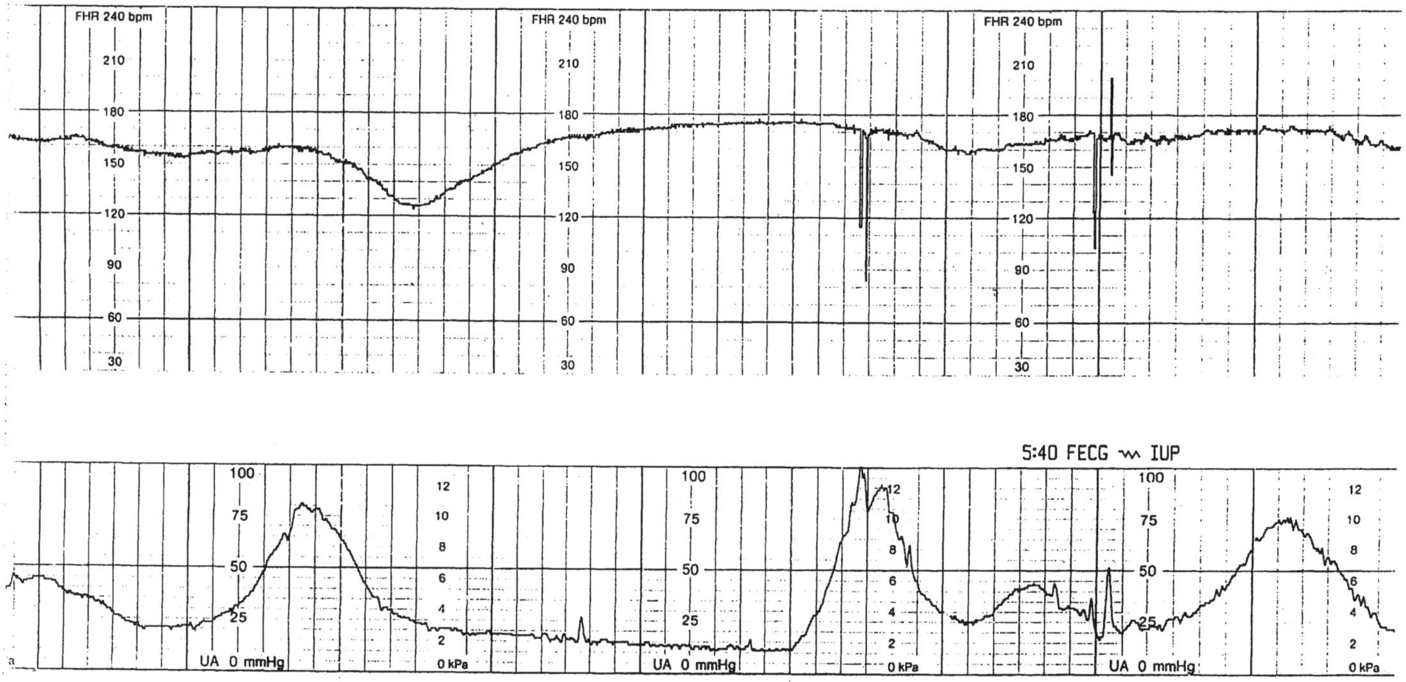

13.6 Strip 6.

24. What kind of decelerations are these? ____________________

25. What is the contraction frequency? every ______ minute(s)

26. What is the contraction duration? _______-_______ seconds

27. What is the contraction strength/peak intrauterine pressure? _______-_______ mm Hg

28. What is the resting tone? _______-_______ mm Hg

29. What is this uterine activity called? ______________________

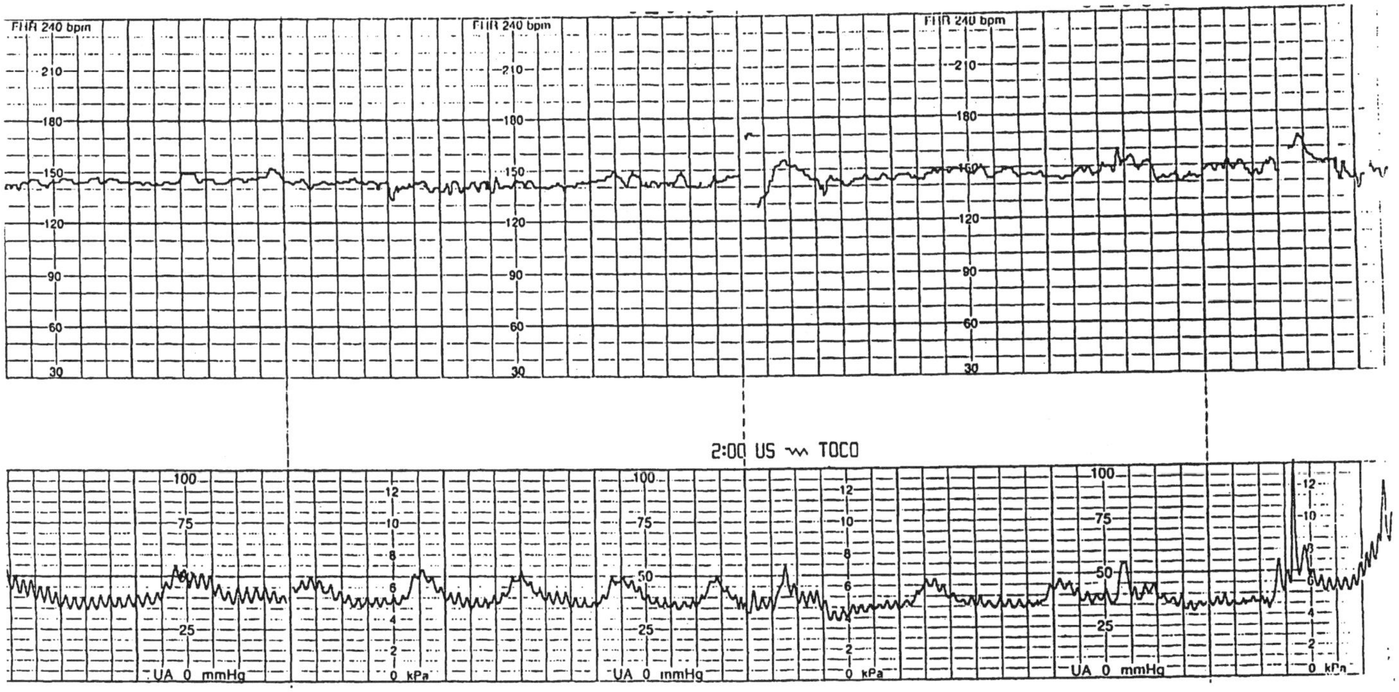

13.7 Strip 7.

30. What would you record as the baseline? ________-________ bpm

31. Classify STV. STV is ______________________________

32. Classify LTV. LTV is ______________________________

33. Are there any accelerations?______________________________

34. Are there any decelerations?______________________________

35. Is this normal UA?______________________________

36. If no, what is this called? ______________________________

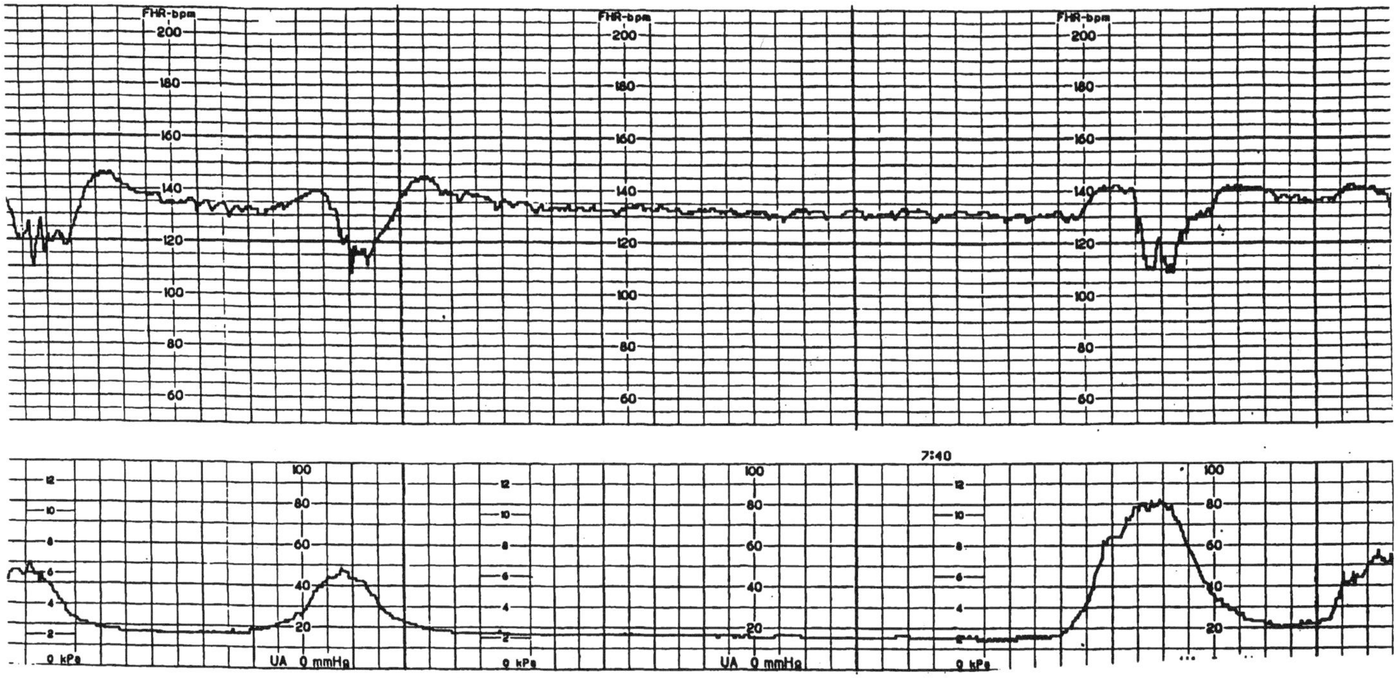

13.8 Strip 8.

37. Fill in each box for Tracing 8

BL	STV	LTV	Accels	Decels
			ht _____ bpm duration ________ sec	type ________________ duration _________ sec depth __________ bpm

38. What is the most likely cause of this pattern?

a. head compression

b. cord compression

c. inadequate uteroplacental perfusion

39. What actions would you take in response to this pattern? (Circle the letter of all that apply)

a. do nothing, it's a normal fetal response
b. turn the woman
c. discontinue pitocin®
d. increase IV fluids
e. observe the pattern
f. apply oxygen by mask
g. notify the midwife or doctor
h. perform a vaginal examination
i. take maternal blood pressure

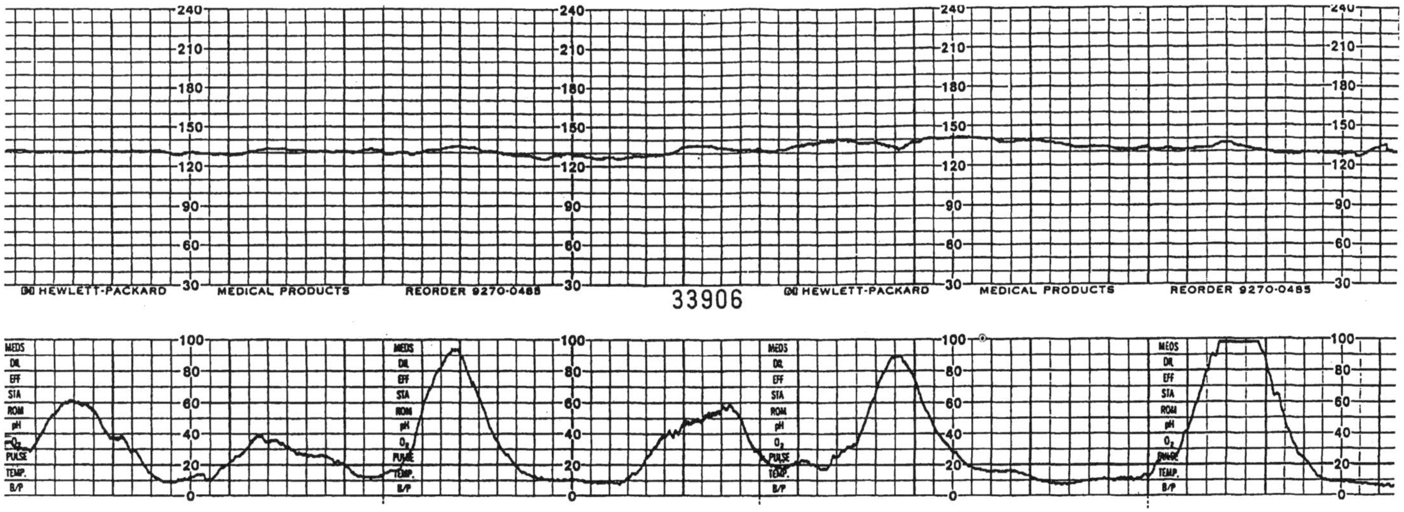

13.9 Strip 9.

Fill in each box for strip 9. Demerol 25 mg IV push was administered 10 minutes ago. Prior to the pattern the fetal heart rate pattern was reassuring.

BL	STV	LTV	Accels	Decels
			ht _____ bpm duration ________ sec	type ________________ duration ________ sec depth __________ bpm

41. What is the most likely cause of this pattern? ______________________________

42. What actions would you take in response to this pattern?

a. do nothing
b. turn the woman
c. discontinue pitocin®
d. increase IV fluids
e. observe the pattern
f. apply oxygen by mask
g. notify the midwife or doctor
h. perform a vaginal examination
i. take maternal blood pressure

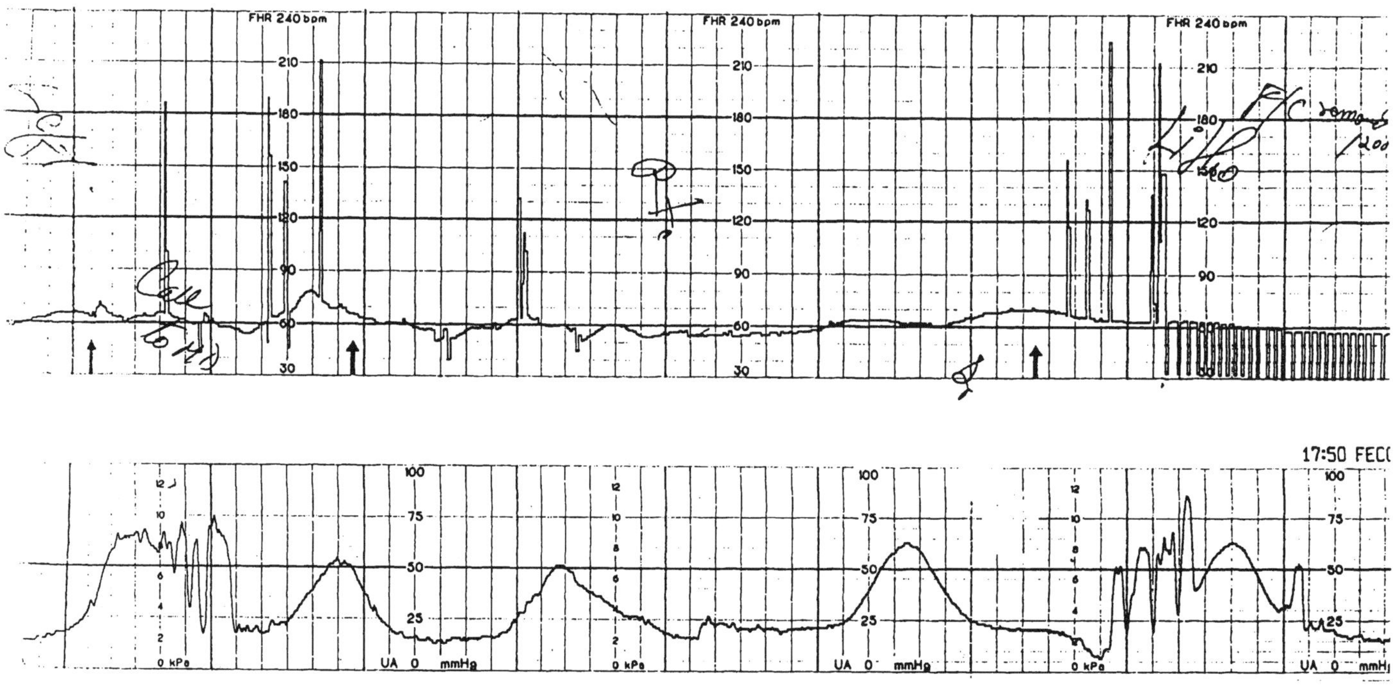

13.10 Strip 10: This fetal heart rate pattern occurred within 7 minutes of the epidural test dose. The maternal blood pressure is 75/35.

43. What 3 immediate actions would you take?

____

____

____

44. If the FHR recovered to a rate greater than 160 bpm would the fetus be out of jeopardy? __________

45. Is the fetal heart rate adequate to perfuse the fetal brain? ______

ANSWERS

Answers To Strip Evaluation

Strip 1

1. 120-125
2. less than
3. 40-50
4. early

Strip 2

5. 25-90
6. 75-100
7. 20-50
8. variable

Strip 3

9. 25-45
10. 45-60
11. 40-45
12. late

Strip 4

13. 120-130
14. present
15. average
16. 145-150
17. 25-45
18. yes
19. no

Strip 5

20. episodic/nonperiodic
21. 5
22. 66 (this is European-scaled paper)
23. umbilical cord compression, uterine hyperstimulation

Strip 6

24. late
25. 1-4
26. 50-90
27. 75-100
28. 10-20
29. possible coupling at 0539-0540

Strip 7

30. 140-150
31. probably present, but this is an external ultrasound tracing
32. minimal to average
33. yes (see last minute)
34. no
35. no
36. LAHF waves or low amplitude high frequency waves or uterine irritability

Strip 8

37. 130-135 bpm (European-scaled paper), present STV, minimal LTV, no accels, only shoulders on variable decelerations, variable decels x 30 sec ⇓ 110-115 bpm
38. b
39. b, e, g if the pattern is unrelieved by your actions or she has a scarred uterus as variable decelerations are the most common deceleration pattern when the uterus is tearing (rupturing)

Strip 9

40. 125-140 bpm, 0 STV, 0 LTV, 0 accels, 0 decels
41. Demerol and uterine hyperstimulation with possible fetal hypoxia
42. b, c, d, e, f, g; remove oxygen once signs of fetal well-being return and the uterus is contracting normally

Strip 10

43. discontinue pitocin®; call the surgeon, anesthesia provider, operating room crew, and pediatrician stat; provide an IV bolus of a non-glucose solution and ephedrine as ordered
44. no, that would be a rebound tachycardia which is highly unlikely with such profound bradycardia, suspect it's maternal heart rate doubling
45. no

A score of 40 correct is excellent. If you scored less than 40 correct, go back and reevaluate the images.

Now it's time to validate your skills in Section 14.

SECTION 14
Skills Validation

Name: ____________________

ID Number: ____________________

Date: ____________________

Skills Validation Sheet for External Fetal Monitor Application

	Level
1. Positions woman to optimize fetal perfusion.	
2. Prior to application, inspects tocotransducer and ultrasound transducer for damage.	
3. Manually tests ultrasound transducer.	
4. Manually tests tocotransducer.	
5. Observes auto test or manually tests fetal monitor. Confirms monitor is properly printing and digital display is complete.	
6. Performs Leopold's Maneuvers.	
7. Properly places tocotransducer on the abdomen based on fetal gestational age.	
8. Evaluates tracing quality and sets the uterine activity baseline as needed.	
9. Properly places ultrasound transducer over the fetal back.	
10. Evaluates tracing quality.	
11. Documents patient identifying information on tracing.	
12. Verbalizes limitations of external fetal monitoring to instructor.	

Levels

I. Hesitates, needs assistance to complete task

II. Requires verbal cues, motions fluid

III. Proceeds accurately and independently without cues

Name: ____________________

ID Number: ____________________

Date: ____________________

Skills Validation Sheet
for Auscultation of Fetal Heart Rate and Palpation of Uterine Activity

	Level
1. Performs Leopold's Maneuvers to determine fetal lie and position of fetal back. 2. Correctly uses and places fetoscope over fetal back. 3. Listens with the fetoscope for ≤ 1 minute. In labor, listens before, during, and after a contraction. 4. Determines fetal heart rate with fetoscope or hand-held doppler. If doppler is used, simultaneously determines maternal heart rate (pulse). 5. Records signs of fetal well-being: • baseline; verbalizes normal range for gestational age • highest rate of audible acceleration(s) • deceleration(s) and lowest rate • palpates fetal movement. 6. Palpates and records frequency, duration, strength, and relaxation of contractions.	

Levels

I. Hesitates, needs assistance to complete task

II. Requires verbal cues, motions fluid

III. Proceeds accurately and independently without cues

Name: ____________________

ID Number: ____________________

Date: ____________________

Troubleshooting EFM equipment

	Level
• Verbalizes procedure to diminish gaps in the printed fetal heart rate or uterine activity tracing and protocol if the printout is too dark or too light. • Knows and can state procedure of when and where to send the monitor for repair.	

Levels

I. Hesitates, needs assistance to complete task

II. Requires verbal cues, motions fluid

III. Proceeds accurately and independently without cues

Name: ____________________

ID Number: ____________________

Date: ____________________

Spiral Electrode (SE) Application

	Level
1. Verbalizes two risks and one benefit for SE use.	
2. Identifies fetal heart rate characteristics that indicate a need for a SE.	
3. Verbalizes placement locations.	
4. Organizes equipment prior to SE placement.	
5. Tests SE cable.	
6. Opens SE package.	
7. Dons sterile glove and applies lubricating gel.	
8. Identifies cervical dilatation and presenting part.	
9. Releases wires from wire lock.	
10. Retracts SE inside outer guide to protect vaginal wall prior to insertion.	
11. Inserts outer guide with retracted SE into vagina.	
12. Verifies fetal presenting part.	
13. Advances outer guide until flush with presenting part.	
14. Advances SE.	
15. Rotates SE 180° clockwise.	
16. Attaches SE to SE cable.	
17. Evaluates quality of tracing.	
18. Inspects insertion site after delivery.	

Verification of Preceptor	Date	Pt ID Number
1. ______________________	__________	________________
2. ______________________	__________	________________
3. ______________________	__________	________________

Levels

I. Hesitates, needs assistance to complete task

II. Requires verbal cues, motions fluid

III. Proceeds accurately and independently, provides patient education, identifies interventions as needed based on tracing

Name: ____________________

ID Number: ____________________

Date: ____________________

Fetal Monitor Scavenger Hunt

Item	Location
1. Fetoscope	
2. Hand-held doppler	
3. Fetal monitor paper	
4. Fetal monitor belts	
5. Tocotransducer	
6. Ultrasound transducer	
7. Ultrasound coupling gel	
8. Spiral electrode	
9. Spiral electrode cable	
10. Intrauterine pressure catheter (IUPC) (read instructions on package, identify brand name)	
11. IUPC cable	
12. Maternal ECG cable for fetal monitor	
13. Electrodes for maternal ECG cable	
14. Maternal pulse oximeter finger probe and cable for fetal monitor	
15. Amniotomy hook	
16. Extra ultrasound transducer	

Item	Location
17. Extra tocotransducer 18. IV tubing 19. Blood tubing 20. Fetal scalp blood sampling kit (if applicable) 21. Cord blood gas kit or 1 ml syringe, heparin (1000 U/ml), ice basin or zip lock bags, and labels 22. Policies and procedures related to fetal monitoring: • Nonstress test • Contraction stress test • Intrapartal fetal monitoring • Amnioinfusion • Other: ____________________ ____________________	

GLOSSARY OF FETAL HEART MONITORING TERMS

A

Ab: number of miscarriages (abortions) and births before 20 weeks' gestation, includes spontaneous (SAB) and therapeutic or elective abortions (TAB/EAB).

Abruptio placentae (placental abruption): premature separation of the placenta prior to delivery of the fetus.

Acceleration: an increase in the fetal heart rate above the baseline level. There are two types: uniform and spontaneous.

Acidemia: abnormal increase in hydrogen ion concentration due to the accumulation of an acid or a loss of base.

Acidosis: the abnormal accumulation of carbon dioxide (respiratory acidosis) or lactic acid (metabolic acidosis).

Agonal pattern: A bradycardic fetal heart rate of a decompensating fetus with a surge of catecholamines. An agonal pattern lacks short-term variability and is less than 100 beats per minute with upward and downward swings that last 20 or more seconds.

Amnioinfusion: instillation of an isotonic, glucose-free solution, such as normal saline, into the uterus.

Amnion: inner membrane of the sac that encloses the fetus.

Amniotomy: breaking the bag of waters, the artificial rupture of fetal membranes (AROM).

Antepartal: before birth, pertaining to the period spanning conception to the onset of labor.

Anoxia: absence of oxygen within the tissues.

Apgar score: system of scoring neonate's physical condition one minute and five minutes after birth. The color or appearance (A), heart rate or pulse (P), response to stimuli or grimace (G), muscle tone or activity (A), and respirations (R) are assessed. Each can receive a maximum of 2 points. The maximum Apgar score is 10.

Arrhythmia: any variation from the normal rhythm of the heart.

Artifact: irregularities on the monitor tracing due to poor reception of the fetal heart signal which appears as scattered dots, gaps on the tracing, or lines.

Asphyxia: a condition due to lack of oxygen resulting in impending or actual cessation of life, from Greek meaning "a stopping of the pulse." Implies a reduction in PO_2 (hypoxia), elevation of $PC0_2$ (hypercapnia), and lowering of blood pH and bicarbonate or mixed acidosis with respiratory and metabolic components. Asphyxia is preceded by anaerobic metabolism. Asphyxia can precede cell damage and/or death.

Auscultation: act of listening for sounds within the body; assisted by use of a stethoscope and/or fetoscope.

B

Ballotable head: A fetal head that has not descended into the pelvis, it floats up when touched.

Baroreceptors: Nerves that respond to changes in arterial diameter and blood pressure. Fetal baroreceptors that affect the fetal heart rate are found in the carotid sinuses and aorta. They are also known as stretch or pressor receptors.

Baseline (BL): the fetal heart rate over a period of time, not including accelerations or decelerations. The BL may be recorded as a range or an average rate.

Beat-to-beat variability (BTBV): The fluctuation or change in the interval between R waves or systole on the fetal electrocardiogram (ECG) measured in milliseconds (msec) by the fetal monitor. The average BTBV is 7.7 msec. When BTBV is present, short-term variability is also present.

Benign sinusoidal: A well fetus pattern with $1^1/2$ or more cycles per minute resembling a pathologic sinusoidal pattern but preceded or followed by fetal movement and accelerations.

Bradycardia: a fetal heart rate less than 100 bpm for 10 or more minutes (term and post-term) or less than 120 bpm for 10 or more minutes (preterm).

C

Caput succedaneum: swelling occurring in and under the scalp of the fetus during labor after rupture of membranes. A localized pitting edema in the scalp of a fetus that may overlie sutures of the skull. It is usually formed during labor as a result of the circular pressure of the cervix on the fetal occiput.

Cervix (Cx): neck of the uterus which protrudes into the vagina.

Chemoreceptors: Chemistry sensitive nerves that line the fourth ventricle near the brainstem and are also found in the aortic and carotid bodies. They respond to changes in pH in the cerebral spinal fluid and pH, PO_2 and PCO_2 in arterial blood.

Compensatory pattern: A classification of a fetal heart rate pattern indicating fetal hypoxia, hypovolemia, hypotension or hypertension. Examples include tachycardia with spontaneous accelerations, end-stage bradycardia with accelerations, a saltatory pattern or marked long-term variability, one prolonged deceleration, accelerations with late decelerations. Compensatory patterns always have accelerations and short-term variability.

Contraction stress test (CST): antepartum surveillance method using induced or spontaneous contractions to evaluate fetal oxygen reserves and placental function. Induced contractions may be from endogenous or exogenous oxytocin.

Cycle: also called a sine wave or complex, the fluctuation of the fetal heart rate above, through and back to the average baseline level.

D

Deceleration: a distinct decrease in the FHR with a return to a baseline with a duration of less than 10 minutes. Decelerations are classified by their shape and/or timing in relation to uterine contractions.

Dilatation: expansion of the opening of the cervix from 1 to 10 cm.

Dip: A drop in the fetal heart rate below the baseline, often before or after a spontaneous acceleration. A dip may have a V shape and be less than 15 seconds in duration. A dip immediately following an acceleration may be a V or U shape and last longer than 15 seconds. A dip is innocuous. Preterm fetuses dip more than term or postterm fetuses.

Doppler ultrasound: instrument that emits and receives sound waves to determine the fetal heart rate.

E

Early deceleration: a deceleration of the fetal heart rate which is caused by compression of the fetal head and characterized by a gradual onset at the beginning of a contraction and a gradual offset or recovery to the baseline soon after the contraction ends. The nadir is < 18 seconds after the contraction peak.

EDD/EDC: expected date of delivery or confinement or due date calculated from the first day of the last menstrual period or estimated by other clinical parameters such as ultrasound measurements of the fetus.

Effacement: shortening or thinning of the cervical canal, usually during the early phase of dilatation, estimated by a percent. For example, 80% effaced indicates the cervix is approximately 4/5th of its original length. The closed cervix is 2.5 to 3 cm long.

Electronic fetal monitor (EFM): computer with paper printout used to show graphically and continuously the relationship between maternal uterine activity and the FHR.

End-stage bradycardia: Also called second-stage bradycardia with a 15 to 30 beats per minute drop from the fetal heart rate baseline level during the second stage of labor when the woman is pushing.

Engagement of the vertex occurs when the biparietal diameter has passed through the pelvic inlet and is clinically diagnosed when the leading bony portion of the fetal head is at or below the level of the ischial spines (station 0 or more)

Epidural: regional anesthesia administered through the back between L3 and L4 via a thin catheter in the epidural space outside of the spinal canal or the dura mater.

Extrinsic factors: Factors outside of the fetus that can affect the fetal heart rate, e.g., cord compression, placental abruption, maternal cardiac or oxygen problems.

F

Fetal distress: An ill-defined term suggesting the fetus has a high risk of asphyxia that can cause fetal brain damage if the asphyxial insult is not relieved. The term should not be used in clinical practice or documentation. Instead, nonreassuring fetus status should be used.

Fetal heart rate (FHR): fetal ventricular rate in beats per minute.

Fetal scalp electrode: see spiral electrode.

Fetal well-being: A nonhypoxic fetus who moves, usually just prior to or during an acceleration, and who has short-term variability and no decelerations.

Fundus: portion of the uterus which lies above the insertion of the fallopian tubes at the top of the uterus. The portion farthest from the mouth of an organ.

G

Gestation: time from conception to birth.

Gestational age: age of the embryo or fetus computed from the first day of the last menstrual period to the present, usually expressed in weeks.

Gravida (G): number of pregnancies.

H

Hematoma: localized collection of blood, usually clotted, caused by a break in the wall of a blood vessel.

Hyperstimulation: Also called tachysystole or hypercontractility. Contraction frequency is less than every two minutes with the contraction interval less than 60 seconds.

Hypertonus: Abnormally high resting tone or when the uterus is firm to palpation between contractions.

Hypoxemia: low blood oxygen content.

Hypoxia: deficiency of oxygen in the cells.

I

Intensity: when an intrauterine pressure catheter is in the uterus, the peak intrauterine pressure minus the resting tone.

Intrapartal: the period of time during labor and birth.

Intrauterine pressure catheter (IUPC): a fluid-filled or solid catheter inserted transvaginally into the uterus. Intrauterine pressure is conducted through the catheter, exerted on a pressure transducer, and transformed to an electronic signal, then printed on the tracing.

Intrinsic factors: Factors within the fetus that can affect the fetal heart rate, e.g., chemoreceptors, baroreceptors, catecholamines, adenosine, arginine vasopressin, the sympathetic nerves, and the vagus nerves or vagi.

Introitus: entrance to the vagina.

Ischial spines: the shortest diameter of the pelvis. Two prominent, palpable bony prominences.

L

Late deceleration: a deceleration of the fetal heart rate caused by uteroplacental insufficiency (low oxygen delivery) and characterized by a gradual, slanted onset after the contraction begins, and *usually* a slow return to baseline. The nadir is always 18 or more seconds after the contraction peak. Late decelerations tend to be similar in shape. They return to baseline after the contraction ends.

Low forceps: The application of forceps when the leading point of the skull is at station +2 or more.

Long-term variability (LTV): the fluctuation of the fetal heart rate above and below an average baseline rate, LTV is evaluated each minute of the baseline by measuring the bandwidth of the baseline when there are 2 or more cycles per minute.

Low amplitude high frequency (LAHF) waves: Also called uterine irritability. The uterine activity waveform shows waves less than 30 seconds in duration with a less than 15 second interval. This is commonly associated with abruption, preterm labor, infection, or ketonuria due to dehydration.

M

Meconium: dark-green mucilaginous material in the intestine of the fetus. The normal contents of the baby's intestines, i.e., 80% water, 20% mucoproteins, mucopolysaccharides, and biliverdin.

Membranes: the sac surrounding the fetus.

Molding: shaping of the fetal head in adjustment to the size and shape of the pelvis and birth canal.

Midforceps: The application of forceps when the head is engaged but the leading point of the skull is above station +2. Application of forceps above station +2 may be attempted while simultaneously initiating preparations for a cesarean delivery in the event that the forceps maneuver is unsuccessful.

Montevideo units: from Uruguay, invented by Drs. Caldeyro-Barcia and Alvarez. The sum of the intensity of contractions in a ten minute period.

Multipara: a woman who has completed two or more pregnancies to the stage of viability.

N

Nadir: Lowest point in a deceleration.

Nonperiodic (pattern): decelerations not related to contractions.

Nonreassuring pattern: A fetal heart rate pattern reflecting a deteriorating fetal status due to hypoxia and the continuing depletion of oxygen reserves which increase the risk of metabolic acidosis. Short-term variability may be absent. Accelerations are absent. There may be decelerations or a pathologic sinusoidal pattern.

Nonstress test (NST): antepartum surveillance method used to evaluate fetal condition by evaluation of the fetal heart rate pattern. An oxygenated, nonacidotic term fetus should have at least 2 accelerations in a 20 minute period with each acceleration peaking 15 bpm above the baseline and lasting 15 or more seconds at its base.

O

Occiput: back part of the head.

Ominous pattern: A fetal heart rate pattern associated with a fetus who has metabolic acidosis or asphyxia requiring immediate delivery. Accelerations and short-term variability are absent. Decelerations, terminal bradycardia, an agonal pattern, or a wandering baseline may be present. Ominous patterns are associated with fetal or neonatal death or poor neonatal outcomes.

Outlet forceps: The application of forceps when a) the scalp is visible at the introitus without separating the labia, b) the fetal skull has reached the pelvic floor, c) the sagittal suture is in the anterior-posterior diameter or in the right or left occiput anterior or posterior position, and d) the fetal head is at or on the perineum.

Overshoot: See variable deceleration.

Oxytocic: agent which acts like the naturally occurring hormone oxytocin, and stimulates contractions of the pregnant uterus.

Oxytocin Challenge Test (OCT): a CST which is conducted by stimulation of uterine contractions with intravenously administered oxytocin. NST criteria also apply to the CST, i.e., a well fetus has a reactive negative test.

P

Para (P) or parity: The number of fetuses delivered who were at least 500 grams or who had a gestational age of 20 weeks. Past obstetric history may be summarized in a series of numbers connected by hyphens. For example, pregnancies (gravida), term infants, premature infants, abortions, number of children currently alive may appear on the prenatal record as 3-2-1-0-3.

Paracervical block: local anesthesia injected around the cervix to relieve the pain of uterine contractions.

Parasympathetic nerves: Includes the 10th cranial nerve or the vagus. The right vagal branch innervates the sinoatrial node and the left vagal branch innervates the atrioventricular node. Vagal stimulation precedes decelerations, bradycardia, and creates short-term variability and a sawtooth pattern.

Periodic pattern: decelerations occurring in relation to contractions.

Pathologic sinusoidal pattern: An undulating baseline with $1^1/2$ to 5 cycles per minute associated with fetal hypoxia, acidosis, and asphyxia. Hypoxia may be associated with severe fetal anemia with a hematocrit less than 20% and the compensatory release of arginine vasopressin from the posterior pituitary gland. Short-term variability will be decreased if the fetus is hypoxic but absent if the fetus is metabolically acidotic or asphyxiated. Fetal movement is decreased or absent. Accelerations are absent.

Pattern: the fetal heart rate plotted on heat sensitive paper in an electronic fetal heart monitor; including baseline rate, variability, accelerations, and decelerations.

Placenta previa: placenta lying partially or totally over the cervical os or opening.

Position: the relation of the presenting part, eg., fetal head or buttocks, to the maternal pelvis.

Presentation: the part of the baby that is over the birth canal.

Presenting part: portion of the fetus which is touched by the gloved examining finger(s) during a vaginal examination. The part of the fetus that is first into the birth canal.

Primigravida: a women pregnant for the first time.

Primipara: a woman who has delivered one fetus weighing 500 or more grams or who is 20 or more week's gestation.

Prolonged deceleration: a nonperiodic deceleration characterized by a drop in the fetal heart rate that lasts at least 2 minutes but less than 10 minutes.

Prostaglandins: hormone-like unsaturated fatty acids that have an effect on blood vessels, smooth muscles, platelets, endocrine glands, the uterus, and the nervous system.

Pseudosinusoidal: See benign sinusoidal pattern.

R

Reactive: An adjective to describe an acceleration that increases 15 beats per minute above the middle of the baseline and lasts 15 seconds at its base. Also a classification term for a nonstress test, or a contraction stress test (CST) that has two reactive accelerations in a 20 minute period, e.g., reactive negative CST.

Reactivity: A vague term with multiple definitions that is not recommended for use.

Reassuring pattern: A fetal heart rate pattern of a nonhypoxic fetus which has spontaneous accelerations and short-term variability. Fetal movement is present.

S

Sawtooth pattern: Small baseline fetal heart rate fluctuations of 20 or more each minute resembling "little teeth" due to stimulation of the vagus in conjunction with stimulation of respiratory nerves in the brainstem. Reflects a fetal respiratory sinus arrhythmia.

Short-term variability (STV): the consecutive beats per minute (bpm) rates plotted on moving fetal monitor paper, which appears as bumps, squiggles or even small lines 9 to 10 bpm long. STV is determined from beat-to-beat variability (BTBV).

Sinusoidal pattern: See pathologic sinusoidal pattern and benign sinusoidal pattern.

Spiral electrode: usually a stainless steel curved wire which is inserted under the fetal skin of the presenting part. It transmits the fetal heart electric current to the fetal monitor.

Station: the level (in centimeters) of the presenting part in relation to the ischial spines. (-) is above the spines, "O" is at the spines, and (+) is below the spines. If the fetal head (vertex) is presenting, station is the relationship of the estimated distance, in centimeters, between the bony portion of the fetal head and the level of the maternal ischial spines.

Sympathetic nerves: Nerves in the autonomic nervous system. When activated, the fetal heart rate increases. There will be accelerations, a rising baseline, or tachycardia.

T

Tachycardia: in the fetus, a heart rate above 160 bpm for 10 or more minutes. Maternal tachycardia is a rate above 100 bpm.

Tocodynamometer/tocotransducer (toco): pressure sensing device applied externally to the maternal abdomen to assess uterine contractions.

Tonus or resting tone: partial contraction of the uterine muscle between contractions, measured in mm Hg by an intrauterine pressure catheter or assessed by palpation.

Tracing: the paper and pattern of the fetal heart rate and/or contractions produced by an electronic fetal monitor. Also called a strip or strip chart.

Transducer: a device which senses a signal for conversion to an electronic form.

True sinusoidal pattern: See pathologic sinusoidal pattern.

U

Uterine contractions (UC): periodic increase in intrauterine pressure. When externally palpated, uterine contractions are classified as mild, moderate, and strong.

Uterine irritability: See low amplitude high frequency waves.

Uterine resting tone: see tonus or resting tone.

Uteroplacental reserve: the amount of blood and oxygen available to support the fetus during contractions.

Uteroplacental insufficiency: an inadequate flow of oxygen from the intervillous space to the fetus, resulting in fetal hypoxemia.

V

Variability (FHRV): fetal heart rate variability has two components: long-term variability (the slow rhythmic fluctuations above and below an average baseline rate) and short-term which are instantaneous fluctuations in the fetal heart rate. The combination of these two types of variability reflects the interaction between parasympathetic and sympathetic branches of the central nervous system.

Variable deceleration: a deceleration of the fetal heart rate caused by umbilical cord compression and/or head compression (especially in the second stage of labor with pushing), characterized by a rapid onset and return to baseline, and a variable relationship to the contraction (may occur at any time in the contraction phase). Variable decelerations may be preceded or followed by acceleratory phases or shoulders.

Shoulders: brief increases in the fetal heart rate (usually less than 20 seconds in duration) preceding or following a variable deceleration and attached to the variable deceleration in response to umbilical vein compression. Shoulders are a compensatory sign.

Overshoot: immediately following a variable deceleration, a high increase (> 20 bpm above the baseline) or a long increase (> 20 seconds in duration). Neither a shoulder or an overshoot is classified as an acceleration. Rather, this acceleratory phase suggests a fetal response to hypoxia with release of catecholamines. Overshoots are a nonreassuring sign.

Variation: computer-generated analysis of the fetal heart rate over 1/16th of a minute (short-term variation) and each minute (long-term variation). Variation is calculated in milliseconds and is determined with an ultrasound transducer in place using specialized computer software.

Viable: a reasonable potential for subsequent survival if the fetus were delivered. In determining parity, viability is considered to be 500 grams or 20 weeks' gestation. A reasonable potential for subsequent survival appears to be delivery at 23 or more weeks' gestation, if neonatal intensive care facilities are available.